中国康复医学会针灸技术与康复专业委员会推荐用书

河南省特色骨干学科中医学第二批学科建设项目（STG - ZYX03 - 202126）

汉英针灸名词术语规范辞典

Chinese-English Dictionary of Acupuncture and Moxibustion Standard Terminology

主 编 高希言

Chief Editor Gao Xiyan

河南科学技术出版社

·郑州·

图书在版编目(CIP)数据

汉英针灸名词术语规范辞典 / 高希言主编. —郑州：
河南科学技术出版社，2023.7
ISBN 978 - 7 - 5725 - 1228 - 5

Ⅰ.①汉… Ⅱ.①高… Ⅲ.①针灸学-名词术语-汉、英
Ⅳ.①R245 - 61

中国国家版本馆 CIP 数据核字(2023)第 099958 号

出版发行:河南科学技术出版社
　　　　　地址:郑州市郑东新区祥盛街 27 号　　　邮编:450016
　　　　　电话:(0371)65788628　65788859
　　　　　网址:www. hnstp. cn
责任编辑:任燕利　马艳茹
责任校对:李　军
封面设计:张　伟
版式设计:杨　柳
责任印制:张艳芳
印　　刷:洛阳和众印刷有限公司
经　　销:全国新华书店
开　　本:720mm×1 020mm　1/16　印张:26.25　字数:600 千字
版　　次:2023 年 7 月第 1 版　　2023 年 7 月第 1 次印刷
定　　价:198.00 元

如发现印、装质量问题,影响阅读,请与出版社联系并调换。

目　录

CONTENT

前　言

进入 21 世纪，中国针灸在世界上 180 多个国家广泛使用，为人类的健康发挥了巨大作用。为了便于世界针灸工作者进行学术交流和满足人们学习针灸知识的需要，我们编写了《汉英针灸名词术语规范辞典》。

本书收集经络、腧穴、针灸、治疗、针灸医籍和人物，以及与针灸有关的中医名词、西医术语共 2 000 余条，以汉语拼音字母顺序排列而成。针灸名词中，有些词语的词义深奥难懂，有些词语的翻译尚不一致，我们根据通用译法和自己的见解做出相应的英文翻译。书中力求用汉语、英语正确释义。

编者

2023 年 3 月

Preface

In the 21st century，Chinese acupuncture and moxibustion has been widely used in more than 180 countries around the world，playing a huge role in human health．In order to facilitate the academic exchange of acupuncture and moxibustion workers around the world and meet the needs for learning acupuncture and moxibustion knowledge，we have compiled the *Chinese-English Dictionary of Acupuncture and Moxibustion Standard Terminology*．

This dictionary is a collection of more than 2 000 entries from meridians，acupoints，acupuncture and moxibustion，treatments，literatures and figures of acupuncture，as well as TCM terms and western medicine terms related to acupuncture and moxibustion．The content is arranged in alphabetical order of Chinese pinyin．In terms of acupuncture and moxibustion，the meaning of some words is difficult to understand，and the existing translation of some words is not consistent．We make corresponding English translation according to the general translation method and with our own interpretation．This dictionary strives to provide accurate explanations in both Chinese and English．

Editor

March，2023

凡　例

　　一、本辞典共收录辞目 2 000 余条,包括经络,腧穴,针法,灸法,针灸器具,治则治法,取穴处方,常见病针灸治疗,历代针灸人物、著作、歌诀,以及与针灸有关的基本理论术语、解剖名称等。辞目按音序法编排,即以辞目第一个汉字的汉语拼音字母顺序排列,如"阿是穴",在"阿"字的条目下查找;声母相同者,按韵母的顺序排列;字音相同者,按声调排列;字音及声调都相同者,按辞目的第二个汉字的读音排列,依次类推。词目中首字为阿拉伯数字及外语字母者(如 1、2 等),按其后第一个汉字的读音排列。

　　二、释文力求简明、准确,一词多义者,按"①、②、③"的次序排列,如"髋关","①部位名。②经穴名。"同一类型的不同释义,以";"隔开。释义的内容以与针灸学有关的为主,其他从略。

　　三、本书中穴位名称的著录方式参照世界卫生组织总部针灸穴名国际标准化科学组会议审议通过的《标准针灸穴名》和国家技术监督局 2021 年修订版《经穴名称与定位》,耳穴采用 2013 年版《耳穴名称与部位》。

　　四、为增加辞典的信息含量和检索功能,书中采用汉语拼音编序和索引。

Notes on the Use of This Dictionary

　　1. The dictionary collects more than 2 000 entries including meridians and collaterals, acupoints, technique of acupuncture and moxibustion, acupuncture equipments, principles and methods of treatment, point prescription, acupuncture treatment for common disease, ancient acupuncture figures, classics, versified formulas, as well as basic TCM theory terms, and anatomies related to acupuncture. The entries are arranged according to the sequence of Chinese phonetic alphabet which is the sequence of the first alphabet letter of the Chinese character in each entry. For example, the entry "Ashi point" can be found below the item of "A". If the initial consonants are same, the order will be arranged in accordance with vowel. If pronunciations are identical, the order will arranged according to tone. If pronunciation and tone are exactly the same, the next one will be considered according to the sequenee of Chinese phonetic alphabet, analogy in turn. If the first word of the entry is Arabic numerals or foreign letters (such as 1,2, etc.), the order will arranged according to the first Chinese character next to it.

　　2. The editorial staff has been striving for conciseness and accuracy. For the terms

with polysemous connotations，the separate interpretations are listed out with "①，②，③"，etc，to demonstrate that the same term has different explanations. For example，Biguan：①part name；②name of acupoint. Different interpretatiens of the Same type are seperated by "；". The content of paraphrase veiled is mainly on acupuncture subject. The else is omitted.

3. The description method of acupoint names in this dictionary refers to the *Standard Acupuncture and Moxibustion Point Names* approved by the International Standardization Scientific Group Meeting of Acupuncture and Moxibustion Point Names of the World Health Organization Headquarters，and the 2021 revision of the *Namenclature and Location of Meridian Points* of the National Bureau of Technical Supervision. Ear points use the 2013 version of *Namenclature and Location of Ear Point*.

4. In order to increase the information content and search function，the dictionary uses Chinese pinyin to sequence and index.

汉语拼音音序检索

C

X

A

阿是穴 Ashi points

又称天应穴、不定穴等。指既无固定名称，又无固定位置，以压痛点或体表反应点作为针灸施术部位的穴位。

Ashi points, also known as natural reactive points, unfixed points, etc, referring to the points which have neither specific names nor fixed locations. They are selected as points according to patient's reaction of tenderness or other feelings.

艾灸补泻 moxibustion reinforcing and reducing

艾灸时以火力的大小区分补泻,补时让艾慢慢燃烧,泻时宜吹旺艾火。

Reinforcing and reducing in moxibustion are distinguished by the intensity of the fire. For reinforcing, the moxa should be burned slowly while for reducing, the moxa fire should be burned more intensely.

艾绒 moxa

指干燥艾叶经粉碎制成的纤维绒状物质。

Fiber-like substances made by grinding dried leaves of the mugwort (*Artemisia argyi* Levl. et Vant).

艾条 moxa stick

用艾绒制成的圆柱形长条。

Cigar-like roll of moxa.

艾条灸 moxibustion with moxa stick

将艾条点燃后离体表穴位 1～4 cm 进行灸治的方法。

A moxibustion method by administering a burning moxa stick about 1-4 cm over the acupoint on the body surface for treatment.

艾叶 moxa leaf

艾的干燥叶。用于散寒止痛,温经止血,并用于针灸。

Dried leaves of mugwort, used as a herbal medicine to disperse cold and relieve pain, warm the meridians and arrest bleeding, and used for moxibustion.

艾炷 moxa cone

用艾绒压制而成的锥状物。

Cone made of pressed moxa.

艾炷灸 moxibustion with moxa cone

将艾炷直接或间接放在穴位上点燃进行灸治的方法。

Moxibustion with a burning moxa cone put directly or indirectly on an acupoint for treatment.

嗳气 eructation

指胃气从胃中上逆有声,其声沉长的症状。多因脾胃虚弱,或胃有痰、火、食滞,使胃失和降,或因肺气不降所致。治宜温中降逆。取穴:天突、膈俞、中脘、足三里、章门。

The sound of gas is from the stomach, due to weakness of spleen and stomach, or failure of descending of stomach-qi resulting from the accumulation of phlegm, fire and indigested food in the stomach, or due to failure of descending of lung-qi. Treatment principle: Warm the middle jiao to lower the adverse flow of stomach-qi. Point selection: Tiantu (CV22), Geshu (BL17), Zhongwan (CV12), Zusanli(ST36), Zhangmen(LR13).

安眠 Anmian

经外奇穴名。在翳风与风池穴连线中点上。主治:失眠,眩晕,头痛,心悸,癫狂等。

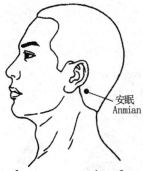

安眠
Anmian

Name of an extra point. Location: At the midpoint of the line between Yifeng (TE17) and Fengchi(GB20). Indications: Insomnia, vertigo, headache, palpitation, mental disorders, etc.

按法 pressing manipulation

针刺手法名,有两种含义:①针刺前用手指按压穴位;②针刺时将针插入深部。

Name of an acupuncture manipulation, which implies:①pressing the point with fingers before insertion;②thrusting the needle into the deeper part during acupuncture.

按摩 massage

①又称推拿,是在人体一定部位上,运用各种按摩手法和进行特定的肢体被动活动来防治疾病的方法。②正骨八法之一,包括按法和摩法,用以舒筋散瘀和消肿。

①Also called Tuina. It is a method to prevent and treat diseases by using various massage manipulations, and specific passive limb activities on a certain part of the human body. ②One of the eight manipulations of bone setting, which contains pressing and rubbing manipulation, used for relaxing the muscles, dissipating blood stasis, and reducing swelling.

按跷 pressing therapy

指一种按捏穴位的治病方法。

A kind of therapy by pressing and kneading the points.

按神经取穴 selecting points by the nerve distribution

取穴法之一。指按照神经的分布选取有关的穴位。

One of the point-selecting methods, i. e., selecting the relevant points in accordance with the nerve distribution route.

B

八风 Bafeng(EX-LE10)

经外奇穴名，又名八冲。在足背侧，第1～5趾间，趾蹼缘后方赤白肉际处，一侧4穴，左右共8穴。主治：脚气，趾痛，足背肿痛等。操作：斜刺0.5～0.8寸，或用三棱针点刺出血；可灸。

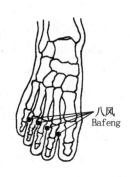

八风 Bafeng

Name of extra points, also named Bachong. Those points are on the dorsal side of the foot, between the toes, on the dorso-ventral boundary of the foot behind the margins of the webs, 4 points on each side, and total 8 points on both sides. Indications: Beriberi, toe pain , swelling and pain of the dorsum of the foot, etc. Method: Puncture obliquely 0.5-0.8 cun or prick with a three-edged needle to cause bleeding. Moxibustion is applicable.

八纲辨证 syndrome differentiation by the eight principles

辨证的基本方法之一。把疾病复杂的临床表现用阴、阳、表、里、寒、热、虚、实八个纲领进行分析归纳，以说明病变的部位、性质及正邪盛衰等情况，进而对疾病做出诊断。

One of the basic methods of differential diagnosis, i. e. , to determine the nature and site of the disease and the confliction between the body's vital qi and the evil, using the eight principle syndromes, which contains yin and yang, exterior and interior, cold and heat, deficiency and excess to represent complicated clinical symptoms in order to provide diagnosis.

八关 Baguan

经外奇穴八邪的别名。

The other name of Baxie(EX-UE9).

八会穴 eight influential points

指脏、腑、气、血、筋、脉、骨、髓的精气汇聚的8个穴位，即气会膻中穴、血会膈俞穴、骨会大杼穴、筋会阳陵泉穴、髓会绝骨穴、脉会太渊穴、脏会章门穴、腑会中脘穴。

The eight important acupoints where essential qi of eight tissues of the body infuses. They include influential point of qi—Danzhong(CV17),influential point of blood—Geshu(BL17), influential point of bones—Dazhu(BL11),influential point of muscles—Yanglingquan(GB34),influential point of veins—Taiyuan(LU9), influential point of the zang organs—Zhangmen(LR13), and influential point of the fu organs—Zhongwan(CV12).

八髎 Baliao

指上髎、次髎、中髎、下髎的合称，双侧共8穴，位于腰尻间。主治：腰部疾患。

Bilateral Shangliao (BL31), Ciliao (BL32), Zhongliao(BL33), and Xialiao (BL34), eight points in total, located between the loins and buttock. Indications: Lumbar diseases.

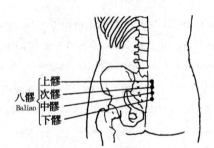

八脉交会穴 eight confluence points

奇经八脉与十二经脉之气相通的八个腧穴。

The eight acupoints where the qi of the eight extra meridians connected with the qi of the twelve regular meridians.

八溪 eight joints

指肘、腕、膝、踝关节。

Joints of the elbows, wrists, knees and ankles.

八邪 Baxie(EX-UE9)

经外奇穴名。在手背侧,微握拳,第1~5指间,指蹼缘后方赤白肉际处,左右共8穴。主治:烦热,手指麻木、手臂拘

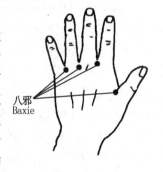

挛、手背红肿等。操作:向上斜刺0.5~0.8寸,或用三棱针点刺出血;可灸。

Name of extra points. They are on the dorsal side of the hands, between the fingers, on the dorso-ventral boundary of the hand behind the margins of the webs. eight in all. Indications: Dysphoria with feverish sensation, finger numbness, spasm and contracture of the arms, redness and swelling of the dorsum of hand, etc.

Method: Puncture obliquely upward 0.5-0.8 cun or prick with a three-edged needle to cause bleeding. Moxibustion is applicable.

八虚 eight fossae

指两侧肘、腋、股、腘的凹陷部,五脏患病时可出现异常反应。

The bilateral elbow, axillary, femoral and popliteal fossae which can manifest abnormal symptoms when the five zang-organs suffer from diseases.

拔罐法 cupping

指以竹罐或玻璃罐为工具,利用热力排出罐内空气而造成负压,使罐吸附于体表的穴位或患处的治疗方法。

The application to an acupoint or an affected area of the body by a bamboo or glass cup in which the air has been expelled with heat to create a negative pressure inside and then produce suction of the cup on the skin.

白带 leucorrhea

阴道分泌的白色黏液,正常情况下,白带量少色淡,无臭;如果白带增多,颜色和气味改变,多属病态。治宜健脾益气、利湿止带。取穴:气海、带脉、白环俞、三阴交、足三里、中极。

The whitish viscid discharge from vagina. It is considered as normal when the discharge is scanty, colourless and odourless, and as pathological when it becomes profuse with ohanges in colour and odour. Treatment principle: Strengthen the spleen and replenish qi, remove dampness and stop leucorrhea. Point selection:

Qihai(CV6), Daimai(GB26), Baihuanshu (BL30), Sanyinjiao (SP6), Zusanli (ST36), Zhongji(CV3).

白癜风 vitiligo

因风邪袭表、气血失和、血不荣肤所致，以局部皮肤脱色而呈白色为特征的一种皮肤病。表现为白斑边缘清楚，其中的毛发也变白，表面光滑，不痛不痒。治宜疏风和营。取穴：风池、大椎、肩髃、曲池、外关、足三里、三阴交。

A skin disease characterized by local discoloration of the skin, due to attack of wind-evil to the superficies, incoordination between qi and blood, leading to lack of nourishment of the skin. The patches usually have a clear border, with discoloured hair and smooth surface, but without pain or itch. Treatment principle: Dispel wind and regulate the nutrient qi. Point selection: Fengchi (GB20), Dazhui (GV14), Jianyu (LI15), Quchi (LI11), Waiguan(TE5), Zusanli(ST36), Sanyinjiao(SP6).

白附子 baifuzi

一种灸用隔垫物，为黄花乌头的干燥根。

A kind of herbal medicine used as moxibustion partition material, i. e. , the dry tuber of *Aconitum coreanum* (Levl) Raipaics.

白虎摇头 white tiger shaking the head

针刺手法名。飞经走气四法之一，与"青龙摆尾"相对。即进针到适当深度，左右摇动并结合上提动作，反复18次，以行经气。

Name of an acupuncture technique, it is one of the four techniques to promote qi by dreding meridians, which is opposite to "blue dragon wagging the tail". Namely, when the needle is inserted to a certain depth, swing it leftward and rightward while combining with lifting action, this can be repeated 18 times to move the meridian qi.

白环俞 Baihuanshu(BL30)

经穴名。属足太阳膀胱经。定位：在骶部，当骶正中嵴旁 1.5 寸，平第四骶后孔。主治：遗尿，疝气，带下，月经不调，腰骶疼痛等。操作：直刺 0.8～1.5 寸；可灸。

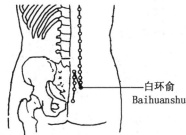

白环俞
Baihuanshu

Name of an acupoint. It belongs to the Bladder Meridian of Foot-Taiyang. Location: On the sacrum and at the level of the 4th posterior sacral foramen, 1. 5 cun lateral to the median sacral crest. Indications: Enuresis, hernia, morbid leucorrhoea, irregular menstruation, lumbosacral pain, etc. Method: Puncture perpendicularly 0. 8-1. 5 cun. Moxibustion is applicable.

白芥子灸 moxibustion with white mustard seed

天灸方法之一。白芥子为草本植物白芥的干燥成熟种子。取白芥子研末，用水调成糊状，敷于选好的腧穴上 3～4 h，待局部皮肤发泡为止。用于治疗肺结核、哮喘、口眼歪斜等病症。

One form of the crude herb moxibustion. Ground the white mustard seed (seed of the *Sinapis alba* L.) into powder, then mix it with water to form a paste and applied to the acupoint. After the blister formation in 3-4 hours, remove the paste. The method is primarily used for pulmonary tuberculosis and asthma, deviation of mouth and eyes, etc..

白肉际 border of white skin

部位名。手足的掌面与背面的交界处。

Name of a body part, i. e., the boundary between the palm and the dorsal side of the hand or foot.

白苔 whitish fur

舌体表面色白,其厚薄及湿润度的变化反映不同的病变。苔白而薄是正常的舌苔;若苔薄白而干,多因津液不足引起。

A sign suggestes different pathological changes according to the thickness and moisture of the fur. For instance, a thin whitish fur is normal while a thin whitish and dry fur suggests insufficiency of body fluid.

白屑风 seborrheic dermatitis

因风邪侵入毛孔,郁久血燥,肌肤失养所引起的一种皮肤病。多见于年轻人,好发于头皮,呈弥漫而均匀的糠秕干燥白屑,痒甚,搔抓时白屑脱落,而且毛发易脱,相当于脂溢性皮炎。治宜补肺健脾、补益气血。取穴:太溪、肺俞、膏肓、太渊、足三里、三阴交。

A skin disease due to invasion of wind-evil through the hair follicles and stagnation of the evil leading to blood-dryness and lack of nourishment of the skin; mostly seen in the young, usually occurring on the scalp with exfoliation of dry and whitish dandruff, falling of hairs, and intense itching. Treatment principle: Tonify the lung and strengthen the spleen, reinforce the qi and blood. Point selection: Taixi (KI3), Feishu (BL13), Gaohuang (BL43), Taiyuan (LU9), Zusanli (ST36), San yinjiao (SP6).

白针 simple acupuncture

指单纯的针刺方法。又称冷针,与温针相对。

A kind of simple needling, also known as cold acupuncture by contrast with warm acupuncture.

百虫窝 Baichongwo(EX-LE3)

①经外奇穴名。定位:屈膝,在大腿内侧,髌底内侧端上3寸,即血海上1寸。主治:风疹,痒疹,虫证等。②血海的别名。

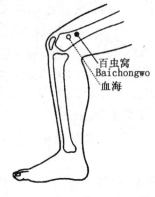

①Name of an extra point. Location: In the medial side of the thigh, 3 cun above the medial superior and of the patella when the knee flexed, i. e., 1 cun above Xuehai(SP10). Indications: Rubella, prurigo, gastro-intestinal parasitic diseases, etc. ②The other name of Xuehai(SP10).

百会 Baihui(GV20)

经穴名,属督脉。定位:在头部,当前发际正中直上 5 寸,或两耳尖连线的中点处。主治:头痛,眩晕,耳鸣,鼻塞,中风失语,昏迷,癫狂,脱肛,阴挺等。操作:平刺0.5～0.8 寸;可灸。

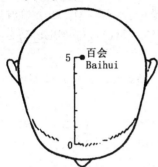

Name of an acupoint. It belongs to the Governor Vessel. Location:On the head, 5 cun directly above the anterior hairline or the midpoint of the line connecting the apexes of both ears. Indications:Headache, vertigo, tinnitus, nasal obstruction, aphasia due to apoplexy, coma, mental disorders, prolapse of rectum and uterus, etc. Method:Puncture horizontally 0. 5-0. 8 cun. Moxibustion is applicable.

百劳 Bailao(EX-HN15)

经外奇穴名。定位:当大椎直上 2 寸,后正中线旁开 1 寸。主治:瘰疬,咳喘,项强等。

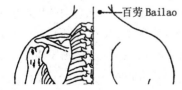

Name of an extra point. Location:2 cun above Dazhui(GV14) and 1 cun la-teral to the posterior midline. Indications:Scrofula, cough, asthma, neck rigidity, etc.

百日咳 whooping cough

一种流行于冬季的传染病,多见于 5 岁以下婴幼儿。临床以阵发性、痉挛性咳嗽和咳后伴有特殊的吸气性回声为特征。治宜健脾补肺。取穴:大椎、丰隆、尺泽、身柱。

An infectious disease prevalent in winter, mostly seen in children under 5 years old; characterized by paroxysmal spasmodic cough with an special inspiratory wheezing sound. Treatment principle:Strengthen the spleen and reinforce the lung. Point selection:Dazhui(GV14), Fenglong(ST40), Chize(LU5), Shenzhu(GV12).

斑秃 alopecia areata

又称油风。指在短期内发生头发成片脱落,皮红光泽或伴有瘙痒的一种疾病。多由血虚生风、风盛火燥、发失濡养所致。治宜养血祛风、活血化瘀。取穴:阿是穴、百会、风池、膈俞、足三里、三阴交。

Also called oily wind. Patchy loss of hair on the scalp occurring in a short time accompanied by itching; caused by deficiency of blood with production of wind-evil, fire-evil and dryness leading to undernourishment of the hair. Treatment principle:Nourish the blood to expel wind, promote blood circulation and remove stasis. Point selection:Ashi points,Baihui(GV20), Fengchi(GB20), Geshu(BL17), Zusanli(ST36), Sanyinjiao(SP6).

瘢痕灸 scarring moxibustion

指将艾炷直接放在体表穴位的皮肤上点燃施灸，促使局部化脓，产生水疱，最后结痂，形成瘢痕的灸法。

A moxa cone is burnt directly on the skin of the acupoint so that small blisters will be formed. As a result, a scar will be formed after the lesion is healed.

半刺 extreme shallow needling

五刺法之一。即刺入很浅，并很快拔针，不伤肌肉的一种针法。古代用于治疗与肺病有关的咳嗽、痰喘等。

One of the five needling techniques, i. e., insert the needle very superficially and withdraw it very swiftly so that the muscles are not injured. It was used for treating cough, asthma due to excessive phlegm and other diseases related to lung diseases in ancient times.

半身不遂 hemiplegia

一侧肢体瘫痪的病症，多见于中风后遗症。治宜通经活络、补益肝肾。取穴：肩髃、曲池、合谷、阳溪、髀关、梁丘、足三里、解溪、肝俞、肾俞。

Paralysis on one side of the body, commonly seen after stroke. Treatment principle：Clear and activate the meridians and collaterals, tonify the liver and kidney. Point selection：Jianyu (LI15), Quchi (LI11), Hegu(LI4), Yangxi(LI5), Biguan (ST31), Liangqiu (ST34), Zusanli (ST36), Jiexi(ST41), Ganshu(BL18), Shenshu(BL23).

半身麻木 hemianesthesia

身体半边或上下半身麻木的症状。治宜通经活络。取穴：内关、水沟、极泉、少海、委中、三阴交。

Numbness of either one side, or the upper part or the lower part of the body. Treatment principle：Clear and activate the meridians and collaterals. Point selection：Neiguan (PC6), Shuigou(GV26), Jiquan(HT1), Shaohai (HT3), Weizhong (BL40), Sanyinjiao (SP6).

傍针刺 perpendicular and lateral needling

十二刺法之一。用于治疗慢性风湿病。刺法是在患部直刺和旁刺各一针。

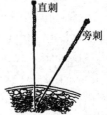

One of the twelve needling techniques for chronic rheumatic diseases. It means to puncture the affected part perpendicularly with a needle and laterally with another needle.

胞 fetus

①指子宫。②指膀胱。

①The uterus；②The urinary bladder.

胞肓 Baohuang(BL53)

经穴名。属足太阳膀胱经。定位：在臀部，平第二骶后孔，骶正中嵴旁开 3 寸。主治：肠鸣，腹胀，腰痛，癃闭等。

Name of an acupoint. It belongs to the Bladder Meridian of Foot-Taiyang. Location：On the buttocks, at the level of the 2nd posterior sacral foramen, 3 cun later-

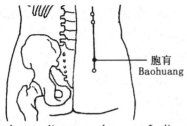

胞肓
Baohuang

al to the median sacral crest. Indications: Borborygmus, abdominal distension, lumbago, retention of urine, etc.

胞脉 uterus meridians

联系子宫的经脉，主要指冲脉，也包括任脉。

The meridians connecting with the uterus, mainly refers to the Thoroughfare Vessel, also includes the Conception Vessel.

胞门、子户 Baomen, Zihu

女子经外奇穴名。位于关元穴左、右各2寸处。左为胞门，右为子户。与水道穴同位。直刺或灸治疗妇女不孕、胎漏下血、腹痛、难产、白带过多等。

Name of extra points in females. Location: 2 cun lateral to Guanyuan (CV4) with the point on the left called Baomen and on the right called Zihu. The location of the two points is the same as Shuidao (ST28). Vertical acupuncture or moxibustion is used to cure infertility, vaginal bleeding during pregnancy, abdominal pain, difficult labour, excessive leukorrhea, etc.

保健灸 health maintenance moxibustion

指以增强人体抗病能力，保健强身为目的的灸法。常用穴有足三里、关元、气海、膏肓等。

A kind of moxibustion with the pur-pose of increasing the resistance to the diseases and improving the health. The commonly used acupoints are Zusanli (ST36), Guanyuan(CV4), Qihai(CV6), Gaohuang(BL43), etc.

报刺 sucessive trigger needling

十二刺法之一。用于治疗没有固定部位的疼痛。刺法：找到痛处，直刺一针，并留针不拔，以左手揣按局部，找到另一个痛处后，先将前针拔出，再在第二个痛处刺针。

One of the twelve needling techniques, used for treating pains without fixed part. Method: Locate the pain trigger point, puncture it directly, retain the needle there and pinch or press local skin until another pain trigger point is found, then withdraw the needle and puncture the second pain point.

报灸 repeated moxibustion

指多次或多壮反复灸治。

Multiple moxibustion or mixibustion with a great number of cones.

豹文刺 leopard-spot needling

中国古代五刺法之一。即在患病部位的周围多处刺破小血管，排出瘀血。用于治疗与心脏有关的血脉瘀阻等病症。

One of the five needling techniques in ancient China, i. e., to pierce small blood vessels around the affected area to drain the stagnated blood. It is an needling technique for treating of heart-related blood stasis, etc.

暴病者取之太阳 select Taiyang meridians to treat acute diseases

针灸治则之一,即对急性病症的治疗,可以从太阳经着手。

One of the acupuncture and moxibustion principles, i. e. , the Taiyang meridians can be first selected to treat the acute diseases.

暴盲 sudden blindness

平日素无他病,突然目不见物,眼廓和瞳神外观正常。多因肝气上逆、气滞血瘀或元气大虚所致。多见于急性视神经炎、视网膜中央动脉栓塞、眼底出血、视网膜剥离等。治宜清肝明目。取穴:睛明、太冲、瞳子髎、光明。

A condition of sudden loss of vision with normal appearance of the eyes, commonly due to adverse rising of liver-qi, stagnation of qi and blood, or exhaustion of primordial qi; seen in cases of acute optic neuritis, embolism of central retinal artery, fundus bleeding, retinal detachment, etc. Treatment principle: Remove the liver-fire to improve eyesight. Point selection: Jingming (BL1), Taichong (LR3), Tongziliao (GB1), Guangming(GB37).

暴喑 sudden aphonia

即突然失音,常见于声带急性炎症、水肿等病。治宜通络开窍。取穴:哑门、廉泉、通里。

A sudden loss of voice, usually seen in acute inflammation and edema of the vocal cord. Treatment principle:Dredge collaterals and open orifices. Point selection:Yamen (GV15),Lianquan(CV23), Tongli(HT5).

《备急千金要方》Essential Prescriptions for Worth Thousand Gold Emergencies

又名《千金要方》,由孙思邈撰写于7世纪。论述医理、药物、妇产、小儿、针刺、饮食、摄生等医学各科及方剂。

A medical book, also known as *Essential Prescriptions Worth Thousand Gold for Emergency*, including different branches of Chinese Medicine such as general medical theory, materia medica, gynecology and obstetrics, pediatrics, acupuncture, diet, health care, and prescription, compiled by Sun Simiao in the 7th century.

背第二侧线 the second lateral line on the back

经穴定位线,距背正中线3寸,为足太阳膀胱经循行处。

Point-locating line, 3 cun lateral to the posterior median line, where the Bladder Meridian of Foot-Taiyang passes.

背第一侧线 the first lateral line on the back

经穴定位线,距背正中线1.5寸,为足太阳膀胱经循行处。

Point-locating line, 1. 5 cun lateral to the posterior median line, where the Bladder Merdian of Foot-Taiyang passes.

背痛 backache

因风寒侵袭足太阳经,造成经脉涩滞所致的病症。症见背部拘紧疼痛,牵连肩项,兼有恶寒等。治宜调气活血、舒筋散寒。取穴:大椎、膈俞、风池、天柱、后溪。

A disorder caused by the blockage of the Foot-Taiyang meridian after exposure to wind-cold evil，manifested as stiffness and pain of the back involving the shoulder and nape，accompanied with chilliness. Treatment principle：Regulate qi and activate blood circulation，relax muscles and dispel cold. Point selection：Dazhui(GV14)，Geshu(BL17)，Fengchi(GB20)，Tianzhu(BL10)，Houxi(SI3).

背阳关 Beiyangguan
腰阳关别名。

The other name of Yaoyangguan(GV3).

背俞穴 back-shu points
①经穴分类名，指脏腑经气输注于背腰部的腧穴，位于背部膀胱经第一侧线上，与脏腑生理、病理反应密切相关，共 12 个。②泛指背部各经穴。

①Name of a group of acupoints，refers to the points where meridian qi of zang-fu infuses in the back. The total 12 points are located on the first lateral line of the Bladder Meridian，which closely related to the physiological and pathological reactions of the zang-fu organs. ②A general term for all the acupoints on the back.

背正中线 median line on the back
经穴定位线，又称后正中线，为督脉循行处。

Point-locating line，also known as posterior median line where passes the Governor Vessel.

贲 ben
部位名。指膈。

Name of a body part，i. e.，the diaphragm.

贲门 cardiac；Benmen
①胃的上口，七冲门之一。②耳穴名。在耳轮脚下后 1/3 处。主治：胃炎，胃及十二指溃疡等。

①The upper opening of the stomach，one of the seven important openings of the digestive system. ② Name of an ear point. It is at the lower 1/3 of the posterior aspect of helix crus. Indications：gastritis，gastroduodenal ulcer，etc.

本池 Benchi
廉泉穴别名。

The other name of Lianquan (CV23).

本节 distal joints
骨骼部位名。手指或足趾的基节部。

Name of body parts，referring to the basal joint parts of the fingers or toes.

本经取穴 selecting points on the diseased meridian
取穴法之一。指本经脉脏腑疾病，选本经穴位进行治疗的方法。包括近取和远取两种。

One of the point-selecting methods which means selecting points along the course of the diseased meridians. It includes adjacent selection and distant selection.

本神 Benshen(GB13)
经穴名。属足少阳胆经。定位：在头部，当前发际上 0.5 寸，神庭旁开 3 寸，神庭与头维连线的外 1/3 与内 2/3 的交点处。主治：头痛，失眠，眩晕，癫痫等。操作：平刺 0.3～0.5 寸；可灸。

Name of an acupoint. It belongs to the Gallbladder Meridian of Foot-Shaoyang. Location：On the head，0. 5 cun above the anterior hairline，3 cun lateral to Shen-

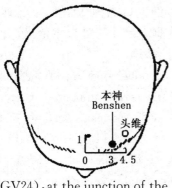

ting (GV24), at the junction of the lateral 1/3 and medial 2/3 of the line between Shenting(GV24) and Touwei(ST8). Indications: Headache, insomnia, vertigo, epilepsy, etc. Method: Puncture horizontally 0.3-0.5 cun. Moxibustion is applicable.

崩漏 metrorrhagia and metrostaxis

女性不在月经期，突然阴道大量出血或持续淋漓不断出血的病症。多发生于青春期及更年期妇女。以冲任不固为基本病理。多因血热气虚、肝肾阴虚、血瘀等所致。治宜清热凉血、祛瘀止崩。取穴：气海、三阴交、隐白、血海、水泉、地机。

Uterine bleeding occurring at menstrual interval, appearing as sudden profuse bleeding or prolonged scanty flow, commonly seen in women in puberty and menopause; due to debility of the Conception Vessel and the Throughfare Vessel resulting from blood-heat, deficiency of qi, deficiency of liver-yin and kidney-yin, stagnation of blood, etc. Treatment principle: Clear heat and cool blood, remove blood stasis and arrest uterine bleeding. Point selection: Qihai (CV6), Sangyinjiao(SP6), Yinbai(SP1), Xuehai (SP10), Shuiquan(KI5), Diji(SP8).

鼻 nose

五官之一，是嗅觉器官，被认为是肺的门户，和脾、胆也有密切的关系。

One of the five sense organs, serving as olfactory organ. It is considered as the orifice of the lung and closely related to the spleen and gallbladder.

鼻穿 Bichuan

上迎香别名。

The other name of Shangyingxiang (EX-HN8).

鼻孔 nostril

七窍之一。指鼻下部的两个外孔道。

One of the seven orifices, i. e., the two external openings of the lower part of the nose.

鼻衄 epistaxis

指鼻中出血。多因肺热上壅，迫血妄行；或胃热熏蒸；或肝火偏旺；或肺肾阴虚；或头风、伤风所致。治宜清热凉血、止血。取穴：合谷、风池、行间、风府。

Bleeding from the nose, due to ascending lung-heat forcing the blood out of the vessels, or attack of stomach-heat, or hyperactivity of liver-fire, or deficiency of lung-yin and kidney-yin, or head cold. Treatment principle: Clear heat, cool and arrest blood. Point selection: Hegu(LI4), Fengchi(GB20), Xingjian(LR2), Fengfu (GV16).

鼻塞 nosal obstruction

鼻塞不通。多由风寒或风热引起肺气不宣所致。常可伴有其他表证。治宜宣肺开窍。取穴：列缺、合谷、迎香、印堂。

A condition due to stagnation of lung-qi resulting from the attack of wind-cold or wind-heat evil, usually accompanied by with other manifestations of superficies-syndrome. Treatment principle: Ventilate the lung-qi to dredge nasal orifice. Point selection: Lieque (LU7), Hegu (LI4), Ying-xiang (LI20), Yintang (GV29).

鼻通 Bitong

经外奇穴名。在鼻唇沟上端尽处。主治：鼻塞，鼻渊，鼻部疮疖等。

Name of an extrapoint. It is located at the upper end of the nasolabial groove. Indications: Nasal obstruction, sinusitis, nasal boils, etc.

鼻渊 sinusitis

因风寒或风热、胆热移于脑，或兼气虚所致的病症。症见鼻塞，不闻香臭，涕色黄、味腥臭，头晕，头痛，健忘等，相当于鼻窦炎。治宜清热开窍。取穴：太冲、上星、列缺、合谷、迎香、印堂。

A condition due to attack of wind-cold or wind-heat evil or gallbladder-heat to the brain, or accompanied by deficiency of qi; manifested as nasal obstruction, loss of smell, yellowish and foul nasal discharge, dizziness, headache, amnesia, etc. Treatment principle: Clear heat to dredge nasal orifice. Point selection: Taichong(LR3), Shangxing(GV23), Lieque (LU7), Hegu(LI4), Yingxiang(LI20), Yintang(GV29).

鼻针 nase acupuncture

指在鼻周围进行针刺以治疗疾病的方法。

It refers to puncture the acupoints around the nose to treat disease.

鼻柱 nosal septum

部位名。即鼻梁。

Name of a body part, i. e. , the nose bridge.

鼻准 bizhun

①部位名，指鼻尖。可作为诊察脾病的参考。②素髎穴别名。

①Name of a body part, i. e. , the nose tip. It can be used as a reference for diagnosing spleen disease. ②The other name of Suliao(GV25).

闭经 amenorrhea

又称经闭。包括原发性闭经和继发性闭经。因肝肾亏损，精血不足，气血虚弱，致冲任失养；或气滞血瘀，痰湿内阻，致经络受阻，胞脉不通。治宜滋补肝肾。取穴：肝俞、肾俞、膏肓、然谷、命门、阴谷。

A condition including primary and secondary amenorrhea, usually due to asthenia of the liver and kidneys, insufficiency of essence and blood, and deficiency of qi and blood, resulting in failing to nourish the Conception Vessel and Thoroughfare Vessel; or due to stagnation of qi and blood, and accumulation of phlegm-dampness, resulting in the obstruction of the uterus vessels. Treatment principle: Nourish the liver and kidney. Point selection: Ganshu (BL18), Shenshu (BL23), Gaohuang (BL43), Rangu (KI2), Mingmen(GV4), Yingu(KI10).

闭证 sthenia-type coma

由于邪气内陷,闭阻心神所致。以神昏为主症,伴有牙关紧闭、两手握拳、痰涎壅盛、脉弦滑或脉洪数为主要临床表现的证候。治宜熄风开窍、清心豁痰。取穴:水沟、十二井、太冲、丰隆、劳宫。

A syndrome with loss of conscious as the major symptom, due to mental disorder resulting from the retention of evils, accompanied with lock jaw, clenching of fists, salivation and profuse phlegm accumulation, wiry and slippery pulse or surging and rapid pulse, etc. Treatment principle: Calm the endopathic wind and regain consciousness, remove heart-heat and eliminate phlegm. Point selection: Shuigou (GV26), the twelve Jing-well points, Taichong (LR3), Fenglong (ST40), Laogong(PC8).

蓖麻子灸 castor seed moxibustion

天灸方法之一。将蓖麻子研末,用水调糊,敷于穴位上。

One form of the crude herb moxibustion. Grind the castor seed into powder, mix it with water to make paste and apply it on the acupoint.

髀关 Biguan(ST31)

①穴位名。属足阳明胃经。定位:在大腿前面,当髂前上棘与髌底外侧端的连线上,屈股时,平会阴,居缝匠肌外侧凹陷处。主治:腿痛,下肢痿痹等。操作:直刺1～2.5寸;可灸。②指股部前上方。

① Name of an acupoint. It belongs the Stomach Meridian of Foot-Yangming. Location: On the anterior side of the thigh and on the line connecting the anterior superior

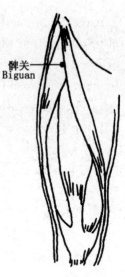

iliac spine and the lateleral end of the pathella base, at the level of the perineum when the thigh is flexed, in the depression lateral to the sartorius muscle. Indications: Leg pain, weakness and paralysis of the lower limbs, etc. Method: Puncture perpendicularly 1-2.5 cun. Moxibustion is applicable. ②The anterior superior part of the thigh.

髀枢 bishu

①位于股部外侧的最上方,股骨向外方显著隆起处,即股骨大转子的部位。②髋臼的部位。

①On the uppermost part of the lateral aspect of the thigh where exists the prominence of femur, i. e. , the site of the greater trochanter. ②The site of the acetabulum.

臂骨 arm bones

指尺骨和桡骨。

It refers to ulna and radius.

臂臑 Binao(LI14)

经穴名。属手阳明大肠经。定位:在臂外侧,三角肌止点处,当曲池与肩髃连线上,曲池上7寸。主治:肩臂痛,颈项挛急,瘰疬等。操作:直刺或向上斜刺1～1.5寸;可灸。

Name of an acupoint. It belongs to the Large Intestine Meridian of Hand-Yang-

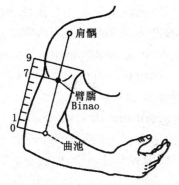

ming. Lacation: On the lateral side of the arm, at the termination of the deltoid muscle, on the line connecting Quchi(LI11) and Jianyu(LI15), 7 cun above Quchi(LI11). Indications: Pain in the shoulder and arm, contracture and rigidity of the neck, scrofula, etc. Method: Puncture perpendicularly or obliquely upward 1-1.5 cun. Moxibustion is applicable.

臂五里 Biwuli

手五里的别名。

The other name of Shouwuli(LI13).

臂中 Bizhong

经外奇穴名。在腕横纹至肘横纹的中点,尺、桡骨之间。主治:上肢偏瘫/痉挛,前臂痛。

Name of an extra point. It is at the midpoint between the transverse crease of the wrist and elbow, between the ulna and the radius. Indications: Paralysis, spasm and contracture of the upper extremities, forearm pain, etc.

砭石 stone needle

又称砭针,是我国古代用尖石制成的医用针具。可用于排脓放血,治疗痈肿及止痛等。

A kind of acupuncture needle made of sharp flint in ancient China, also known as flint needle. It is used for discharging pus and blood to treat carbuncles, furuncles and for relieving pains.

砭针 flint needle

指古代用尖石制成的针。

It is an ancient needle made of flint.

扁鹊 Bian Que

古代名医(公元前 5 世纪)。原名秦越人,精通医术,能治多种疾病,尤精脉诊和针术,著作已佚。

A famous physician in the 5th century B. C., formerly called Qin Yueren. He was proficient in medicine, especially in pulse taking and acupuncture, and can treat various diseases. He was believed to have authored some works which had been lost.

扁桃体 Biantaoti

耳穴名。在耳垂 8 区正中。主治:扁桃体炎,咽炎等。

Name of an ear point. It is in the 8th section of the ear lobe. Indications: Tonsillitis, pharyngitis, etc.

便秘 constipation

指大便干燥坚硬,排出困难;或排便次数少,两天以上不大便。多因气虚推动无力,或阴虚血少、大肠燥结,或胃中实热、气滞不行所致。治宜清热保津、补气养血。取穴:合谷、曲池、足三里、大肠俞、上巨虚、承山。

A condition of infrequency or difficulty in defecation with discharge of dry and impacted feces, due to inability of promoting peristalsis resulting from the deficiency of qi, or dryness of the large intestine resulting from the deficiency of yin and blood, or stagnation of qi resulting from the retention of excessive heat in the stomach. Treatment principle: Save the body fluid by clearing heat, benefit qi and nourish blood. Point selection: Hegu (LI4), Quchi (LI11), Zusanli (ST36), Dachangshu(BL25), Shangjuxu(ST37), Chengshan(BL57).

便溏 loose stool

指大便稀烂不成形。常伴有食欲不佳、疲乏、腹隐痛、脉濡弱等。多因脾虚不能运化水谷精微和水湿所致。有时湿热下注也可引起，以伴有腹痛、肛门灼热感、尿黄短、舌苔黄腻、脉滑数为特点。治宜健脾益气、升阳止泻。取穴：脾俞、胃俞、中脘、章门、足三里、商丘。

Thin and shapeless stool accompanied with poor appetite, fatigue, dull abdominal pain, and floating, soft and weak pulse, usually due to disorder of transportation of food and water resulting from the hypofunction of spleen; while accompanied with abdominal pain, burning sensation over the anus, oliguria with yellowish urine, yellowish and greasy fur on the tongue, and slippery and rapid pulse, due to damp-heat in lower jiao. Treatment principle: Strengthen spleen and benefit qi, elevate yang to arrest diarrhea. Point selection: Pishu (BL20), Weishu (BL21), Zhongwan (CV12), Zhangmen (LR13), Zusanli(ST36), Shangqiu(SP5).

辨络脉 observe the collateral

运用视觉观察患者浮行于浅表的小静脉丛的色泽、充盈度等进行诊断的方法。

Inspecting small superficial venules for their color and extent of filling as a reference for diagnosis.

辨证 syndrome differentiation

将四诊所搜集的临床资料，运用脏腑、经络、病因等基础理论，加以分析归纳，从而对疾病的病位、病性等做出判断的诊断思维过程。

Clinical observation for making a diagnosis based on the analysis and comprehension of the clinical data collected through the four methods of examination with the basic theories of viscera, meridian and etiology.

辨证论治 treatment based on syndrome differentiation

将四诊所搜集的临床资料，运用脏腑、经络、病因等基础理论，加以分析归纳以确定证候，并确立治则、治法及方药的思维和实践过程。

Making a diagnosis and selecting the treatment based on the analysis and comprehension of the clinical data collected by the four methods of examination with the basic theories of viscera, meridian and etiology.

表里 exterior and interior

是辨别疾病的部位和病势深浅的两个纲领。一般以病变在皮毛、经络属表，病较轻浅；病变在脏腑属里，病较深重。

A pair of principles for estimating the site and severity of a disease. In general, a disease involving the skin, hair and meridian is considered as a mild form impairing the exterior, while involving the viscera is considered as a more serious form impairing the interior.

表里配穴法 exterior-interior points combination

配穴法之一。即按照十二经脉阳经与阴经的表里关系配穴的方法。

One of the point-combining methods, i. e., the combination according to the exterior-interior relationship between yang meridian and yin meridian of the twelve regular meridians.

表实证 exterior excess syndrome

表证的一种。多因外邪侵入后,正邪相争于肌表,腠理密闭所表现出的证候。除有表证的症状外,常以恶寒、无汗、头痛、身痛、脉浮有力为特点。

A type of exterior syndrome caused by the confliction between the healty qi and the pathogenic evil in the superficies while the superficies is strong; characterized by aversion to cold, anhidrosis, headache, general aching, and floating, vigorous pulse in addition to the common manifestations of exterior syndrome.

表虚证 exterior deficiency syndrome

表证的一种。是正邪相争于肌表而卫外的阳气不足,腠理不密而出现的一种证候。除有表证的症状外,以自汗或汗出恶风、脉浮缓无力等为特征。

A type of exterior syndrome caused by the confliction between the healthy qi and the pathogenic evil in the superficies while the protective yang-qi is insufficient and the superficies is weak; characterized by spontaneous sweating, aversion to wind while sweating, and floating, slow and weak pulse in addition to the common manifestations of superficies syndrome.

表证 exterior syndrome

病邪在浅表的证候,多见于外感病的初期。症见恶寒发热、头痛、鼻塞、咳嗽、舌苔薄白、脉浮等。

A syndrome caused by the attack of evil to the superficies, usually seen in the primary stage of exogenous diseases; manifested as aversion to cold with fever, headache, nasal obstruction, cough, thin and whitish fur on the tongue, floating pulse, etc.

标本 manifestation and root cause

标本是个相对概念。临床上应用标本关系辨别病症的主次、本末、轻重、缓急,以确定治疗原则。

Two concepts existing with opposite relation, such as primary and secondary, major and minor, mild and severe, chronic and acute; the differentiation between them would be helpful to determine the therapeutical principle in clinical practice.

别穴 biexue

即经外奇穴。

The extra points.

冰台 bingtai

艾的别名。

The other name of moxa.

秉风 Bingfeng(SI12)

经穴名。属手太阳小肠经。定位:在肩

胛部,冈上窝中央,天宗直上,举臂有凹陷处。主治:肩胛痛,上肢痛麻,肩臂不举等。操作:直刺 0.5～1 寸;可灸。

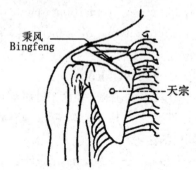

秉风
Bingfeng

天宗

Name of an acupoint. It belongs to the Small Intestine Meridian of Hand-Taiyang. Location:On the scapula, in the center of the supraspinous fossa, when raising arm, it is in the depression directly above Tianzong(SI11). Indications:Pain in the scapular region, numbness and pain of the upper limbs, motor impairment of the shoulder and arm, etc. Method:Puncture perpendicularly 0. 5-1 cun. Moxibustion is applicable.

病候 manifestations of a disease

指疾病反映出来的外在现象。包括症状和体征。

The external reflections of a disease, including symptoms and signs.

病机 pathogenesis

指病因、病位、证候、脏腑气血虚实变化的机制。

The mechanism of a disease including its etiology, location, manifestations, and the changes of difficiency or excess of qi and blood of the viscera.

病入膏肓 diseases beyond cure

指疾病由轻转重,发展到了危重阶段,此时患者往往形体消瘦、神色衰败。

A critical stage of a disease manifested as emaciation and seriously sick complexion.

病因辨证 syndrome differentiation of etiology

根据疾病的不同临床表现,了解疾病的原因及其病理变化的一种辨证方法。

A diagnostic method by observing the various clinical manifestations of the disease to detect its etiology and pathological changes.

病在中旁取之 treating internal diseases by needling limbs

身体内在的脏腑发生病变,可以取分布于四肢经络的穴位来治疗。

A treatment for the diseased viscera by puncturing the points of the meridians distributed on the limbs.

剥苔 peeled fur

舌苔全部或部分脱落,若舌苔长期剥脱如地图样,多属虫积。若在热性病中,舌苔在短时间内全部剥脱,且舌质深红或光如镜面,是肝肾真阴亏损、正虚病邪内陷的重症。

The tongue fur is partially or completely peeled off. Map-like tongue fur existing for a long time indicates parasitic amassment. If the fur peels completely in a short time during a febrile disease, and the tongue is smooth like a mirror or has a deep red color, it indicates a serious disease due to exhaustion of liver-yin and kidney-yin and invasion of evil due to deficiency of vital qi.

补法 tonifying method

补养人体阴阳气血不足,治疗各种虚证的方法。通常分补气、补血、补阴、补阳等。

A therapy for various types of asthenia syndrome due to insufficiency of yin, yang, qi and blood; generally classified into invigorating qi, enriching blood, tonifying yin and yang.

补气 invigorating qi

又称益气。补法之一。适用于气虚病证,症见倦怠无力、精神不振、呼吸少气、面色㿠白、自汗怕风、大便稀薄或泄泻、脉弱或虚大无力等。治宜补脾益气。取穴:足三里、关元、气海、三阴交、脾俞。

Also called benefiting qi. One of the tonifying methods. A treatment for the deficiency of qi, applicable to the case manifested as weakness, lassitude, shortness of breath, pale complexion, spontaneous sweating, aversion to wind, loose stools or diarrhea, weak pulse or feeble and large pulse, etc. Treatment principle: Tonify spleen and benefit qi. Point selection: Zusanli (ST36), Guanyuan(CV4), Qihai (CV6), Sanyinjiao (SP6), Pishu(BL20).

补肾 tonifying kidney

补益肾脏的方法。一般分为补肾阴和补肾阳。治宜补肾益精。取穴:肾俞、太溪、命门、关元、三阴交。

A treatment for invigorating the kidney, usually classified into invigoration of kidney-yin and invigoration of kidney-yang. Treatment principle: Tonify kidney and essence. Point selection: Shenshu (BL23), Taixi (KI3), Mingmen (GV4), Guanyuan(CV4), Sanyinjiao(SP6).

补生泻成 reinforcing the growing and reducing the grown

针刺补泻法之一。以针刺深浅结合生成数分补泻。针刺深度0.1~0.5寸为补,0.6~1寸为泻。

One of the reinforcing and reducing acupuncture methods. The reinforcing and reducing are distinguished by the needling depths, 0.1-0.5 cun is reinforcing while 0.6-1 cun is reducing.

补泻手法 reinforcing and reducing method

各种具有扶助正气或祛除病邪作用的针刺手法。

Manipulations used in acupuncture to strengthen body resistance and eliminate pathogenic factors.

补血 enriching blood

治疗血虚证的方法。适用于症见面色苍白或萎黄、头晕目眩、心悸气短、唇舌色淡、脉细等血虚证。治宜滋阴养血。取穴:足三里、肾俞、关元、血海、三阴交、脾俞。

A treatment for blood deficiency, applicable to the case manifested as pallor or sallow complexion, dizziness, palpitation, shortness of breath, pale lips and tongue, thin pulse, etc. Treatment principle: Nourish yin and blood. Point selection: Zusanli (ST36), Shenshu (BL23), Guanyuan(CV4), Xuehai(SP10), Sanyinjiao(SP6), Pishu(BL20).

补阳 tonifying yang

治疗阳虚证的方法,多指补肾阳。适用

于腰膝酸冷、软弱无力、阳痿遗精、小便频数、舌淡苔白、脉沉细等。治宜补肾壮阳。取穴：大椎、命门、肾俞、气海、关元。

A treatment for the syndrome of yang deficiency, usually refering to the tonification of kidney yang, applicable to the case manifested as soreness and cold feeling in the waist and knees, lassitude, impotence, emission, frequent urine, pale tongue with whitish fur, deep and thin pulse, etc. Treatment principle：Tonify kidney and strengthen yang. Point selection：Dazhui（GV14）, Mingmen（GV4）, Shenshu（BL23）, Qihai（CV6）, Guanyuan（CV4）.

补阴 nourishing yin

治疗阴虚证的方法。适用于阴虚液亏的各种疾病。治宜滋养阴液。取穴：太溪、肾俞、三阴交、足三里、关元。

A treatment for the syndrome of yin deficiency, applicable to various diseases caused by yin deficiency and fluid consumption. Treatment principle：Nourish yin and fluid. Point selection：Taixi（KI3）, Shenshu（BL23）, Sanyinjiao（SP6）, Zusanli（ST36）, Guanyuan（CV4）.

不定穴 indefinite point

即阿是穴，也称天应穴。

Ashi point or Tianying point.

不容 Burong(ST19)

经穴名。属足阳明胃经。定位：在上腹部，当脐上 6 寸，距前正中线 2 寸。主治：腹胀，呕吐，胃痛等。操作：直刺 0.5～0.8 寸；可灸。

Name of an acupoint. It belongs to the Stomach Meridian of Foot-Yangming.

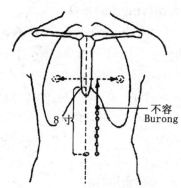

Location：On the upper abdomen, 6 cun above the center of the umbilicus and 2 cun lateral to the anterior midline. Indications：Abdominal distension, vomiting, gastric pain, etc. Method：Puncture perpendicularly 0.5-0.8 cun. Moxibustion is applicable.

不锈钢针 stainless steel needle

现代针具，强韧而不易锈蚀，为针灸临床上所常用。

Modern needles which are strong, flexible and erosion-preventing and so are widely used in clinic.

不育症 infertility in male

通常指男子无生育能力的一种病症。可因先天性生殖器官发育不全或其他疾病引起肾气亏损、精气虚冷所致。治宜补益肾精。取穴：肾俞、气穴、然谷、关元、三阴交、足三里。

A disorder in male with lack of reproductive function, caused by the congenital malformations of reproductive organs, or deficiency of kidney-qi and deficiency cold of essential qi resulting from other diseases. Treatment principle：Tonify the essence of the kidney. Point selec-

tion：Shenshu(BL23),Qixue(KI13),Ran-
gu(KI2), Guanyuan（CV4）, Sanyinjiao
(SP6),Zusanli(ST36).

不孕症 infertility in female

由于先天缺陷或其他各种疾病而致不
能受孕的一种疾病。治宜补益肾气、调理
冲任。取穴：肾俞、气穴、然谷、关元、三阴
交、足三里。

The inability to conceive resulting from
congenital defect or other diseases. Treat-
ment principle：Tonify the kidney-qi and
regulate the Conception Vessel and the
Thoroughfare Vessel. Point selection：
Shenshu（BL23）, Qixue（KI13）, Rangu
（KI2）, Guanyuan （CV4）, Sanyinjiao
(SP6),Zusanli(ST36).

步廊 Bulang(KI22)

经穴名。属足少阴肾经。定位：在胸部，
当第五肋间隙，前正中线旁开 2 寸。主治：
咳嗽，气喘，胸胁胀满，呕吐，厌食等。操作：
直刺或平刺 0.5～0.8 寸；可灸。

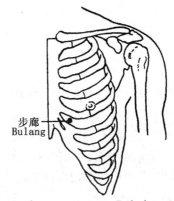

步廊
Bulang

Name of an acupoint. It belongs to the
Kidney Meridian of Foot-Shaoyin. Loca-
tion：On the chest, in the 5th intercostal
space, 2 cun lateral to the anterior midline. Indications：Cough, asthma, distension and fullness in the chest and hypochondriac region, vomiting, anorexia,
etc. Me thod：Puncture perpendicularly
or horizontally 0. 5-0. 8 cun. Moxibustion
is applicable.

苍龟探穴 green tortoise exploring point

针刺手法名。飞经走气四法之一，与"赤凤迎源"相对。即先进针到深部，再退到皮下，依次斜向上、下、左、右，分别用三进一退的手法行针，有通行经脉的作用。

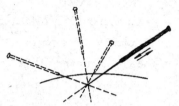

One of the four acupuncture techniques of moving qi throughout the meridians, contrasted with the technique of "phoenix greeting the source", i. e. , first, insert the needle into the deep part, then lift it beneath the skin and follow three-thrusting and one-lifting method in the upward, downward, leftward and rightward directions to open and dredge the meridians.

苍龙摆尾 green dragon shaking the tail

针刺治疗手法之一。其法有两种。①进针得气后，使针尖朝向病所，不提不插，也不捻动。以右手拇指和示指扳倒针柄约45°角，如此轻轻地左右往来拨动针柄，促使经气流动。②进针得气后，将针提至浅部，摇动针柄，以疏通气血。

A method of acupuncture manipulations. It has two forms: ①Following insertion of the needle with sensation, point the needle tip towards the disease location without twirling, lifting and thrusting. Use the thumb and the index finger gently move the needle left and right at a 45°angle to impel the flow of qi. ②Following insertion of the needle with sensation, life the needle to the superficial tissue and then shake the needle handle left and right to induce the flow of qi and blood.

插花 chahua

经外奇穴名。位于两额角发际直上 1.5 寸处。沿皮刺或灸，治疗头面疔疮、偏头痛等。

Name of extra points. Located 1. 5 cun directly above the hairline of the frontal angles. Horizontal puncture or moxibustion can used to cure the deep-rooted sore on the head and face, migraine, etc.

镵针 shear needle

古代九针之一。针的头部膨大而末端锐利。用于浅刺治疗热病、皮肤病。

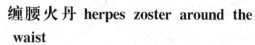

One of the nine needles in ancient times. Its head is large but its tip is sharp. It is used for superficial pricking in treating febrile and skin diseases.

缠腰火丹 herpes zoster around the waist

生于腰肋间的疱疹性疾病。由心经、肝经火邪湿毒凝结而成。初起患处刺痛发红，继而出现米粒样透明水疱，累累如串珠，呈束带状排列，即带状疱疹。治宜清热利湿。取穴：外关、内庭、侠溪、阴陵泉。

Herpetic disease starting with local redness and pain, following rice grain like blisters arranged in bundles in the waist and hypochondrium, accompanied by neuralgic pain; caused by the stagnation of fire and dampness-evils in the Heart and Liver Meridians. Treatment principle: Clear heat and promote diuresis. Point selection: Waiguan (TE5), Neiting (ST44), Xiaxi (GB43), Yinlingquan (SP9).

产后大便难 postpartum constipation

即产后大便秘结。多因产后血虚津少, 不能滋润大肠, 或气虚大肠传送无力所致。治宜养血润燥。取穴:脾俞、胃俞、大肠俞、天枢、支沟、足三里。

A condition in puerperium due to dryness of the large intestine resulting from deficiency of blood and body fluid, or due to weak peristalsis of the large intestine resulting from deficiency of qi. Treatment principle: Nourish the blood and moisten dryness. Point selection: Pishu (BL20), Weishu (BL21), Dachangshu (BL25), Tianshu (ST25), Zhigou (TE6), Zusanli (ST36).

产后乳汁自出 postpartum galactorrhea

产后不吸吮而乳汁自动流出。多因脾胃气虚不能固摄, 乳汁失约而自溢;或因肝火亢盛, 迫乳外溢。治宜健脾温肾。取穴:脾俞、肾俞、气海、太溪、足三里。

Spontaneous flow of milk in puerperium, caused by qi deficiency of the spleen and stomach leading to inability to hold the milk, or by the hyperactivity of liver-fire which forces the milk to over-

flow. Treatment principle: Tonify the spleen and warm the kidney. Point selection: Pishu (BL20), Shenshu (BL23), Qihai (CV6), Taixi (KI3), Zusanli (ST36).

产后水肿 postpartum edema

产后四肢或全身浮肿。因患者平素脾肾虚弱, 产后阳气更虚, 水湿不能运化敷布, 溢于肌肤所致。治宜健脾温肾、助阳利水。取穴:脾俞、肾俞、水分、气海、太溪、足三里。

A disorder due to disturbance of body fluid metabolism with the retention of fluid in the skin and the subcutaneous tissues resulting from the debility of the spleen and kidney which is aggravated by childbirth. Treatment principle: Tonify the spleen and warm the kidney. Point selection: Pishu (BL20), Shenshu (BL23), Shuifen (CV9), Qihai (CV6), Taixi (KI3), Zusanli (ST36).

产后血崩 postpartum metrorrhagia

产后子宫大量出血的危症。

A serious condition with profuse uterine bleeding after childbirth.

产后腰痛 postpartum lumbago

孕妇在分娩后腰部隐痛, 伴乏力、耳鸣等。多因分娩伤肾, 腰无所主所致;也有因败血瘀阻带脉而引起。治宜温阳补肾。取穴:肾俞、命门、三阴交、足三里、腰阳关。

A condition in puerperium usually accompanied with fatigue and tinnitus, due to impairment of the kidney during labour, or due to the obstruction of the Belt Vessel by blood stasis. Treatment principle: Warm the yang and tonify the kidney. Point selection：Shenshu(BL23)，Mingmen(GV4)，Sanyinjiao（SP6），Zusanli(ST36)，Yaoyangguan(GV3).

产后遗尿 postpartum enuresis

产后出现小便不能控制，容易遗出的病症。多因产后肾气虚弱，运化失职，气机不畅所致。治宜温补下焦。取穴：肾俞、三焦俞、气海、委阳、百会、中极。

Involuntary discharge of urine in puerperium, due to asthenia and hypofunction of the kidney, or injury of the bladder during labour. Treatment principle：Warm and strengthen the lower jiao. Point selection：Shenshu（BL23），Sanjiaoshu（BL22），Qihai（CV6），Weiyang（BL39），Baihui(GV20)，Zhongji(CV3).

长谷 Changgu

经外奇穴名。又名循际、长平。定位：神阙穴旁开 2.5 寸处。主治：泄利，不嗜食，食不消等。直刺或灸治。

Name of an extra point, also called Xunji or Changping. Location：2. 5 cun transversely away from Shenque(CV8). Indications：Diarrhea, dysentery, lack of appetite, indigestion, etc. Perpendicular acupuncture and moxibustion are applicable.

长窌 Changliao

口禾髎别名。

The other name of Kouheliao (LI19).

长平 Changping

章门别名，又指经外奇穴长谷。

The other name of Zhangmen (LR13); it also refers to the extrapoint Changgu.

长强 Changqiang(GV1)

经穴名。属督脉，本经络穴。定位：在

尾骨下，当尾骨端与肛门连线的中点处。主治：泄泻，便血，痔疾，脱肛，便秘，腰痛，癫痫等。操作：斜刺，针尖向上，与骶骨平行刺入 0.5～1 寸，直刺易伤直肠；可灸。

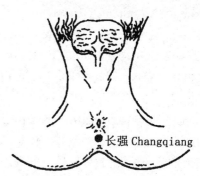

长强 Changqiang

The acupoint, Luo-Connecting point, belongs to the Governor Vessel. Location：Below the tip of the coccyx, at the midpoint of the line between the tip of the coccyx and the anus. Indications：Diarrhea, bloody stool, hemorrhoids, prolapse of rectum, constipation, pain in the lower back, epilepsy, etc. Method：Puncture obliquely upward 0. 5-1 cun closely along the anterior border of the sacrum. The rectum may be easily injured if puncturing perpendicularly. Moxibustion is applicable.

长蛇灸 long snake moxibustion

间接灸的一种，即取大蒜适量，去皮捣成泥糊状，平铺于脊柱（大椎至腰俞）上，直径、厚各约 6 mm，周围用厚纸固定，再用小型艾炷 2 枚，分别置于大椎及腰俞上点燃施灸，灸至患者自感口鼻内有蒜味为止，民间用此治疗虚痨等病证。

One form of indirect moxibustions, by placing a layer of garlic paste about 6 mm in diameter and thickness along the spinal column from Dazhui (GV14) to Yaoshu

(GV2), and fixing it with thick papers a- round, then burn a small moxa cone on top of the garlic paste at the two ends. The treatment is completed when the pa- tient has experienced a garlic taste in the mouth and nose. The method is used for consumptive diseases.

长溪 Changxi

天枢别名。

The other name of Tianshu(ST25).

长夏 long summer

夏季的最后 1 个月。

The last month in summer.

长针 long needle

古代九针之一。针体较长,一般为 6～7 寸(相当于 20～23 cm)或更长一些。多用 于深刺,以治疗慢性风湿病、坐骨神经痛等。

One of the nine needles in ancient times. Its body is long, usually 20-23 cm, or slightly longer. It is often used for deep acupuncture to treat chronic rheumatism and sciatica, etc.

肠鸣 borborygmus

指肠蠕动声。因中气虚或邪在大肠所 致。治宜疏通肠胃气机。取穴:大肠俞、 气海、中脘、上巨虚、天枢。

The sound caused by the propulsion of qi through the intestines, due to qi defi- ciency of spleen and stomach or the at- tack of evil to the large intestine. Treat- ment principle: Regulate the movement of qi in the intestine and stomach. Point se- lection: Dachangshu (BL25), Qihai (CV6), Zhongwan (CV12), Shangjuxu (ST37),Tianshu(ST25).

肠痈 periappendicular abscess

由湿热之邪留注肠中,气血瘀阻所致的 病证,以右下腹痛、明显压痛及反跳痛为 特征,伴有发热、恶寒、恶心等症。相当于 急性阑尾炎、阑尾脓肿等。治宜清热导 滞、活血散结。取穴:曲池、天枢、上巨虚、 地机。

A disorder due to stagnation of qi and blood in intestines affected by damp-heat evil; marked by pain in the lower right quadrant of the abdomen with intense lo- cal tenderness and rebound tenderness, accompanied with fever, aversion to cold, nausea, etc. ; corresponding to a- cute appendicitis, appendiceal abscess, etc. Treatment principle: Clear away heat and resolve stagnation,activate blood and remove obstruction. Point selection: Qu- chi (LI11), Tianshu (ST25), Shangjuxu (ST37),Diji(SP8).

潮热 tidal fever

指发热如潮汛有定时。以阴虚和血虚 者为多。常在午后或夜间发热,早晨热退 至正常。实证则多为阳明里实证,热退不 清,每至下午 3～5 点钟热势增高,常伴大 便不通等症。治宜滋阴清热。取穴:三阴 交、地机、足三里、照海、阴陵泉。

A fever recurring daily at certain time. In case of asthenia syndrome, mostly yin deficiency and blood deficiency, the tem- perature is usually high in the afternoon or at night, and becomes normal in the morning. In case of sthenia syndrome, mostly internal sthenia syndrome of yang- ming, from 3-5 o'clock in the afternoon, the temperature is higher with recurrent fever and is usually accompanied with constipation. Treatment principle: Nourish yin and clear yang. Point selection: Sanyinjiao (SP6), Diji (SP8), Zusanli (ST36), Zhaohai (KI6), Yinlingquan (SP9).

臣觉 Chenjue

经外奇穴名。位于肩胛骨上角边际。斜刺或灸治疗精神疾病。

Name of an extra point. Located at the margin of the upper corner of the scapula. Oblique puncture or moxibustion is used to treat mental diseases.

沉脉 deep pulse

脉搏深沉，轻按不应、重按才得的一种脉象。主病在里。沉而有力为里实；沉而无力为里虚。

A pulse condition in which the beats are located deeply and palpable only by heavy pressure, indicating that the disease located in the interior. The deep but strong pulse indicates an internal sthenia syndrome, while the deep but weak pulse indicates an internal asthenia syndrome.

承扶 Chengfu(BL36)

经穴名。属足太阳膀胱经。定位：在大腿后面，臀下横纹的中点。主治：腰臀部疼痛。操作：直刺1～2寸；可灸。

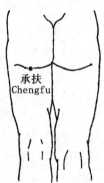

承扶 Chengfu

Name of an acupoint. It belongs to the Bladder Meridian of Foot-

Taiyang. Location: On the posterior side of the thigh, at the midpoint of the transverse gluteal crease under the buttocks. It is used for treating pain in lower back and gluteal region. Method: Puncture perpendicularly 1-2 cun. Moxibustion is applicable.

承光 Chengguang(BL6)

经穴名。属足太阳膀胱经。定位：在头部，当前发际正中直上2.5寸，旁开1.5寸。主治：头痛，视物不清，鼻塞等。操作：斜刺0.3～0.5寸；可灸。

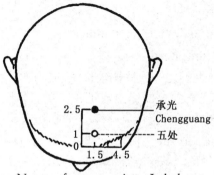

承光 Chengguang
五处

Name of an acupoint. It belongs to the Bladder Meridian of Foot-Taiyang. Location: On the head, 2.5 cun directly above the midpoint of the anterior hairline and 1.5 cun lateral to the midline. Indications: Headache, blurred vision, nasal obstruction, etc. Method: Puncture obliquely 0.3-0.5 cun. Moxibustion is applicable.

承浆 Chengjiang(CV24)

经穴名。属任脉。定位：在面部，当颏唇沟的正中凹陷处。主治：面肿，齿龈肿痛，齿痛，流涎，癫狂，口眼歪斜等。操作：斜刺0.3～0.5寸；可灸。

Name of an acupoint. It belongs to the Conception Vessel. Location: On the face,

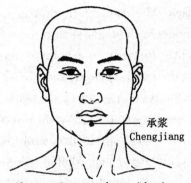

承浆
Chengjiang

in the depression at the midpoint of the mentolabial sulcus. Indications：Facial swelling, swelling and pain of the gums, toothache, salivation, mental disorders, deviation of the eyes and mouth，etc. Method：Puncture obliquely 0.3-0.5 cun. Moxibustion is applicable.

承筋 Chengjin(BL56)

经穴名。属足太阳膀胱经。定位：在小腿后面，当委中与承山连线上，腓肠肌肌腹中央，委中下 5 寸。主治：小腿痛，痔疾，急性腰痛等。操作：直刺 1～2 寸；可灸。

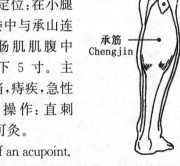

承筋
Chengjin

Name of an acupoint. It belongs to the Bladder Meridian of Foot-Taiyang. Location：On the posterior side of the leg, on the line connecting Weizhong (BL40)and Chengshan(BL57)，at the center of the gastrocnemius muscle belly,5 cun below Weizhong（BL40）. Indications：Leg pain, hemorrhoids, acute lower back pain, etc. Method：Puncture perpendicularly 1-2 cun. Moxibustion is applicable.

承灵 Chengling(GB18)

经穴名。属足少阳胆经。定位：在头部，当前发际上 4 寸，头正中线旁开 2.25寸。主治：头痛，眩晕，目痛，鼻塞，鼻衄等。操作：平刺 0.3～0.5 寸；可灸。

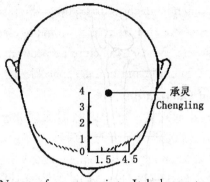

承灵
Chengling

Name of an acupoint. It belongs to the Gallbladder Meridian of Foot-Shaoyang. Location：On the head，4 cun above the anterior hairline and 2.25 cun lateral to the midline of the head. Indications：Headache, vertigo, eye pain, nasal obstruction, epistaxis, etc. Method：Puncture horizontally 0.3-0.5 cun. Moxibustion is applicable.

承满 Chengman(ST20)

经穴名。属足阳明胃经。定位：在上腹部，当脐中上 5 寸，距前正中线 2 寸。主治：胃痛，腹胀，呕吐，食欲不振等。操作：直刺 1～1.5 寸；可灸。

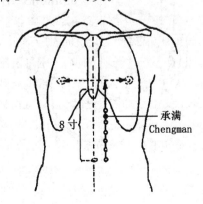

承满
Chengman

8 寸

Name of an acupoint. It belongs to the Stomach Meridian of Foot-Yangming. Location: On the upper abdomen, 5 cun above the center of the umbilicus and 2 cun lateral to the anterior midline. Indications: Stomachache, abdominal distension, vomiting, anorexia, etc. Method: Puncture perpendicularly 1-1.5 cun. Moxibustion is applicable.

承命 Chengming

经外奇穴名。位于内踝后太溪穴上 3 寸。直刺或灸治狂邪癫痫病。

Name of an extra point. Located 3 cun above Taixi(KI3) behind the medial ankle. Perpendicular puncture or moxibustion is adopted to cure mania, epilepsy, etc.

承泣 Chengqi(ST1)

经穴名。属足阳明胃经。定位:在面部,目正视,瞳孔直下,当眼球与眶下缘之间。主治:目赤肿痛,流泪,夜盲,眼球瞤动,面瘫等。操作:左手拇指向上轻推眼球,紧靠眶下缘缓慢直刺 0.5~1 寸,不宜提插,以防刺破血管引起血肿;禁灸。

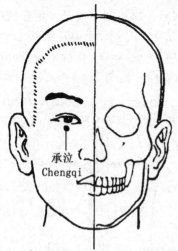

承泣
Chengqi

Name of an acupoint. It belongs to the Stomach Meridian of Foot-Yangming. Location: On the face, with the eyes look straightly forward, the point is directly below the pupil, between the eyeball and the infraorbital margin. Indications: Redness, swelling and pain of the eyes, lacrimation, night blindness, twitching of eyelids, facial paralysis, etc. Method: Push the eyeball gently upwards with the thumb of the left hand, insert the needle closely to the infraorbital margin, puncture perpendicularly 0.5-1 cun. It is not allowed to lift or thrust the needle so as to avoid injuring the blood vessels and causing hematoma. Moxibustion is prohibited.

承山 Chengshan(BL57)

经穴名。属足太阳膀胱经。定位:在小腿后面正中,委中与昆仑之间,当小腿或足跟上提时,腓肠肌肌腹下出现尖角凹陷处。主治:腰痛,腿痛转筋,痔疾,便秘,脚气等。操作:直刺1~1.2 寸;可灸。

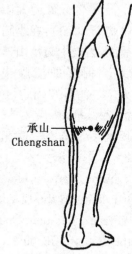

承山
Chengshan

Name of an acupoint. It belongs to the Bladder Meridian of Foot-Taiyang. Location: In the middle of the posterior side of the leg, between Weizhong(BL40) and Kunlun(BL60), in the depression below the gestrocnemius mucle belly when the leg is stretched or the heel is lifted. Indications: Lower back pain, spasm and pain of the gastrocnemius, hemorrhoids, constipation, beriberi, etc. Method: Puncture perpendicularly 1-1. 2 cun. Moxibustion is applicable.

迟脉 slow pulse

脉率缓慢,通常指每分钟脉搏在 60 次以下的一种脉象。一般常见于寒证,也可因阳气被实邪阻滞所引起。久经锻炼的运动员也可见迟缓有力的脉象,此不属病脉。

A pulse condition with less than 60 beats per minute, commonly seen in the case of cold syndrome and also stagnation of yang-qi by excessive pathogen. A slow but vigorous pulse occurring in a well trained athlete is considered as normal.

持针法 needle grasping

针刺时夹持针具的方法。一般用右手拇、示指夹持针柄或针身,露出针尖,以便刺入穴位;若针身较长,多夹持针身下部进行针刺。

The way of holding the needle during acupuncture therapy. Usually the thumb and index grasp the handle or body of the needle, exposing the needle tip so as to puncture. The longer needle usually be grasped the lower part to puncture.

尺泽 Chize(LU5)

经穴名。属手太阴肺经,本经合穴。定位:在肘横纹中,肱二头肌肌腱桡侧凹陷处。主治:咳嗽,咯血,午后潮热,气喘,咽喉肿痛,胸满,小儿惊风,肘臂挛痛等。操作:直刺 0. 5～1 寸。

The acupoint, He-Sea point, belongs to the Lung Meridian of Hand-Taiyin.

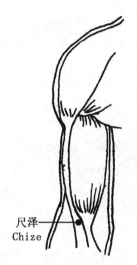

Location: In the cubital crease, in the depression of the radial side of the biceps brachii tendon. Indications: Cough, hemoptysis, tidal fever in the afternoon, asthma, sore throat, fullness in the chest, infantile convulsion, spasm and pain of the elbow and arm, etc. Method: Puncture perpendicularly 0. 5-1 cun.

尺泽 Chize

齿 teeth

又名牙。为口腔内嚼食物的器官,属足少阴肾经,为肾所主。手阳明大肠经与足阳明胃经分别入下、上齿。

A set of small hard structures in the jaws used for mastication of food, belonging to the Kidney Meridian of Foot-Shaoyin, and administered by the kidney. The Large Intestine Meridian of Hand-Yangming and the Stomach Meridian of Foot-Yangming pass through the lower and upper jaw respectively.

齿衄 gingival hemorrhage

血从齿缝、牙龈处渗出,甚至流血不止。多因胃腑积热上乘,或肾阴不足、虚火上炎,或脾不统血所致。治宜清胃火、止血。取穴:内庭、胃俞、地机、隐白。

A disorder due to upward attack of the heat-evil accumulated in the stomach, or insufficiency of kidney-yin leading to the hyperactivity of asthenia fire, or failure of controlling blood by the spleen. Treatment principle: Clear stomach-fire and stop bleeding. Point selection: Neiting (ST44), Weishu(BL21), Diji(SP8), Yinbai(SP1).

豉饼灸 fermented soybean cake moxibustion

间接灸的一种。取豆豉适量,捣烂,用水或黄酒调和制成 6 mm 厚的药饼,如疮口大,用细针穿刺数孔,置疮面上,放艾炷点燃施灸。适用于痈疽发背、顽疮等症。

A form of the indirect moxibustions. Method: Take a proper amount of fermented soybean and mash it, mix it with water or rice wine, then make cakes about 6 mm thick each, just the size of the opening sore. Punch several holes in the cake with a small needle, then place it on the surface of a sore. Put the ignited moxa cone on the cake for moxibusion. It is used for carbuncle on the back, cellulitis, etc.

赤白肉际 dorso-ventral boundary of the hand or foot

指手足掌面与背面的交界处。

Boundary between the sole-palmar side and the dorsal side of the hand or foot.

赤凤迎源 red phoenix greeting the source

针刺手法名。飞经走气四法之一,与"苍龟探穴"相对。即先进针至深部,再提至浅部,得气后进入中部进行提插捻转,有通经行络的作用。

A kind of acupuncture technique, one of the four techniques of moving qi throughout the meridians, by contrast with the technique of "green tortoise exploring point", namely, first insert the needle into the deep site, then lift it to the shallow site after having got the sensation, thrust the needle into the middle site and perform the lifting, thrusting, twisting and twirling manipulations to open and dredge the meridians and collaterals.

瘈脉 chimai (TE18)

经穴名。属手少阳三焦经。定位:在头部,耳后乳突中央,当角孙与翳风之间,沿耳轮连线的中、下 1/3 的交点处。主治:头痛,耳鸣耳聋,小儿惊风。操作:平刺0.3～0.5 寸;可灸。

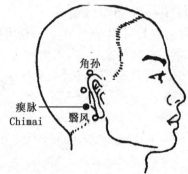

Name of an acupoint. It belongs to the Sanjiao Meridian of Hand-Shaoyang. Location: On the head, at the center of the mastoid process, and at the junction of the middle third and lower third of the line connecting Jiaosun (TE20) and Yifeng(TE17) along the curve of the ear helix. Indications: Headache, tinnitus, deafness, infantile convulsion, etc. Method: Puncture horizontally 0.3-0.5 cun. Moxibustion is applicable.

冲道 Chongdao

神道穴别名。

The other name of Shendao(GV11).

冲脉 the Thoroughfare Vessel

奇经八脉之一。起于小腹(胞中)内,沿脊柱内部上行。同时由阴部的两侧开始,夹脐两旁向上,到胸部而止。本经发病,主要有哮喘、腹痛、肠鸣、月经不调、不孕症等病症。

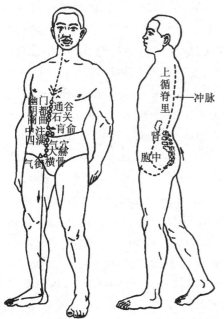

One of the eight extra meridians. It originates in the lower abdomen(uterus) and runs upwards along the interior side of the spine; at the same time, starts from the sides of the genitalia and passes by both sides of umbilicus, and ends at the chest. When this meridian is diseased, the main symptoms are asthma, abdominal pain, borborygmus, irregular menstruation, infertility, etc.

冲脉穴 the Thoroughfare Vessel points

①指冲脉与十二正经、任脉、督脉的交会穴。②指公孙穴,为八脉八穴之一。

①All the crossing points of the Thoroughfare Vessel with the twelve regular meridians, the Conception Vessel and the Governor Vessel. ②Gongsun(SP4). One of the eight crossing points of the eight extra meridians.

冲门 Chongmen(SP12)

经穴名。属足太阴脾经。定位:在腹股沟外侧,距耻骨联合上缘中点 3.5 寸,当髂外动脉搏动处的外侧。主治:腹痛,疝气,小便不利等。操作:直刺 0.5～1 寸;可灸。

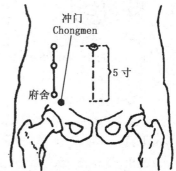

Name of an acupoint. It belongs to the Spleen Meridian of Foot-Taiyin. Location: At the lateral end of the inguinal groove, 3.5 cun lateral to the midpoint of the superior margin of the symphysis pubis, outside the point where the pulsation of the external iliac artery is palpable. Indications: Abdominal pain, hernia, dysuria, etc. Method: Puncture perpendicularly 0.5-1 cun. Moxibustion is applicable.

冲阳 Chongyang(ST42)

经穴名。属足阳明胃经,本经原穴。定位:在足背最高处,当姆长伸肌腱与趾长伸肌腱之间,足背动脉搏动处。主治:上牙痛,足背红肿,面瘫,足肌萎缩无力等。操作:避开动脉,直刺0.3~0.5寸。

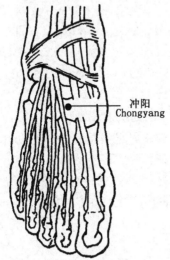

冲阳
Chongyang

The acupoint, Yuan-Primary point, belongs to the Stomach Meridian of Foot-Yangming. Location: At the top of the dorsum of foot, between the extensor pollicis longus tendon and the extensor digitorum longus tendon, at the point where the pulsation of the dorsal artery of the foot is palpable. Indications: Pain of the upper teeth, redness and swelling of the dorsum of foot, facial paralysis, muscular atrophy and motor impairment of the foot, etc. Method: Puncture perpendicularly 0. 3-0. 5 cun, avoiding the artery.

重舌 sublingual swelling

舌下静脉瘀血致舌下组织肿胀。常并见头项疼痛、发热等症状。常因心脾积热所致。治宜清泄心热。取穴:少府、大都、少海、内庭。

A sign of swelling of the hypoglossal tissues due to congestion of the sublingual vein, usually accompanied by neck pain, headache and fever, indicating the accumulation of heat-evil in the heart and spleen. Treatment principle: Clear heart heat. Point selection: Shaofu (HT8), Dadu (SP2), Shaohai (HT3), Neiting (ST44).

抽添法 lifting and pressing method

针刺抽按法之一。类似于纳气法。即先紧按慢提九阳之数,得气后转换针向向病所,行提按法使气至病所,最后直针下按纳气。多用于瘫痪、半身不遂等症。

A kind of lifting and thrusting acupuncture method, similar to the Qi-receiving method, i. e., first fast thrust and slowly lift the needle nine times, after getting the sensation, turn the needle towards the location of the disease and perform the pressing-lifting manipulations to make the sensation reach the diseased part, and finally thrust the needle perpendicularly to receive qi. The method is mostly used to treat paralysis, hemiplegia, etc.

出针 withdraw the needle

针刺手法之一。即针刺完毕后,将针拔出体外的方法。

One of the acupuncture techniques, i. e., pulling the needle out after needling.

触电感 electrical sensation

针刺入后,针下产生酸麻、胀痛感,并沿经络循行部位走窜,如同触电,是得气的反应。

The feeling of soreness, numbness,

swelling and pain like an electric shock runs along the meridians after acupuncture is the reflection of obtaining qi.

揣法 search and select

手指揣摸寻找穴位的方法。

Identification of a point by massage local tissue with fingers.

川椒饼灸 pepper cake moxibustion

取花椒研细末,用醋调和,制药饼,贴痛处,上置艾炷,施灸。适用于心痛、胸痛、腹痛、腰痛。

Grind a certain mount of Sichuan pepper into powder,then mix it with vinegar to make cakes,on which moxibustion is performed. Indications:Pains of the heart,chest,abdomen,waist,etc.

穿鼻 Chuanbi

经外奇穴,上迎香别名。位于鼻骨下凹陷中。主治:鼻炎、鼻窦炎、久流冷泪、烂弦火眼等。

The other name of the extra point Shangyingxiang(EX-HN8). Located at the inferior depression of the nasal bone. Indications: Rhinitis, sinusitis, dacryorrhea, marginal blepharitis,etc.

喘鸣 bronchial wheezing

指呼吸急促,喉间有痰鸣声的症状,为哮喘主证。治宜宣肺、化痰、平喘。取穴:列缺、大椎、丰隆、尺泽、肺俞、定喘。

The major symptom of asthma, manifested as rapid respiration with wheezing. Treatment principle:Ventilate lung-qi and disperse phlegm to relieve asthma. Point selection: Lieque (LU7), Dazhui (GV14),Fenglong(ST40),Chize(LU5),

Feishu(BL13),Dingchuan(EX-B1).

喘息 chuanxi

经外奇穴名。又名定喘穴。位于第七颈椎棘突旁开 0.5～1 寸间压痛明显处。直刺或灸治疗哮喘、咳嗽、落枕、荨麻疹等。

Name of an extra point, also known as Dingchuan(EX-B1). Located at the sensitive points 0.5-1 cun lateral to the spinous process of the 7th cervical vertebra. Vertical acupuncture or moxibustion is adopted to cure asthma, cough, stiff neck, urticaria, etc.

喘证 asthma

指以呼吸急促、困难,甚则张口抬肩、鼻翼煽动、不能平卧为特征的一种病症。因风寒痰饮,邪火壅肺,肺失肃降;或肺肾虚弱,肺虚气无所主,肾虚摄纳无权所致。治宜化痰平喘。取穴:列缺、大椎、丰隆、尺泽、肺俞、定喘。

A symptom characterized by rapid and difficult respiration, patient could not lie flat with open mouth, lifting shoulder and flaring nostrils. It is caused by the inability to purificate and descend qi by the lung due to wind-cold evils, phlegm and fire, and inability to grasp qi by the lung and kidney resulting from deficiency of them. Treatment principle:Disperse phlegm to relieve asthma. Point selection:Lieque (LU7),Dazhui (GV14),Fenglong (ST40), Chize (LU5), Feishu (BL13), Dingchuan(EX-B1).

《串雅内外篇》 Treatises on Internal and External Folk Medicine

赵学敏撰(1759),《串雅》分内、外篇,各

4 卷,《内篇》收集铃医方药及其他验方编成;《外篇》载录验方、针灸、熏洗、熨贴等法,保存了不少民间医药、针灸的经验。

A book compiled by Zhao Xuemin in 1759, in which records various kinds of healing methods and remedies collected from among folk healers.

窗笼 chuanglong

①指耳部。②天窗穴别名。

①The ear. ②The other name of Tianchuang(SI16).

疮疡 sore

是体表上有形证可见的外科及皮肤科疾病的总称。包括痈疽、疔疮、流注、瘰疬、溃疡等。治宜散热解毒。取穴:曲池、解溪、委中、风门。

A general condition seen in external medicine and dermatology, including carbuncle, deep-rooted carbuncle, furuncle, deep multiple abscess, scrofula, ulcer, etc. Treatment principle: Dispel heat and remove toxicity. Point selection: Quchi (LI11), Jiexi(ST41), Weizhong(BL40), Fengmen(BL12).

疮疡灸法 moxibustion for sore

灸疗的一种,临床所见疮疡,不论阴证、阳证,初期均可先施灸法。

Use of moxibustion in treating sores from various etiology at the early stage for either yin type or yang.

垂浆 Chuijiang

承浆穴别名。

The other name of Chengjiang(CV24).

垂前 Chuiqian

耳穴名。又称神经衰弱点、拔牙麻醉点,在耳垂四区。主治:牙痛,神经衰弱。也用于拔牙麻醉。

Name of an ear point. This point is also known as neurasthenic point, or anesthetic point for tooth extraction. It is in the 4th section of ear lobe. Indications: Toothache, neurasthenia, anesthetic for tooth extraction.

垂手 Chuishou

风市穴别名。

The other name of Fengshi (GB31).

唇 lips

七冲门之一。口唇分上、下唇,为脾的外候,中医临床上常通过诊察口唇来帮助诊断脾病。

One of the seven important openings, the flesh margins of the mouth, composed of lower and upper lips. Spleen manifests in lips. The inspection of the lips is helpful to diagnose disorders of the spleen.

唇里 Chunli

经外奇穴名。位于下唇黏膜中点,外对承浆。直刺或三棱针点刺出血,主治黄疸、瘟疫、口噤、牙龈炎、口腔炎等。

Name of the extra point that located at the center of the lower lip mucosa, externally opposite to Chengjiang(CV24). Perpendicular puncture or letting out blood with a three-edged needle is used to cure jaundice, pestilence, lockjaw, gum inflammations, stomatitis, etc.

唇针 lip acupuncture

针刺口唇周围的穴位以治疗疾病的方法。

To puncture the acupoints around the lips for therapy.

唇肿 swelling of lips

即口唇肿胀,甚则痛痒并作。多由脾胃湿热所致。治宜清泄脾胃湿热。取穴:大都、行间、阴陵泉、内庭。

A disorder accompanied with pain and itching of the lips, caused by the accumulation of the damp-heat in the spleen and stomach. Treatment principle: Clear the heat and dampness in the spleen and stomach. Point selection: Dadu (SP2), Xingjian (LR2), Yinlingquan (SP6), Neiting(ST44).

淳于意 Chunyu Yi

西汉著名医家(公元前216—公元前150年),又名仓公。他重脉法,治病针药并用,是第一个在史书上留有病案的医家。

An renowned physician in the Western Han Dynasty(B. C. 216-B. C. 150), also known as Cang Gong. He was particularly adept in pulse palpation and in treating disease with both acupuncture and herbal medicine. He was the first to keep records of clinical cases.

瓷针 porcelain needle

用于砭刺出血的瓷器碎片。

The porcelain pieces used to let out blood.

慈宫 Cigong

①冲门别名。②经外奇穴名。位于耻骨联合中点旁开 2.5 寸处。直刺或灸治泄泻、痢疾、月经不调等。

① The other name of Chongmen (SP12). ②Name of the extra point located 2.5 cun lateral to the midpoint of the symphysis pubis, vertical acupuncture or moxibustion is used to cure diarrhea, dysentery, irregular menstruation, etc.

磁疗 magnetotherapy

利用磁场作用于人体经穴达到治疗目的的一种方法。

A therapeutic technique applying the magnetic field on the acupoints.

磁针 magnetic needle

①用带有磁性的铁针或钢针进行针刺。②即瓷针,用于放血排脓的瓷器碎片。

①Use a magnetic iron or steel needle for acupuncture. ② Porcelain needle, i. e., the porcelain pieces used to let out blood or dredge pus.

磁珠疗法 magnetic bead therapy

现代疗法之一。用磁珠按压一定部位,代替针刺的一种疗法,体穴和耳穴均可用,主要用于治疗慢性疾病。

A recently developed method of therapy that uses magnetic beads to press certain parts instead of acupuncture. This technique is applicable to both body and ear points, primarily used in treating chronic diseases.

次髎 Ciliao(BL32)

经穴名。属足太阳膀胱经。定位:在骶部,当髂后上棘内下方,适对第二骶后孔处。主治:腰痛,疝气,月经不调,白带,痛经,梦遗,阳痿,遗尿,小便不利等。操作:直刺 0.8～1.2 寸;可灸。

Name of an acupoint. It belongs to the Bladder Meridian of Foot-Taiyang. Location: On the sacrum, medial and inferior to the

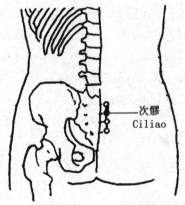

次髎
Ciliao

posterior superior iliac spine just opposite to the 2nd sacral foramen. Indications: Lumbago, hernia, irregular menstruation, leukorrhea disease, dysmenorrhea, nocturnal emission, impotence, enuresis, dysuria, etc. Method: Puncture perpendicularly 0. 8-1. 2 cun. Moxibustion is applicable.

次门 Cimen

关元穴别名。

The other name of Guanyuan(CV4).

刺激参数 stimulation parameters

指针刺时对穴位施加的刺激条件、刺激量等各项数据。记录和分析这些数据对研究针刺原理及提高疗效具有重要意义。

All the data collected during the acupuncture process including stimulus conditions and stimulus amount. Collecting and analyzing these data are of great importance in acupuncture mechanism research and in increasing the therapeutic effects.

刺激强度 stimulus intensity

指针灸刺激的强度,分强、中、弱三种。刺激的强度与多种因素有关,如手法的轻重、针刺的深浅、针的粗细和数量、针刺频率的快慢和持续时间的久暂等。

The intensity of the stimulus of acupuncture or moxibustion, which is classified into three degrees, i. e. , the intense, the middle and the weak stimulus. The intensity of the stimulus is depended upon many factors, such as the force of the manipulations, the depth of the puncture, the size and number of the needles, the frequency and the duration of the acupuncture, etc.

刺禁 acupuncture prohibitions

指针刺的禁忌,包括某些特殊的部位(重要脏器、大血管、脑、脊髓)和某些特殊情况(过饥、过饱、过劳、激动)下的禁针等。

The contraindications of acupuncture, for example, some special parts (important viscera, large vessels, brain and spinal cord) or some special conditions(hunger, overeating, overwork, over excitement), etc.

刺络 puncturing the collaterals

针刺方法名。即用三棱针或皮肤针在浅表小络脉上点刺或散刺出血。

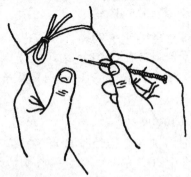

Name of an acupuncture method, i. e. , puncturing the shallow, small collaterals to let out blood with a three-edged needle （pointed puncture）or dermal needles (scattered puncture).

刺络拔罐 pricking and cupping

针刺与拔罐相结合的一种疗法。先于皮肤上做浅刺，后拔罐，以吸出少量血液。

A kind of therapy method combining cupping and acupuncture, i. e., first puncture the skin superfically and then use cupping method to suck out a small amount of blood.

刺手 puncturing hand

进针时两手同时操作，持针手（一般为右手）称为刺手，配合做按压穴位动作的手（一般为左手）称为押手。

During acupuncture, two hands operate at the same time; the hand(usually the right hand) holding the needle is called puncturing hand, while the other hand (usually the left hand) pressing the points is called pressing hand.

刺血拔罐 cupping combined with bleeding

同刺络拔罐，见该条。

The same as the therapy of pricking and cupping.

刺血疗法 bleeding therapy

指用三棱针刺破体表穴位或浅静脉，使之流出少量血液而达到治疗目的的一种方法。

The therapeutic technique to prick an acupoint or the superficial veins to draw a small amount of blood out with a three-edged needle.

从卫取气 obtaining qi from the wei

刺法用语，与"从营置气"相对。为针刺补法的要领，意指针刺补法，须于浅部候气并向下接纳。

A term of acupuncture, contrasted with "discharging qi from ying". It is an important principle in reinforcing acupuncture technique which means collecting qi from the shallow part.

从阳引阴 guiding qi in yang meridian to expel pathogen in yin meridian

《黄帝内经》取穴法则之一，指病在阴经而先刺阳经，以引导之。

One of the point-selecting principles in *Huangdi's Canon of Medicine*, which means to expel pathogens in the yin meridians by needling the yang meridians first.

从阴引阳 guiding qi in yin meridians to expel pathogen in yang meridian

《黄帝内经》取穴法则之一。指病在阳经而先刺阴经，以引导之。

One of the point-selecting principles in *Huangdi's Canon of Medicine*, which means to expel the evil pathogens in the yang meridians from needling the yin meridians first.

从营置气 discharging qi from ying

刺法用语，与"从卫取气"相对，为针刺泻法的要领。即泻法的操作要于深部候气，并向浅部引提。

A term of acupuncture, contrasted with "obtaining qi from wei". It is an important principle in reducing acupuncture technique which means collecting qi from the deep part and then leading it outward to the shallow part.

丛刺 cluster puncturing

在同一部位上多针并刺的方法。

Several needles inserted simultaneously on the same part.

丛毛 clustered hair

生于足大趾第一节背面皮肤上的毛。

Cluster of hairs growing on the back of the proximal phalange of the big toe.

丛针 bundled needles

将若干枚等长的毫针并列地捆扎在一起,使针尖平齐,此称为"丛针"。可用此针在皮肤表面进行浅刺。

Several filiform needles of the same length are bundled together with the tips at the same level. It can be used for superficial acupuncture on the surface of the skin.

腠理 striae

即皮肤、肌肉的纹理及皮肤与肌肉之间的间隙,是气血流通的门户和液体排泄的途径之一,也是防御外邪内侵的屏障。

The grain of the skin and muscles, and the space between the skin and muscles. It serves as a portal for the flow of qi and blood and one of the routes for the excretion of body fluid, and also as a barrier against the exogenous evils.

攒竹 Cuanzhu(BL2)

经穴名。属足太阳膀胱经。定位:在面部,当眉头陷中,眶上切迹处。主治:头痛,视物不明,流泪,眉棱骨痛,目赤肿痛,眼球瞤动等。操作:向眉中平刺 0.3~0.5寸;禁灸。

Name of an acupoint. It belongs to the Bladder Meridian of Foot-Taiyang. Location: On the face, in the depression of the

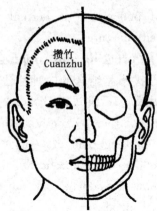

medial end of the eyebrow, at the supraorbital notch. Indications: Headache, blurring vision, lacrimation, pain in the supraorbital bome, redness, swelling and pain of the eyes, twitching of eyelids, etc. Method: Puncture horizontally 0.3-0.5 cun towards the middle of the eyebrow. Moxibustion is contraindicated.

催气 promoting arrival of qi

指针刺未得气时运用各种行针手法以取得针感。

Applying different manipulations during acupuncture when the sensations haven't occur.

焠刺 fire puncture

九刺法之一。也就是"火针"。

One of the nine needling techniques to puncture with a fire needle.

搓法 rubbing method

①推拿手法之一。用双手掌面夹住一定部位,相对用力,来回快速搓揉。用于四肢及胁肋部,有疏通经络、行气活血的作用。②针刺术语。同搓针。

① One of the manipulations of massage. It refers to manipulation using both palms to knead and press a certain part of the body, often used in limbs and costal region. It has the effect of dreging meridians and promoting qi and blood circulation. ②A term of acupuncture manipulation, same as needle twisting.

搓针 needle twisting

针刺手法之一。即将针刺入体内后,用右手拇指、示指向一个方向捻转,以加强针感的方法。

One of the acupuncture techniques, i. e. , to rotate the inserted needle towards one direction with the thumb and index finger of the right hand to strengthen the needling sensation.

D

大包 Dabao(SP21)

经穴名。属足太阴脾经,脾之大络。定位:在侧胸部,腋中线上,当第六肋间隙处。主治:胸胁胀痛,气喘,全身疼痛,四肢无力等。操作:斜刺 0.5~0.8 寸,不可直刺、深刺,以防刺伤肺脏;可灸。

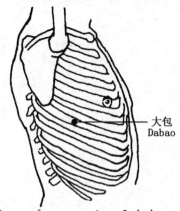

大包
Dabao

Name of an acupoint. It belongs to the Spleen Meridian of Foot-Taiyin. It is the large collateral of the spleen. Location: On the lateral side of the chest and on the midaxillary line, in the 6th intercostal space. Indications: Pain in the chest and hypochondrium, asthma, general aching and weakness, etc. Method: Puncture obliquely 0.5-0.8 cun. Perpendicular and deep puncture is prohibited, so as to prevent injuring the lung. Moxibustion is applicable.

大便干结 dry stool

指粪便干燥成粒,排便极难的症状,与便秘不同。湿热结于大肠,热邪入里,肠中津液耗伤;或肺脾气虚,大肠传送无力;或阴血耗损、肠失滋润等,均可引起本症。治宜清热保津、补气益血。取穴:合谷、曲池、足三里、大肠俞、上巨虚、承山。

A symptom different from comstipation which is characterized by dry and pebble stool that is dilicult to discharge. It is caused by the accumulation of damp-heat-evil in the large intestine, leading to consumption of the intestinal fluid, or by the hypofunction of the large intestine resulting from the qi deficiency of lung and spleen, or by the loss of moisture of the intestine resulting from the consumption of yin-blood. Treatment principle: Save the body fluid by clearing heat, benefit the qi and blood. Point selection: Hegu (LI4), Quchi (LI11), Zusanli (ST36), Dachangshu(BL25), Shangjuxu(ST37), Chengshan(BL57).

大补大泻 strong reinforcing-reducing method

针灸手法之一,指手法较重、刺激较强的补泻方法。如烧山火、透天凉皆属此法。与小补小泻(平补平泻)相对。

One of the acupuncture methods which consists in strong manipulations and intense stimulations to reinforce or reduce. Mountain-burning method and heaven-penetrating cooling method are examples of this method, contrary to slight reinforcing-reducing method (even reinforcing-reducing method).

大肠 large intestine; Dachang

①六腑之一。大肠上接小肠,下接肛门,有接纳小肠输送下来的食糜并吸收其

中的水分和营养物质,把糟粕形成粪便,最后从肛门排出体外的功能。②耳穴名。在耳轮脚上方前 1/3 处。主治:腹泻,便秘,咳嗽等。

①One of the six fu-organs, starting from the small intestine, extending to the anus. It receives the chyme from the small intestine, discharges the residue as feces from the anus after further absorption. ②Name of an ear point. It is at the anterior 1/3 of the upper part of the helix crus. Indications: Diarrhoea, constipation, cough, etc.

大肠经 Large Intestine Meridian

手阳明大肠经的简称。

Abbreviation for the Large Intestine Meridian of Hand-Yangming.

大肠俞 Dachangshu(BL25)

经穴名。属足太阳膀胱经,大肠背俞穴。定位:在腰部,当第 4 腰椎棘突下,后正中线旁开 1.5 寸。主治:腰痛,肠鸣,腹胀,泄泻,便秘等。操作:直刺 1～1.2 寸;可灸。

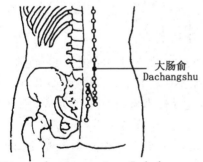

大肠俞
Dachangshu

Name of an acupoint. It belongs to the Bladder Meridian of Foot-Taiyang. It is the Back-Shu point of the large intestine. Location: On the low back, below the spinous process of the 4th lumbar vertebra, 1.5 cun lateral to the posterior midline.

Indications: Low back pain, borborygmus, abdominal distension, diarrhea, constipation, etc. Method: Puncture perpendicularly 1-1.2 cun. Moxibustion is applicable.

大冲 Dachong

太冲穴别名。

The other name of Taichong(LR3).

大都 Dadu(SP2)

经穴名。属足太阴脾经,本经荥穴。定位:在足内侧缘,当足大趾本节前下方,赤白肉际凹陷处。主治:腹胀,胃痛,便秘,热病无汗等。操作:直刺 0.3～0.5 寸;可灸。

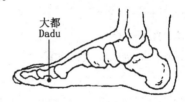

大都
Dadu

The acupoint, Ying-Spring point, belongs to the Spleen Meridian of Foot-Taiyin. Location: On the medial border of the foot, in the depression of the dorsoventral boundary of the foot, anterior and inferior to the 1st phalange of the big toe. Indications: Abdominal distension, gastric pain, constipation, febrile diseases with anhidrosis. Method: Puncture perpendicularly 0.3-0.5 cun. Moxibustion is applicable.

大敦 Dadun(LR1)

经穴名。属足厥阴肝经,本经井穴。定位:在足大指末节外侧,距趾甲角 0.1 寸。主治:疝气,遗尿,崩漏,阴挺,癫痫等。操作:浅刺 0.1～0.2 寸;可灸。

The acupoint, Jing-Well point, belongs to the Liver Meridian of Foot-Jueyin. Location: On the lateral side of the distal segement of the big toe, 0. 1 cun from the corner of the toenail.

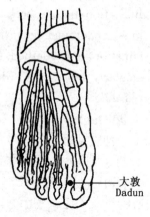

大敦
Dadun

Indications: Hernia, enuresis, uterine bleeding, prolapse of the uterus, epilepsy, etc. Method: Puncture shallowly 0. 1-0. 2 cun. Moxibustion is applicable.

大谷 large valley

部位名。指肌肉间大的凹陷处。

Name of an anatomical part, referring to the deep depression between the muscles.

大骨空 Dagukong(EX-UE5)

经外奇穴名。位于拇指背侧,指节横纹中点,屈指取之。用艾炷灸,主治目痛、目翳、内障、鼻衄、吐泻等。

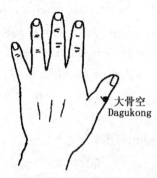

大骨空
Dagukong

Name of an extra point. Location: On the dorsal thumb, at the midpoint of the transverse crease of the knuckle. Take the point when the thumb flexes. Moxibustion with moxa cones can be used to treat pain of the eyes, cloudiness of cornea, cataract, rhinorrhagia, vomiting, diarrhea, etc.

大骨枯槁 bones becoming dry and brittle

极度消瘦衰弱,全身骨节显露的垂危病状,见于慢性消耗性疾病后期及恶液质患者。不宜针灸。

A critical condition which marked by muscular atrophy and bony appearance, usually seen in the later stage of chronic consumptive diseases and cachexia. Acupuncture is not adapt to this type of patient.

大赫 Dahe(KI12)

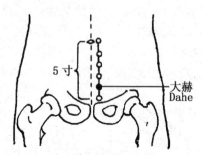

5 寸

大赫
Dahe

经穴名。属足少阴肾经。定位:在下腹部,当脐中下 4 寸,前正中线旁开 0.5 寸。主治:遗精,阳痿,白带,外阴痛,阴挺等。操作:直刺 1～1.5 寸;可灸。

Name of an acupoint. It belongs to the Kidney Meridian of Foot-Shaoyin. Location: On the lower abdomen, 4 cun below the center of the umbilicus and 0. 5 cun lateral to the anterior midline. Indications: Nocturnal emission, impotence, leukorrhea disease, pain in the external genitalia, prolapse of uterus, etc. Method: Puncture perpendicularly 1-1. 5 cun. Moxibustion is applicable.

大横 Daheng(SP15)

经穴名。属足太阴脾经。定位:在腹中部,距脐中 4 寸。主治:腹痛,腹胀,泄泻,痢疾,便秘等。操作:直刺 1～2 寸;可灸。

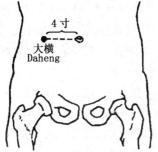

Name of an acupoint. It belongs to the Spleen Meridian of Foot-Taiyin. Location: On the middle abdomen, 4 cun from the center of the umbilicus. Indications: Abdominal pain and distension, diarrhea disease, dysentery, constipation, etc. Method: Puncture perpendicularly 1-2 cun. Moxibustion is a-pplicable.

大接经法 method of connecting the meridians

配穴法之一。有"从阳引阴"和"从阴引阳"两种方法,皆取十二经井穴。

One of the methods of points combination. There are two ways, one is called "start from yang to connect yin", the other is called "start from yin to connect yang". In the methods all the points are selected from the Jing-Well points of the twelve regular meridians.

大经 large meridians

全身经脉中粗大者。

The larger meridians of the body.

大巨 Daju(ST27)

经穴名。属足阳明胃经。定位:在下腹部,当脐中下 2 寸,距前正中线 2 寸。主治:小腹胀满,小便不利,疝气,遗精,早泄等。操作:直刺1～1.5寸;可灸。

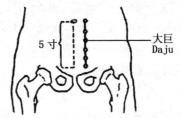

Name of an acupoint. It belongs to the Stomach Meridian of Foot-Yangming. Location: On the lower abdomen, 2 cun below the center of the umbilicus and 2 cun lateral to the anterior midline. Indications: Lower abdominal distension, dysuria, hernia, nocturnal emission, premature ejaculation, etc. Method: Puncture perpendicularly 1-1. 5 cun. Moxibustion is applicable.

大陵 Daling(PC7)

经穴名。属手厥阴心包经,本经输、原穴。定位:在腕掌横纹的中点处,当掌长肌腱与桡侧腕屈肌腱之间。主治:心痛,心悸,胃痛,呕吐,癫、狂、痫,胸闷胁痛。操作:直刺 0.3～0.5寸;可灸。

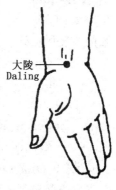

The acupoint, Shu-Stream and Yuan-Primary point, belongs to the Pericardium Meridian of Hand-Jueyin. Location: At the midpoint of the carpometacarpal transverse crease, between the palmaris longus tendon and flexor carpi radialis tendon. Indications: Heart pain, palpitation, stomachache, vomiting, mental disorders, epilepsy, stuffy chest, pain in the hypochondriac region, etc. Method: Puncture perpendicularly 0.3-0.5 cun. Moxibustion is applicable.

大络 large collateral
即全身最大的络脉。

The largest collateral of the body.

大门 Damen
经外奇穴名。位于头部中线,后发际上3.5寸,脑户穴上1寸。主治半身不遂。沿皮刺或灸治。

Name of an extra point. Located on the midline of the head, 3.5 cun from the posterior of the hairline or 1 cun above Naohu(GV17). Main indication is hemiplegia. Applying subcutaneous acupuncture or moxibustion.

大泉 Daquan
①太渊穴别名。②经外奇穴名。位于腋前皱襞尽头处。主治胸胁痛、肩臂痛。

①The other name of Taiyuan(LU9). ②Name of an extra point. Located at the end of the front axillary fold. Main indications are pains in the shoulders, arms, chest and hypochondrium, etc.

大肉陷下 emaciation
骨肉极度瘦削的病态,多见于慢性消耗性疾病后期及恶液质患者。不宜针灸。

A morbid state manifested as excessive thinness, usually seen in the late stage of chronic consumptive diseases and cachexia. Acupuncture is not adapt to this type of patient.

大腧 Dashu
大杼穴别名。

The other name of Dazhu(BL11).

大泻 vigorous reducing
针刺手法中泻法之一。即针刺入穴位后,用一手紧按并固定针刺部位周围的皮肤,另一手持针柄向左右前后大幅度地摇动。

One of the reducing methods in acupuncture technigues. After inserting the needle into an acupoint, one hand presses and tightens the skin around the point and the other hold the needle handle and shake it back and forth, left and right in a large range.

大泻刺 evacuation puncture
九刺法之一。指利用铍针切开脓疡,排出脓血。

One of the nine needling techniques, i. e., to drain the pus and blood from an abscess by incising it with a sword shaped needle.

大阴脉 dayin meridian
早期经脉名,指足太阴经。

The ancient name of a meridian. It refers to the Meridian of Foot-Taiyin.

大迎 Daying(ST5)
经穴名。属足阳明胃经。定位:在下颌角前方,咬肌附着部的前缘,当面动脉搏动处。主治:面瘫,口噤,颊肿,牙痛等。操作:直刺0.2~0.3寸;可灸。

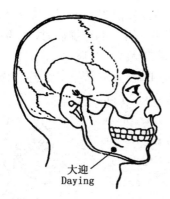

大迎
Daying

Name of an acupoint. It belongs to the Stomach Meridian of Foot-Yangming. Location: Anterior to the mandibular angle, on the anterior border of the masseter muscle where the pulsation of the facial artery is palpable. Indications: Facial paralysis, lockjaw, swelling of the cheek, toothache, etc. Method: Puncture perpendicularly 0.2-0.3 cun. Moxibustion is applicable.

大羽 Dayu

强间穴别名。

The other name of Qiangjian(GV18).

大针 big needle

古代九针之一，状如小竹片，多用于关节水肿。后人将其在火上烧红针刺病灶，也称火针。

One of the nine needles in ancient times shaped like a small bamboo piece, mostly used to cure the edema of joints. In modern times, the needle is heated on the fire to puncture the diseased site, so also called the fire needle.

大钟 Dazhong(KI14)

经穴名。属足少阴肾经，本经络穴。定位：在足内侧，内踝后下方，当跟腱附着部的内侧前方凹陷处。主治：腰脊强痛，癃闭，便秘，足跟痛，呆痴等。操作：直刺0.3～0.5寸；可灸。

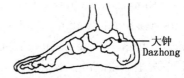

大钟
Dazhong

The acupoint, Luo-Connecting point of the Kidney Meridian of Foot-Shaoyin. Location: On the medial side of the foot, posterior and inferior to the medial malleolus, in the depression of the medial side and anterior to the attachment of the Achilles tendon. Indications: Stiffness and pain of the lower back and spine, retention of urine, constipation, pain in the heel, dementia, etc. Method: Puncture perpendicularly 0.3-0.5 cun. Moxibustion is applicable.

大杼 Dazhu(BL11)

经穴名。属足太阳膀胱经，八会穴之一，骨会于大杼。定位：在背部，当第一胸椎棘突下，后正中线旁开1.5寸。主治：头痛，项背痛，肩胛酸痛，咳嗽，发热，项强。操作：斜刺0.5～0.8寸，不宜深刺，以免伤及肺脏；可灸。

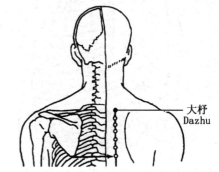

大杼
Dazhu

Name of an acupoint. It belongs to the

Bladder Meridian of Foot-Taiyang. It is the influential point of bone. Location: On the back , below the spinous process of the 1st thoracic vertebra, 1.5 cun lateral to the posterior midline. Indications: Headache, pain in the neck and back, soreness in the scapular region, cough, fever, neck rigidity. Method: Puncture obliquely 0.5-0.8 cun, don't puncture deeply, or the lung may be injured. Moxibustion is applicable.

大眦 big canthus

亦名内眦,为上下眼睑联结部靠近鼻侧处。该处血络丰富,和心有密切关系。

Also named inner canthus, it is the place near the nasal side of the upper and lower egelid junction, where a number of blood vessels are exist and are closely related with the heart.

带脉 Daimai(GB26); Belt Vessel

①经穴名。属足少阳胆经。定位:在侧腹部,章门下1.8寸,当第十一肋游离端下方垂线与脐水平线的交点上。主治:月经不调,经闭,白带,腹痛,疝气,腰胁痛

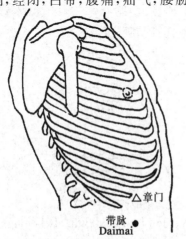

带脉
Daimai

△章门

等。②奇经八脉之一。起于季肋部,横行环绕腰部一周。本经发病时,主要有腹部胀满、腰部无力、下肢软弱不能走路、怕冷、月经不调、赤白带下等病症。操作:直刺0.5~0.8寸;可灸。

①Name of an acupoint. It belongs to the Gall-bladder Meridian ofFoot-Shaoyang. Location: On the lateral side of the abdomen, 1.8 cun below Zhangmen (LR13), at the crossing point of the vertical line drawing from the free end of the 11th rib and the

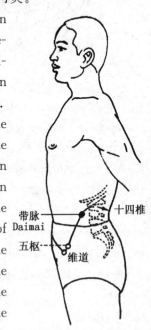

带脉
Daimai

五枢

十四椎

维道

horizontal line drawing from the umbilicus. Indications: Irregular menstruations, amenorrhea, leukorrhea disease, abdominal pain, hernia, pain in the lumbar and hypochondriac regions, etc. ②One of the eight extra meridians. It runs from the hypochondrium transversely around the waist. When this meridian is diseased, the main symptoms are abdominal distension, lumbar weakness, inability to walk due to weakness of the lower limbs, fear of cold, irregular menstruation, red and white vaginal discharge, etc. Method: Puncture perpendicularly 0.5-0.8 cun. Moxibustion is applicable.

丹毒 erysipelas

由热毒邪气引起的急性皮肤感染。以患处皮肤红如涂丹为特点，边缘清楚，灼热疼痛，并伴有发热恶寒、头痛、全身酸痛、局部淋巴结肿大等症状。治宜散热解毒。取穴：曲池、解溪、委中、风门、阿是穴。

A disorder caused by heat-evil; marked by redness of skin with a clear outline and burning pain; accompanied by fever, aversion to cold, headache, general soreness and enlargement of local lymph nodes. Treatment principle: Clear heat and toxic material. Point selection: Quchi (LI11), Jiexi(ST41), Weizhong(BL40), Fengmen(BL12), Ashi points.

丹田 Dantian

①指石门穴。②指关元穴。③指气海穴。④指肚脐与耻骨联合中点连线的上2/3处，有人将此处称为下丹田。⑤心窝部，又名中丹田。⑥脐下正中之处。

①Shimen(CV5). ②Guanyuan(CV4). ③Qihai(CV6). ④The upper 2/3 of the line connecting the umbilicus and the midpoint of the symphesis pubis. This part is called lower dantian. ⑤The precordial region, also called middle dantian. ⑥The cental area below the navel.

单手进针法 single-hand needle insertion

针刺进针法之一。以右手拇、示指持针体与针尖之间向下迅速刺入穴位而不加捻转。

A method of needle insertion in which the needle is grasped by the thumb and index finger of the right hand and inserted rapidly into the point without twirling.

胆 gallbladder

六腑之一。胆合肝，贮存胆汁，与消化及勇气有关。足少阳胆经属胆。其背俞穴为胆俞，募穴为日月，合穴为阳陵泉。

One of the six fu-organs paired with liver, stores bile, and is related to digestion and courage. The Gallbladder Meridian of Foot-Shaoyang belongs to it, with the Back-Shu point Danshu(BL19) the Front-Mu point Riyue(GB24) and the He-Sea point Yanglingquan(GB34).

胆经 Gallbladder Meridian

足少阳胆经的简称。

Abbreviation for the Gallbladder Meridian of Foot-Shaoyang.

胆囊 Dannang(EX-LE6)

经外奇穴名。在小腿外侧上部，当腓骨小头前下方凹陷处，在阳陵泉下2寸。主治：急、慢性胆囊炎，胆石症，胆道蛔虫病，下肢痿痹等。操作：直刺1～1.5寸；可灸。

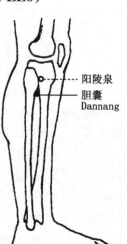

阳陵泉
胆囊
Dannang

Name of an extra point. Location: On the upper part of the lateral side of the leg, in the depression anterior and inferior to the head of the fibula, i. e., 2 cun below Yang-lingquan(GB34). Indications: Acute or chronic cholecystitis, cholelithiasis, biliary ascariasis, muscular atrophy and numbness of the lower extremities. etc. Method: Puncture perpendicularly 1-1. 5 cun. Moxibustion is applicable.

胆俞 Danshu(BL19)

经穴名。属足太阳膀胱经,胆的背俞穴。定位:在背部,当第十胸椎棘突下,后正中线旁开 1. 5 寸。主治:黄疸,口苦,胸胁痛,肺痨,潮热 等。操作:向内斜刺 0. 5~0. 8寸;可灸。

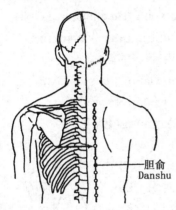

胆俞
Danshu

Name of an acupoint. It belongs to the Bladder Meridian of Foot-Taiyang. It is the Back-Shu point of the gallbladder. Location: On the back, below the spinous process of the 10th thoracic vertebra, 1. 5 cun lateral to the posterior midline. Indications: Jaundice, bitter taste of the mouth, pain in the chest and hypochondriac region, pulmonary tuberculosis, tidal fever, etc. Method: Puncture obliquely 0. 5-0. 8 cun towards the interspace of the spines. Moxibustion is applicable.

膻中 Danzhong(CV17)

经穴名。属任脉,心包的募穴,八会穴之一,气会膻中。定位:在胸部,当前正中线上,平第四肋间,两乳头连线的中点。主治:气喘,胸闷,胸痛,心悸,乳汁少,呃逆,吞咽困难等。操作:平刺 0. 3~0. 5 寸;可灸。

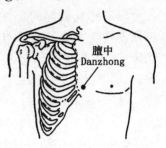

膻中
Danzhong

Name of an acupoint. It belongs to the Conception Vessel. It is the Front-Mu point of the pericardium and the influential point of qi. Location: On the chest, at the anterior midine, on the lever of 4th intercostal space, at the midpoint of the line connecting both nipples. Indications: Asthma, fullness in the chest, pain in the chest, palpitation, insufficient lactation, difficulty in swa-llowing, etc. Method: Puncture horizontally 0. 3-0. 5 cun. Moxibustion is applicable.

当容 Dangrong

经外奇穴名。即太阳穴。主治眼部炎症、头痛等。

Name of the extra point, i. e. , Taiyang (EX-HN5) with main indications of eye inflammations, headache, etc.

当阳 Dangyang(EX-HN2)

奇穴名。位于头前部,瞳孔直上入发际 1 寸处,即头临泣后 0. 5 寸。主治:头痛,头晕,感冒,鼻塞,目赤肿痛等。平刺或灸治。操作:平刺 0. 3~0. 5 寸;可灸。

Name of extra points. Location: On the

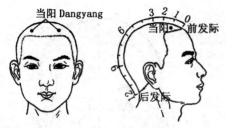

当阳 Dangyang

当阳·　前发际

后发际

forehead, directly above the pupil and 1 cun above the anterior hairline, 0. 5 cun behind Toulinqi（GB15）. Indications: Headache, dizziness, common cold, nasal obstruction, redness, swelling and pain of the eyes, etc. , treated with horizontal acupuncture or moxibustion. Method: Puncture horizontally 0. 3-0. 5 cun. Moxibustion is applicable.

导气 inducing qi

指通过各种针刺手法操作, 促使针感产生。

To produce and enhance the needle sensation by performing various manipulations during acupuncture therapy.

导引 breathing exercise

古代的一种健身方法。即运动肢体、调节呼吸及自我按摩相结合。通过行气活血、养筋壮骨, 达到消除疲劳、祛病延年的目的。

Physical exercise in ancient times consisting of special movements, respiratory regulation and self massage, which can relieve fatigue, cure diseases, prolong life by activating qi and blood circulation, and strengthening muscles and bones.

捣针 thrusting the needle

针刺手法之一。即将刺入体内的针反复上下捣动, 但不拔出皮肤外。

One of the acupuncture techniques, i. e. , repeatedly thrust the inserted needle without taking it out completely.

盗汗 night sweating

指入睡后出汗, 醒后即止。多属虚劳之证, 尤以阴虚者多见。治宜滋阴降火。取穴:少海、肾俞、复溜、合谷、阴郄。

It refers to sweating after falling asleep and stopping after waking up, mostly seen in consumptive diseases, especially the yin deficiency syndrome. Treatment principle:Nourish yin to reduce fire. Point selection: Shaohai （HT3）, Shenshu （BL23）, Fuliu（KI7）, Hegu（LI4）, Yinxi （HT6）.

得气 obtaining qi

指针刺时患者出现酸、麻、胀、重等感觉反应, 行针者则觉得针下有沉紧的感觉。

During acupuncture, the patient may feel soreness, numbness, distension, heaviness, etc. , and the acupuncturist may feel a heavy and tight sensation from the needle.

灯草灸 lamp moxibustion

即灯火灸。

The other name of burning rush moxibustion.

灯火灸 burning rush moxibustion

灸法的一种。即用灯心草吸麻油点火后灸灼穴位。主治小儿惊风昏迷, 以及头风、腮腺炎、呃逆、呕吐、腹痛、消化不良、功能失调性子宫出血、手足厥冷等。

One of moxibustion methods, i. e. , soak a stem of rush in sesame oil, then ignite it and place it over the points to cure infantile convulsion and coma, inter-

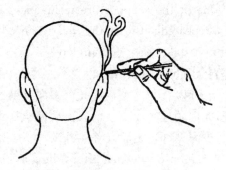

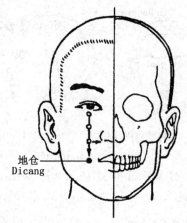

地仓
Dicang

mittent headache, mumps, hiccup, vomiting, abdominal pain, indigestion, dysfunctional uterine bleeding, cold extremities, etc.

锃针 spoon needle

古代九针之一。针体粗大而针尖钝圆。多用于治疗血脉病及热病。

One of the nine needles in ancient times. Its body is thick and its tip is blunt and raund. It is often used for vascular and febrile diseases.

地部 earth level

指穴位的深部,筋骨之间。

It refers to the deep level of the point between the tendons and the bones.

地仓 Dicang(ST4)

经穴名。属足阳明胃经。定位:在面部,口角外侧,上指瞳孔。主治:口㖞流涎,眼睑瞤动等。操作:直刺 0.2 寸,或向颊车方向平刺 0.5～0.8 寸;可灸。

Name of an acupoint belongs to the Stomach Meridian of Foot-Yangming. Location:On the face,directly below the pupil,beside the corner of the mouth. Indications:Mouth deviation, salivation, twitch-ing of eyelids, etc. Method:Punc-

ture perpendicularly 0.2 cun, or horizontally 0.5-0.8 cun towards Jiache(ST6). Moxibustion is applicable.

地合 Dihe

经外奇穴名。位于下颌骨正中向前突起之高点。斜刺主治头面疔疮、牙痛等。

Name of an extra point. Located at the top of the prominence of the mandible center, oblique puncture is used to cure boils on head and face, toothache, etc.

地机 Diji(SP8)

经穴名。属足太阴脾经,本经郄穴。定位:在小腿内侧,当内踝尖与阴陵泉的连线上,阴陵泉下 3 寸。主治:腹痛腹胀,泄泻,水肿,小便不利,遗精,月经不调,痛经等。操作:直刺 1～1.5 寸;可灸。

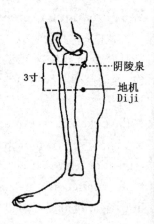

阴陵泉

3寸

地机
Diji

The acupoint, Xi-Cleft point belongs to the Spleen Meridian of Foot-Taiyin. Location: On the medial side of the leg, on the line connecting the tip of the medial malleolus and Yinlingquan(SP9), 3 cun below Yinlingquan (SP9). Indications: Abdominal pain and distension, diarrhea, edema, dysuria, nocturnal emission, irregular menstruation, dysmenorrhea, etc. Method: Puncture perpendicularly 1-1.5 cun. Moxibustion is applicable.

地卫 Diwei

涌泉穴别名。又称地冲。

The other name of Yongquan(KI1), also known as Dichong.

地五 Diwu

地五会的别名。

The other name of Diwuhui(GB42).

地五会 Diwuhui(GB42)

经穴名。属足少阳胆经。定位:在足背外侧,当足四趾本节的后方,第四、五跖骨之间,小趾伸肌内侧缘。主治:目眦痛,耳鸣,乳胀痛,足背肿痛等。操作:直刺 0.5～0.8 寸;可灸。

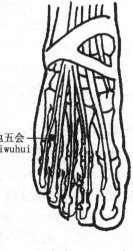

地五会 Diwuhui

Name of an acupoint. It belongs to the Gallbladder Meridian of Foot-Shaoyang. Location: On the lateral side of the dorsum of foot, posterior to the proximal segment of the 4th toe, between the 4th and 5th metatarsal bones, on the medial side of the extensor muscle of the little toe. Indications: Pain of the canthus, tinnitus, distending pain of the breast, swelling and pain of the dorsum of foot, etc. Method: Puncture perpendicularly 0.5-0.8 cun. Moxibustion is applicable.

地支 earthly branches

十二地支。古代表时、序的一种方法。与天干配合,用于时间配穴方法中。

Twelve earthly branches. They were used in ancient China to designate time and order, and combined with the heavenly stems to select points in the time-based point-combining method.

颠 top

部位名。指头顶部。

Name of the body part, i. e. , the top of the head.

颠顶痛 parietal headache

头痛以颠顶部为甚,多属太阳经病。治宜平肝疏风。取穴:百会、太冲、太阳、风池。

Headache most severe at the top of the head, usually related to the disorder of Taiyang meridian. Treatment principle: Calm the liver and dispel the wind. Point selection: Baihui (GV20), Taichong (LR3), Taiyang (EX-HN5), Fengchi (GB20).

颠上 Dianshang

百会穴别名。

The other name of Baihui(GV20).

癫 epilepsy

精神病的一种类型。多由痰气郁结所致。症见精神抑郁,表情淡漠或幻想幻觉,言语错乱,不思饮食,舌苔薄腻,脉弦滑等。治宜调气化痰、清心安神。取穴:

神门、大陵、印堂、膻中、丰隆、三阴交。

A psychiatric syndrome caused by stagnation of phlegm and qi; manifested as depression, apathy, illusion, hallucination, paraphasia, poor appetite, thin and greasy fur on the tongue, wiry and slippery pulse, etc. Treatment principle: Resolve phlegm by regulating the flow of qi, and tranquilize mind by clearing away heart-fire. Point selection: Shenmen (HT7), Daling(PC7), Yintang(GV29), Danzhong(CV17), Fenglong(ST40), Sanyinjiao(SP6).

癫狂 mania-depressive syndrome

指精神错乱的一类疾病。癫属阴，多偏于虚，患者多静默；狂属阳，多偏于实，患者多躁动。治宜清肝泻火、清心豁痰。取穴：劳宫、水沟、丰隆、大钟、内庭、行间。

Generally refers to psychosis, in which the depressive state is attributed to the disorder of yin, manifested as asthenia syndrome, the patients are usually quiet, while the manic state is attributed to the disorder of yang, manifested as sthenia syndrome, the patients are usually restless. Treatment principle: Clear the liver-fire, clear the heart-fire and eliminate phlegm for resuscitation. Point selection: Laogong(PC8), Shuigou(GV26), Fenglong (ST40), Dazhong(KI4), Neiting(ST44), Xingjian(LR2).

点刺 peck needling

指用针（多用三棱针）连续刺皮下浅层静脉，并挤出数滴血液的治疗方法。

Repeatedly pricking the superficial veins underneath the skin (often with a three-edged needle) and squeezing out a few drops of blood.

点穴 mark or press the points

①在人体上点定穴位。②用手指按压穴位。

①Marking the location of the points on the body. ②Pressing the points with fingers.

电热灸 electric moxibustion

近代利用电能发热代替艾灸，多用于风湿痹痛等症。

In modern times the electric heat is used to replace the mugwort moxibustion mostly to cure rheumatic arthralgia.

电兴奋疗法 electroexcitation therapy

指用感应电或直流电刺激患者体表的一定部位或穴位的治疗方法。

The therapeutic technique for stimulating a certain area of patient's body or acupoints with induced or direct electric current.

电针法 electroacupuncture

针刺结合电流刺激治病的方法。系在针刺留针过程中，于有关穴位上通以由电针机输出的脉冲电流刺激穴位的方法。

A therapy of acupuncture combined with electric stimulation, i. e., the relevant acupoints are stimulated by the pulse current generated by the electric acupuncture device during the retention of needle in acupuncture.

电针机 electric acupuncture device

应用脉冲电流加强穴位针刺作用的电子治疗仪器。

A kind of therapeutic electric device used to strengthen the acupuncture effect on the points with the pulse current generated by the device.

顶门 Dingmen

即囟会穴。

The other name of Xinhui(GV22).

顶上回毛 Dingshanghuimao

经外奇穴名。位于头顶发旋中;有人指百会穴。灸治小儿惊痫、癫痫、脱肛等。

Name of an extra point. Located at the center of the twirling hairs on the vertex; someone regard it as Baihui (GV20). Moxibustion is used to cure infantile convulsion, epilepsy, anal prolapse of rectum, etc.

定喘 Dingchuan(EX-B1)

经外奇穴名。定位:大椎穴旁开 0.5 寸处。主治:气喘,咳嗽,项强,肩背痛,荨麻疹等。操作:直刺或向内斜刺 0.5~0.8寸;可灸。

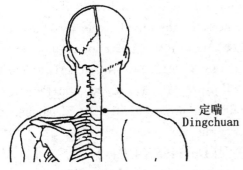

定喘
Dingchuan

Name of an extra point. Location：0.5 cun lateral to Dazhui (GV14). Indications：Asthma, cough, neck rigidity, pain in the shoulder and back, urticaria, etc. Method：Puncture perpendicularly or obliquely inward 0.5-0.8 cun. Moxibus-

tion is applicable.

东医宝鉴 *Treasure Compendium of Eastern Medicine*

医书名。朝鲜许浚编著,全书 25 卷,成书于 1610 年。

Name of an medical book compiled by Xujun of Korea, 25 volumes in all, finished in 1610.

动而伸之 rotating-lifting technique

刺法用语。意思是取得感应后,将针转动而上提,是为泻法。

A kind of acupuncture technique, i. e., after obtaining the needle sensation, the needle should be rotated and lifted, which is a reducing method.

斗肘 Douzhou

经外奇穴名。位于曲池正外方骨高点处。灸治臂肘神经痛、偏瘫、神经衰弱等。

Name of an extra point. Located on the top of the bone just outside Quchi (LI11). Moxibustion is used to cure arm and elbow neuralgia, hemiplegia, neurasthenia, etc.

督脊 Duji

经外奇穴名。位于第七颈椎棘突至尾骨端连线中点处。灸治癫痫等。

Name of an extra point. Located at the midpoint of the line between the 7th spinous process of the cervical vertebra and the coccyx tip. Moxibustion is used to cure epilepsy, etc.

督脉 Governor Vessel

奇经八脉之一。起自会阴部,循背部脊柱正中线向上,经过后颈部,越过头顶部,止于颜面部的上齿龈正中(以上均沿正中线分布）。在循行过程中与脊髓、脑和诸阳经相联系,是阳经经脉的总纲。本经发病时,主要有神志不清、癫、狂、癔病、项背强直、角弓反张、咽喉干燥、癃、痔、遗尿、脱肛、疝气、不孕症、体力衰退等病症。

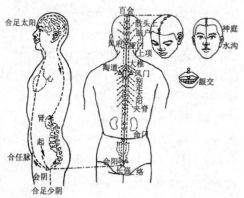

One of the eight extra meridians. It arises at the perineum, runs upwards along the midline of the spinal column, passes through the back of the neck, turns anteriorly over the top of the head to the face and ends at the middle of the upper gum. Along its course, it is connected with the spinal cord, brain, and all the yang meridians. It is the governor of all the yang meridians. When it is diseased, there may chiefly appear such symptoms as unconsciousness, epilepsy, mania, hysteria, stiffness of the neck and back, opisthotonos, dryness of the throat, retention of urine, hemorrhoids, enuresis, prolapse of rectum, hernia, infertility and debility, etc.

督脉络 Governor Vessel collateral

十五络脉之一,名长强,分布于脊旁肌肉,上至头部,下入足太阳经。

One of the fifteen collaterals, named Changqiang, distributed in the muscles lateral to the spinal column, up to the head and down to the meridian of the Foot-Taiyang.

督俞 Dushu(BL16)

经穴名。属足太阳膀胱经。定位:在背部,第六胸椎棘突下,后正中线旁开1.5寸。主治:心痛,胸闷,腹痛,气喘等。操作:向内斜刺0.5~1寸;可灸。

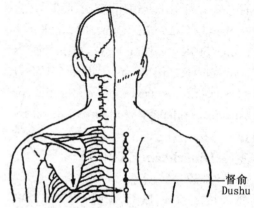

Name of an acupoint. It belongs to the Bladder Meridian of Foot-Taiyang. Location: On the back, below the spinous process of the 6th thoracic vertebra, 1.5 cun lateral to the posterior midline. Indications: Heart pain, stuffy chest, abdominal pain, asthma, etc. Method: Puncture obliquely inward 0.5-1 cun. Moxibustion is applicable.

独阴 Duyin(EX-LE11)

经外奇穴名。定位:在足第二趾跖侧远端趾间关节的中点。主治:疝气,胎盘滞留,月经不调等。

Name of an extra point. Location: On the plantar side of the 2nd toe, on the midpoint of the distal interphalangeal joint. Indications：Hernia，retention of placenta，irregular menstruation，etc.

犊鼻 Dubi(ST35)

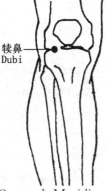

犊鼻
Dubi

经穴名。属足阳明胃经。定位：屈膝，在膝部，髌骨与髌韧带外侧凹陷中。主治：膝痛、麻木、屈伸不利，脚气等。操作：稍向髌韧带内方斜刺 0.5～1.2 寸；可灸。

Name of an acupoint. It belongs to the Stomach Meridian of Foot-Yangming. Location：With the knee flexed，the point is in the depression lateral to the patella and patellar ligament. Indications：Pain，numbness and motor impairment of the knee，beriberi，etc. Method：Puncture obliquely 0.5-1.2 cun slightly towards the medial side of the patellar ligament. Moxibustion is applicable.

短刺 short needling

十二刺法之一。用于治疗骨痹。方法是稍加摇动地将针刺入，深达骨部，并进行提插手法。

One of the twelve needling techniques for treating the bone bi syndrome. It is to insert the needle down to the bone with slightly shaking and then lift and thrust the needle.

对耳轮 antihelix

解剖名称。指耳轮前方与耳轮相对的隆起部分，包括对耳轮上脚、对耳轮下脚及对耳轮体三部分。

Nomina anatomica. An elevated ridge anterior and opposite to the helix. It consists of three parts，i. e.，the superior and inferior antihelix crus and the principal part of antihelix.

对耳轮上脚 superior antihelix crus

解剖名称。指对耳轮向上分叉的一支。

Terminologia anatomica. The upward bifurcation of the antihelix.

对耳轮体 principal part of antihelix

解剖名称。即对耳轮垂直走向的主干部分。

Terminologia anatomica. The roughly vertical part of the antihelix.

对耳轮下脚 inferior antihelix crus

解剖名称。指对耳轮向前分叉的一支。

Terminologia anatomica. The forward bifurcation of the antihelix.

对耳屏 antitragus

解剖名称。在耳垂上部，与耳屏相对的隆起。

Terminologia anatomica. A small tubercle opposite to the tragus and superior to the earlobe.

对屏尖 Duipingjian

耳穴名。又名平喘、腮腺。在对耳屏的尖端。主治：哮喘，腮腺炎，皮肤瘙痒症，附睾炎等。

Name of an ear point. Also called Pingchuan or Saixian. It is at the tip of antitragus. Indications：Asthma，mumps，itchy skin and epididymitis.

对应取穴 corresponding point selection

取穴法之一。指在与病痛部位相对应的远部取穴，包括前后对应、上下对应、左右对应、手足对应等。

One of the point selection methods. It means select the distal points in the parts corresponding to the diseased part, including correspondence between the anterior and posterior, upper and lower, left and right, hand and foot.

兑端 Duiduan(GV27)

经穴名。属督脉。定位：在面部，当上唇的尖端，人中沟下端的皮肤与上唇的移行部。主治：癫狂，唇瞤动，唇胀，齿龈肿痛等。操作：向上斜刺 0.2～0.3 寸；禁灸。

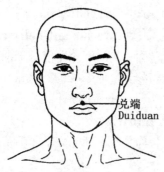

兑端
Duiduan

Name of an acupoint. It belongs to the Governor Vessel. Location：On the face, on the tip of the upper lip, on the border between the philtrum and the upper lip. Indications：Mental disorders, lip twitching, lip swelling, pain and swelling of the gums, etc. Method：Puncture obliquely upward 0.2-0.3 cun. Moxibustion is prohibited.

兑骨 duigu

①颧髎穴别名。②腕部豆状骨。③神门穴别名。

①The other name of Quanliao(SI18). ②Pisiform bones. ③The other name of Shenmen(HT7).

多汗 hyperhidrosis

指不是由于炎热、运动、药物等因素引起的出汗过多。治宜固表止汗。取穴：少海、肾俞、复溜、合谷、阴郄。

Excessive sweating not due to hot weather, sports or drugs. Treatment principle：Consolidate superficies to arrest sweating. Point selection：Shaohai(HT3), Shenshu(BL23), Fuliu(KI7), Hegu(LI4), Yinxi(HT6).

多梦 dreaminess

睡眠不熟，梦扰纷纭。常因情志郁结、肝阳偏亢，或气血虚少、心神不安所致。常见于神经衰弱的患者。治宜滋阴养血、平肝降火、化痰和胃。取穴：神门、三阴交、太溪、太冲、丰隆。

A morbid state due to depression, hyperactivity of liver yang, deficiency of qi and blood, and Uneasiness；usually seen in the patients suffering from neurasthenia. Treatment principle：Nourish yin and blood, calm the liver and clear the liver-fire, resolve phlegm and hormonize the stomach. Point selection：Shenmen(HT7), Sanyinjiao(SP6), Taixi(KI3), Taichong(LR3), Fenglong(ST40).

多针浅刺 multiple-superficial needling

同时应用几枚针进行浅刺。

Insert several needles superficially and simultaneously in an acupoint or a certain part.

夺命 Duoming

经外奇穴名。位于肩髃穴与尺泽穴连线中点。直刺主治昏厥、臂痛、丹毒等。

Name of an extra point. Located at the middle point of the line between Jianyu (LI15) and Chize (LU5). Perpendicular acupuncture is used to cure syncope, arm pain, erysipelas, etc.

顿灸 draught of moxibustion

灸法用语。即一次灸完规定的壮数,与报灸相对。

A term of moxibustion, i. e. , perform moxibustion of all the prescribed cones at one time, as contrasted with repeated moxibustion.

E

鹅口疮 thrush

见于新生儿、婴儿泄泻及营养不良或麻疹等病后期的口腔疾病之一。主症为口腔、舌上满布白色糜点，形如鹅口。多因脾经郁热循经上行，熏于口舌，或胃阴不足所致。治宜清脾胃之热。取穴：内庭、中脘、阴陵泉、脾俞、地机。

Fungus infection of the oral mucous of infants characterized by the formation of whitish spots in the mouth and on the tongue; usually secondary to diarrhea, malnutrition and measles; resulting from stagnation of heat in the Spleen Meridian and heat ascending along the meridian, affecting the mouth and tongue, or from the insufficiency of stomach-yin. Treatment principle: Clear the heat of the spleen and stomach. Point selection: Neiting (ST44), Zhongwan (CV12), Yinlingquan(SP9), Pishu(BL20), Diji(SP8).

额 E

耳穴名。在对耳屏外侧面的前下方。主治：头痛，头晕，失眠，多梦等。

Name of an ear point. At the anterior and inferior corner of the lateral aspect of antitragus. Indications: Headache, dizziness, insomnia, dreaminess, etc.

额角 corner of forehead

前额两端发际下垂所成的角度。

The area formed by the dropping hairline on both ends of the forehead.

额颅 forehead

头部前发际与两眉之间的部位。

The region between the anterior hairline and the eyebrows.

呃逆 hiccup

指胃气冲逆而上，以喉间呃呃有声，声短而频，不能自控为特征的一种证候，多因脾胃虚寒所致。治宜降逆止呃。取穴：天突、中脘、膈俞、内关、足三里、脾俞。

It refers to the adverse rising of stomach qi, characterized by uncontrollable and constant hiccup with short and frequent sound, usually caused by deficient cold of spleen and stomach. Treatment principle: Lower the adverse flow of stomach-qi to stop hiccup. Point selection: Tiantu(CV22), Zhongwan(CV12), Geshu(BL17), Neiguan(PC6), Zusanli(ST36), Pishu(BL20).

饿马摇铃 hungry horse rings the bell

针刺补法。即拇指向前缓缓向左捻针。与"凤凰展翅"相对。

Reinforcing acupuncture technique, i. e., twirling the needle leftwards gently with the thumb forwards, as contrasted with the technique of " the phoenix spreads its wings".

儿枕痛 postpartum abdominal pain

由于产后恶露未尽或风寒侵袭胞脉致使瘀血内停所引起的病证。表现为小腹硬痛拒按或可触及硬块。治宜行气化瘀、通络止痛。取穴：中极、归来、膈俞、血海、太冲。

A condition of retention of blood stasis resulting from postpartum lochiorrhea or wind-cold attacking the uterine vessels; manifested as lower abdominal hard and pain and aversion to pressure or palpable mass. Treatment principle: Activate qi and remove blood stasis, resolve obstruction in the meridians to relieve pain. Point selection: Zhongji (CV3), Guilai (ST29), Geshu (BL17), Xuehai (SP10), Taichong (LR3).

耳 ear

五官之一，为听觉器官。它的功能靠精、髓、气、血的充养，赖肾脏功能的正常。耳的疾病常与肾有关，与心、脾、肝等脏器也有关。此外，小肠经、膀胱经、三焦经、胆经、胃经等也均循行于耳。所以，耳与脏腑经络都有密切关系，全身脏器及肢体常可在耳廓上找到相应的反应点，现在常用这些反应点来诊断和治疗多种疾病。

One of the five sense organs, the auditory organ. Its function is maintained by the nourishment from the essence, marrow, qi and blood, as well as the normal function of the kidney. The disorder of the ear is closely related to the dysfunction of the kidney and also the heart, spleen and liver. In addition, the meridians of the small intestine, bladder, san jiao, gallbladder and stomach all pass through the ear. So, there is a close relationship between the ear and the meridians of the zang-fu organs. Corresponding reaction points of the zang-fu organs and extremities are found on the auricle and are applied to diagnose and treat various diseases.

耳背肺 Erbeifei

耳穴名。在耳背脾的耳根侧。主治：咳喘，皮肤瘙痒症，发热等。

Name of an ear point. On the back of the ear, on the medial side of Erbeipi. Indications: Cough and asthma, skin itching, fever, etc.

耳背肝 Erbeigan

耳穴名。在耳背脾的耳轮侧。主治：胸胁胀满，胆囊炎，胆石症，急性阑尾炎等。

Name of an ear point. On the back of the ear, on the lateral side of Erbeipi. Indications: Distension and fullness of chest and hypochondrium, cholecystitis, cholelithiasis, acute appendicitis, etc.

耳背沟 Erbeigou

耳穴名。又名降压沟。在对耳轮上、下脚沟与对耳轮沟在耳背面呈"Y"字形凹沟处。主治：高血压，皮肤病。

Name of an ear point. Also named Jiangyagou. Through the backside of superior antihelix crus and inferior antihelix crus, in the Y-shaped depression formed by the groove of the superior and inferior antihelix crus and antihelix. Indications: hypertension, skin di-seases.

耳背脾 Erbeipi

耳穴名。在耳背的中间。主治：胃痛，腹胀，泄泻，消化不良等。

Name of an ear point. In the middle of the ear back. Indications: Stomachache, abdominal distension, diarrhea, indigestion, etc.

耳背肾 Erbeishen

耳穴名。在耳背下部。主治：头痛，失

眠,眩晕,月经不调,神经衰弱等。

Name of an ear point. At the lower part of the ear back. Indications：Headache, insomnia, vertigo, irregular menstruation, neurasthenia, etc.

耳背心 Erbeixin

耳穴名。在耳背上部。主治:疮疡,失眠多梦,心悸,高血压,头痛等。

Name of an ear point. At the upper part of the ear back. Indications：Furuncle, insomnia, dreaminess, palpitation, hypertension, headache, etc.

耳垂 earlobe

解剖名称。指耳廓最下部无软骨的皮垂。

Terminologia anatomica. The lowest part of the auricle where there is no cartilage.

耳廓 auricle

外耳道在头部以外的部分。耳廓内侧有脏腑和肢体的反应点,应用于耳针。

The visible part of the ear outside the head. Corresponding reaction points of the zang-fu organs and extremities are distributed on the inside of the auricle and applied in ear acupuncture.

耳廓视诊 inspection of the auricle

通过望耳廓皮肤变色、变形、丘疹、脱屑与相应部位出现的不同反应,以帮助诊断疾病的一种方法。

The diagnostic inspection of the changes of color, deformation, papule and peeling of a particular location of the auricular skin, as diagnostic signs of pathologic conditions of the corresponding parts of the body.

耳和髎 Erheliao(TE22)

经穴名。属手少阳三焦经。定位:在头侧部,当鬓发后缘,平耳廓根之前方,颞浅动脉的后缘。主治:偏头痛,耳鸣,牙关拘急等。操作:斜刺 0.2～0.5 寸;可灸。

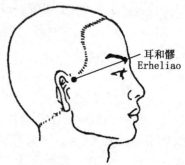

耳和髎
Erheliao

Name of an acupoint. It belongs to the Sanjiao Meridian of Hand-Shaoyang. Location：On the lateral side of the head, on the posterior margin of the temples, anterior to the inferior border of the auricle and posterior to the superficial temporal artery. Indications：Migraine, tinnitus, lockjaw, etc. Method：Puncture obliquely 0.2-0.5 cun. Moxibustion is applicable.

耳后发际 Erhoufaji

经外奇穴名。位于耳后颞骨乳突下缘发际处。灸治瘿气、瘰疬等。

Name of an extra point. Located on the hairline inferior to the mastoid process of temporal bone on the back of the ear with main indications of goiter, scrofula, etc. by moxibustion.

耳甲 auricular concha

解剖名称。指由对耳屏和对耳轮体部及对耳轮下脚围成的凹窝。

Terminologia anatomica. The hollow

formed by the antitragus, principal part of antihelix and inferior antihelix crus.

耳甲腔 cavity of auricular concha

解剖名称。指耳轮脚以下的耳甲部。

Terminologia anatomica. The part of the concha inferior to the crus of helix.

耳甲艇 cymba of auricular concha

解剖名称。指耳轮脚以上的耳甲部。

Terminologia anatomica. The part of the concha superior to the crus of helix.

耳尖 Erjian(EX-HN6)

①耳穴名。在耳轮顶端，与对耳轮上脚后缘相对的耳轮处。主治：发热，高血压，目赤肿痛。②经外奇穴名。折耳向前，在耳廓上端取穴。主治：目赤肿痛，热病，目翳等。

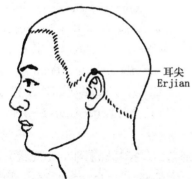

耳尖
Erjian

①Name of an ear point. At the top of the helix, at the point of the helix opposite to the posterior border of the superior antihelix crus. Indications: Fever, hypertension, redness, swelling and pain of the eye. ②Name of an extra point. Fold the auricle, the point is at the top of the auricle. Indications: Redness, swelling and pain of the eyes, febrile diseases, claudiness of cornea, etc.

耳聋 deafness

听力有不同程度障碍的一种病证。可由先天因素或外感、内伤所致。急性耳聋多属实证；慢性耳聋多属虚证。治宜通络开窍。取穴：耳门、听宫、听会。

Lack or loss of hearing. It is congenital or acquired from the attack of exogenous evils or internal damage. Acute Deafness usually manifests sthenia syndrome, while chronic deafness usually manifests asthenia syndrome. Treatment principle: Remove obstruction in the meridians and open orfices. Point selection: Ermen (TE21), Tinggong (SI19), Tinghui(GB2).

耳轮 helix

解剖名称。指耳廓外缘向外卷曲的部分。

Terminologia anatomica. The part of the lateral edge of the auricle that curls outward.

耳轮脚 crus of helix

解剖名称。指耳轮深入耳腔的横行突起。

Terminologia anatomica. The transverse protrusion of the helix into the ear cavity.

耳轮结节 helix tubercle

解剖名称。指耳轮后上方的小突起。

Terminologia anatomica. The small tubercle at the posterior-superior aspect of the helix.

耳轮尾 tail of helix

解剖名称。在耳轮下方，与耳垂交界处。

Terminologia anatomica. At the inferior part of the helix, at the junction of the helix and the earlobe.

耳门 Ermen(TE21)

经穴名。属手少阳三焦经。定位:在面部,当耳屏上切迹的前方,下颌骨髁突后缘凹陷处。主治:耳鸣耳聋,聤耳,齿痛,唇强等。操作:直刺 0.5~1 寸,避开耳前动脉;可灸。

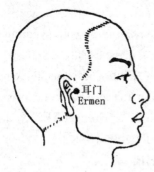

Name of an acupoint. It belongs to the Sanjiao Meridian of Hand-Shaoyang. Location: On the face, anterior to the supratragic notch, in the depression on the posterior border of the condylar process of the mandible. Indications: Tinnitus, deafness, otitis media suppurativa, toothache, stiffness of the lip, etc. Method: Puncture perpendicularly 0.5-1 cun, avoiding the superficial temporal artery. Moxibustion is applicable.

耳迷根 Ermigen

耳穴名。在耳背与耳后乳突交界的耳根部,耳轮脚对应处。主治:胆囊炎,胆石症,胆道蛔虫病,鼻塞,头痛,腹痛,腹泻等。

Name of an ear point. At the part of the ear root where the ear back and mastoid process meets, opposite to the helix crus. Indications: Cholecystitis, choleli-thiasis, biliary ascariasis, nasal obstruction, headache, abdominal pain, diarrhea, etc.

耳鸣 tinnitus

耳内鸣响,其声如蝉鸣、如水击、如钟声等听觉异常的自觉症状。肝胆火气上逆、脾胃痰火上升,或肾精不足,中气下陷均可引起。前者属实证,后者属虚证。治宜补益肾精、平肝泻火。取穴:翳风、听会、肾俞、太溪、太冲。

The noise in the ears, like cicada chirping, water roaring, bell ringing, etc.; usually caused by adverse rising of liver-fire and gallbladder fire and hyperactivity of phlegm fire in the spleen and stomach (in case of sthenia syndrome), or caused by insufficiency of kidney essence and sinking of middle qi (in case of asthenia syndrome). Treatment principle: Tonify the kidney essence, reduce the liver-fire. Point selection: Yifeng (TE17), Tinghui (GB2), Shenshu (BL23), Taixi (KI3), Taichong (LR3).

耳屏 tragus

解剖名称。指耳廓前部的小瓣状突起。

Terminologia anatomica. A small flap bulge in front of the auricle.

耳上 Ershang

经外奇穴名。位于耳尖直上三横指。主治小儿暴痫。

Name of an extra point. Located transverse width of three fingers directly above the auricular tip with the main indication of infantile sudden convulsion.

耳上发际 Ershangfaji

经外奇穴名。位于耳尖直上入发际处。

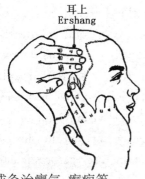

耳上
Ershang

沿皮刺或灸治瘿气、癫痫等。

Name of an extra point. Located at the hairline directly above the auricular tip. It is used to treat goiter, epilepsy, etc. by subcutaneous acupuncture or moxibustion.

耳神门 Ershenmen

耳穴名。在三角窝内,对耳轮上、下脚分叉处稍上方。主治:失眠,多梦,头痛等。

Name of an ear point. In the triangular fossa, slightly above the bifurcation of the superior and inferior antihelix curs. Indications: Insomnia, dreaminess, headache, etc.

耳痛 earache

耳部疾病的一种常见症状。可由肝胆风热、三焦火盛或虚火等引起。治宜清热止痛。取穴:耳门、听宫、听会、合谷。

A common symptom of ear diseases caused by the retention of wind-heat in the liver and gallbladder, or the hyperactivity of fire-evil in Sanjiao, or the asthenic fire. Treatment principle: Clear heat to relieve pain. Point selection: Ermen (TE21), Tinggong (SI19), Tinghui (GB2), Hegu (LI4).

耳心痛 earache

又称耳痛。耳内干痛而痒者,多因肝胆风热所致;耳肿胀痛者,则属三焦相火炽盛;耳内疼痛并见溃烂流水者,多属风邪兼湿热之邪侵入肝胆两经;伴有眩晕者,则多属虚火上炎。治疗见耳痛条。

Pain in the ear. If accompanied by itching but without exudation, it is caused by wind-heat in liver and gallbladder; if accompanied by swelling, it is caused by the hyperactivity of ministerial fire in sanjiao; if accompanied by ulcer and exudation, it is caused by the attack of wind-evil and damp-heat evil of the liver and gallbladder meridians; if accompanied by dizziness, it is caused by flaring up of the asthenic fire. Treatment is the same as the supperior term.

耳穴贴压法 auricular-plaster therapy

根据耳廓变化诊断疾病,然后用胶布将绿豆或王不留行籽等贴到一定耳穴上,通过压按刺激耳穴以治疗疾病的方法。

According to the auricular diagnosis, tape mung bean or vaccaria seed, etc. to a particular ear point with a plastic tape, to stimulate the point with pressure for therapy.

耳针 ear acupuncture

指在耳廓上进行针刺以治疗疾病的方法。

The technique to puncture the auricle with needles to treat diseases.

耳中 Erzhong

耳穴名。又称膈。在耳轮脚上。主治:呃逆,黄疸,咯血,小儿遗尿,皮肤瘙痒症。

Name of an ear point. Also named ge. It is on the crus of helix. Indications: Hiccup, jaundice, hemoptysis, infantile enuresis, itchy skin.

耳舟 scapha

解剖名称。指耳轮与对耳轮之间的凹沟。

Terminologia anatomica. The narrow curved depression between helix and antihelix.

二白 Erbai(EX-UE2)

经外奇穴名。在腕横纹上 4 寸,桡侧腕屈肌腱两侧,一手二穴。主治:脱肛、痔疾等。

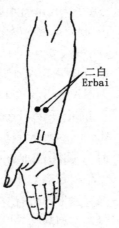

二白 Erbai

Name of extra points. Located 4 cun above the transverse of the wrist crease, on both sides of the flexor carpi radialis tendon, two points on one forearm. Indications: Prolapse of the rectum, hemorroids, etc.

二间 Erjian

经穴名。属手阳明大肠经,本经荥穴。定位:微握拳,当示指桡侧,第二掌指关节前凹陷中。主治:目昏、鼻衄、齿痛、咽喉肿痛、热病等。操作:直刺 0.5～0.8 寸;可灸。

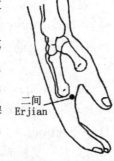

二间 Erjian

The acupoint, Ying-Spring point belongs to the Large Intestine of Hand-Yangming. Location: On the radial side of the index finger, in the depression anterior to the 2nd metacarpophalangeal joint when a loose fist is made. Indications: Blurred vision, epistaxis, toothache, sore throat, febrile diseases, etc. Method: Puncture perpendicularly 0.5-0.8 cun. Moxibustion is applicable.

二十七气 twenty-seven kinds of qi

十二经脉和十五络脉之气的总称。

The general term of qi in the 12 regular meridians and 15 collaterals.

二阳 double yang

经络名,指阳明经。

Name of the meridian, i. e., the Yangming Meridian.

二阴 double yin

①经络名,指少阴经。②指外生殖器(前阴)和肛门(后阴)。

① Name of the meridian, i. e., the Shaoyin Meridian。② The external genitalia (anterior yin) and the anus (posterior yin).

二趾上 Erzhishang

经外奇穴名。位于内庭和陷谷两穴连线的中点处。主治水病。

Name of an extra point. Located at the midpoint of the line between Neiting (ST44) and Xiangu(ST43) with the main indications of edema.

二椎下 Erzhuixia

经外奇穴名。位于后正中线,第二胸椎棘突下凹陷处。主治精神病、癫痫、疟疾。可斜刺或灸治。

Name of an extra point. Located in the depression under the spinous process of the second thoracic vertebra on the posterior midline. Indications: Mental diseases, epilepsy, malaria, etc. Acupuncture or moxibustion can be applied.

发洪 sore bleeding

指灸疮出血。

Bleeding from a sore caused by moxibustion.

发泡 vesiculation

用对皮肤有刺激性的药物,捣烂(鲜药),或研末(干药),以酒、蜜或醋等液体调和,敷在一定部位的皮肤上,使局部起水疱而治疗某些疾病。

Apply certain irritative drugs, mash them up(fresh medical herbs) or grind them into fine powder(dry drugs), mix them with wine, honey or vinegar to form paste, and then apply the paste to the affected part to produce vesicles for treatment.

发泡灸 vesiculating moxibustion

①使灸治穴位的皮肤发泡的治疗方法。②指敷药发泡法。

① A treatment that the skin of the point is vesiculated after moxibustion. ② Vesiculating method with application of herbs.

发热 fever

体温高于正常标准的一种常见症状。治宜清热去火。取穴:大椎、曲池、合谷、外关。

A common symptom with the body temperature higher than the normal standard. Treatment principle: Clear heat to reduce fire. Point selection: Dazhui (GV14), Quchi (LI11), Hegu (LI4), Waiguan(TE5).

发际 Faji

①神庭穴别名。②经外奇穴名。位于前发际中点处。主治:小儿风痫,头痛,目眩等。沿皮刺或灸治。

① The other name of Shenting (GV24). ②Name of an extra point. Located at the midpoint of the anterior hairline. Indications: Infantile wind-convulsion, headache, dizziness, etc. by horizontal acupuncture or moxibustion.

反应点 reaction point

近代对腧穴的一种称谓。又称疾病反应点。

A modern term applied to the acupoint, also called disease-reacting point.

烦躁 irritability

指胸中热郁不安,手足扰动不宁的征象,常因阴虚火旺或外感病汗下后伤津所致。治宜泻心火、滋心阴。取穴:劳宫、少府、阴郄、然谷。

A state of feverish smothering sensation in the chest and restlessness of the limbs, due to yin deficiency and hyperactivity of fire, or consumption of body fluid after sweating in exogeous febrile disease. Treatment principle: Purge pathogenic fire of the heart, nourish the yin-fluid of the heart. Point selection: Laogong (PC8), Shaofu(HT8), Yinxi(HT6), Rangu(KI2).

燔针 fan needle (heated needle)

①指温针,即进针后在针柄施灸。②指火针,即烧针而刺。

①The warm acupuncture, i. e., after needle insertion, moxibustion is performed around the handle of the needle. ②The heated needle, i. e., the needle is heated in the fire to puncture.

返本还原 returning to the root and origin

子午流注针法用语。在按时取用五输穴中的输穴时,需加取与所开井穴同属一经的原穴。

A term used in the point selection following midnight-noon and ebb-flow doctrine. When the five Shu points are selected according to the calculated time, the Yuan-Primary points pertaining to the same meridian as the opened Jing-Well points must be also selected.

飞法 flying method

针刺辅助手法之一。针刺进入一定深度后,先将针做大幅度的捻转,然后松手,拇指、示指张开,一捻一放,如飞鸟状,反复数次。

One of the auxiliary manipulations in acupuncture. After inserting a needle into an acupoint to a certain depth, twirl the needle with thumb and index finger with a large range, then twirl once and release once. The movements of the needle twirling and the finger releasing should be like a flying bird spreading its wings and be repeated for several times.

飞虎 Feihu

支沟别名。

The other name of Zhigou (TE6).

飞经走气 moving qi through out the meridians

刺法用语。指催行经气的一些针刺手法。

A term of the acupuncture methods refers to stimulate qi to move in the meridians.

飞门 flying gate

指唇,为七冲门之一。

The term means lips which are one of the seven outward doors.

飞腾八法 method of eight flight

按时配穴法的一种。系以八脉八穴配合八卦,以每日各个时辰的天干推算开穴。

One of the time points combination, which is to calculate the opening points using the heavenly stems of each day's Chinese ancient hours (each equals today's 2 hours), and to combine the eight points of the eight meridians and the eight Chinese ancient divination trigram.

飞扬 Feiyang(BL58)

经穴名。属足太阳膀胱经,本经络穴。定位:在小腿后面,昆仑直上7寸,承山外下方1寸处。主治:头痛,目眩,鼻塞,鼻衄,背痛,腿痛,痔疾。操作:直刺1~1.5寸;

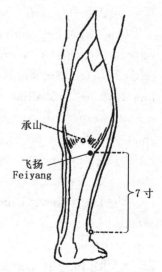
承山
飞扬
Feiyang
7寸

可灸。

The acupoint, Luo-Connecting point belongs to the Bladder Meridian of Foot-Taiyang. Location: On the posterior side of the leg, 7 cun directly above Kunlun (BL60) and 1 cun lateral and inferior to Chengshan (BL57). Indications: Headache, blurred vision, nasal obstruction, epistaxis, pain in the lower back and legs, hemorrhoids, etc. Method: Puncture perpendicularly 1-1.5 cun. Moxibustion is applicable.

腓腨 calf

小腿腓肠肌隆起的部分。

Fleshy part of the back of the leg, formed by the prominence of the gastrocnemius muscle.

肺 lung

①五脏之一。居于胸中，与大肠相表里。其主要功能是主气而司呼吸，主宣发与肃降。开窍于鼻，在液为涕，在志为忧。②耳穴名。在心穴的周围。主治：咳嗽，哮喘，声音嘶哑，皮肤疾病，荨麻疹等。

①One of the five zang organs. It is located in the chest and exterior-interiorly related to the large intestine. Its main functions are controlling qi and respiration, governing dispersing, purification and descending. It opens in the nose and related to melancholy and nasal discharge. ② Name of an ear point. It is near the Heart point. Indications: Cough, asthma, hoarseness of voice, skin diseases, urticaria, etc.

肺合大肠 lung is connected with the large intestine

指肺和大肠之间相互关联、相互影响。它们通过经络的联系互为表里，在生理上互相协调，在病理上互相影响。如肺热可引起大便秘结，这时往往用通大便的方法来清泄肺热。

The paired relationship between the lung and the large intestine which are connected with each other by the meridians. One is involved with another in physical function and pathology of disease. For instance, lung heat may result in constipation, and it can be relieved by facitating feces excretion.

肺经 Lung Meridian

手太阴肺经的简称。

Abbreviation for the Lung Meridian of Hand-Taiyin.

肺募 feimu

脏腑募穴之一，即中府穴。

One of the Front-Mu points, namely, Zhongfu (LU1).

肺肾两虚 deficiency of both the lung and kidney

指肺肾两脏同时出现虚证。多由于久病损伤肺肾两脏所致，通常分肺肾阴虚和肺肾气虚两类。治宜补肺益肾。取穴：肺俞、肾俞、太渊、太溪。

A morbid condition resulting from the damage of both lung and kidney during a chronic disease, classified into two types, i.e., yin deficiency and qi deficiency of lung and kidney. Treatment principle: Strengthen the lung and tonify the kidney. Point selection: Feishu(BL13), Shenshu(BL23),Taiyuan(LU9),Taixi(KI3).

肺俞 Feishu(BL13)

经穴名。属足太阳膀胱经,肺的背俞穴。定位:在背部,当第三胸椎棘突下,后正中线旁开 1.5 寸。主治:咳嗽,气喘,胸痛,吐血,潮热,盗汗等。操作:向内斜刺0.5～0.8 寸;可灸。

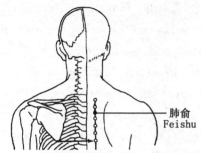

The acupoint, Back-Shu point of the lung, belongs to the Bladder Meridian of Foot-Taiyang. Location: On the back, below the spinous process of the 3rd thoracic vertebra, 1.5 cun lateral to the posterior midline. Indications: Cough, asthma, chest pain, hematemesis, tidal fever, night sweating, etc. Method: Puncture obliquely 0.5-0.8 cun towards the interspace of the spines. Moxibustion is applicable.

肺系 pulmonary system

即呼吸道,包括鼻腔、咽、气管和支气管等。

Referring to the respiratory tract, including the nasal cavity, larynx, trachea, bronchi, etc.

肺主气 lung dominates qi

肺的主要功能之一。一是指肺主呼吸之气,通过肺的呼吸,吸入清气,呼出浊气,进行气体交换。二是指肺主一身之气,体内各种气机活动均与肺有密切关系。

One of the main functions of the lung. One is that the lung controls breathing qi, through which inhale the fresh air and exhale the turbid air, thus exchange gas constantly. Another is that the lung controls qi in the whole body. All the qi activities in the body are related to the lung.

分刺 between muscles puncture

九刺法之一。指直接刺在肌肉的间隙处,以泻邪气。用于治疗肌肉酸痛、肌萎无力等。

One of the Nine Needling techniques, i. e. , to puncture the space between two muscles so as to purge the pathogenic qi. It is used for treating muscular soreness and atrophy, etc.

分娩 delivery

足月胎儿及其附属物从临产至从母体全部产出的过程。针刺合谷、三阴交有助于分娩。

The whole process from the beginning of labor to the delivery of the mature fetus and its attachments. Acupuncture Hegu(LI4) and Sanyinjiao(SP6) may do favor to delivery.

分肉 muscle

①指骨骼肌。②阳辅穴别名。

① The skeletal muscles. ② The other name of Yangfu (GB38).

分中 Fenzhong

环跳穴别名。

The other name of Huantiao (GB30).

丰隆 Fenglong(ST40)

经穴名。属足阳明胃经,本经络穴。定

位：在小腿前外侧，当外踝尖上 8 寸，条口外，距胫骨前缘二横指。主治：头痛，头晕，咳嗽，气喘，痰多，胸痛，便秘，癫狂，下肢肿痛，痿痹等。操作：直刺 1～1.5 寸；可灸。

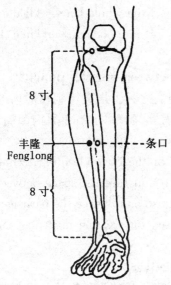

8 寸

丰隆
Fenglong ——— 条口

8 寸

The acupoint, Luo-Connecting point, belongs to the Stomach Meridian of Foot-Yangming. Location：On the anterior lateral side of the leg, 8 cun above the tip of the external malleolus, lateral to Tiaokou (ST38), and two finger breadths from the anterior crest of the tibia. Indications：Headache, dizziness, cough, asthma, excessive phlegm, pain in the chest, constipation, mania, pain, swelling or paralysis of the lower extremities, etc. Method：Puncture perpendicularly 1-1.5 cun. Moxibustion is applicable.

风 wind

①自然界正常的气象之一。②风邪，六淫之一，为外感疾病的致病因素，它往往和其他致病因素合而致病。其致病特点是发病迅速而多变，并呈游走性。常见症状有恶寒、发热、发热。③风证，见内风，指在疾病发展过程中出现风证。表现为眩晕、抽搐、震颤等一类神经症状，因它不同于外感的风，故名。

①One of the climatic factors in the natural world. ②Referring to the wind-evil, one of the six evils which is the common pathogenic factor of the exogenous diseases and usually blends with other factors to attack the human body. Its pathogenic characteristics are sudden onset, rapid changes and tendency of wandering. The chief symptoms caused by wind-evil are aversion to wind, cold and fever. ③ Referring to wind syndrome, see endogenous wind-syndrome, wind-syndrome occurring during the course of a disease, as compared with that resulting from the attack of exogenous evils, manifested with neurological symptoms such as dizziness, convulsion, tremor, etc.

风池 Fengchi(GB30)

经穴名。属足少阳胆经。定位：在头项部，当枕骨之下，与风府相平，胸锁乳突肌与斜方肌上端之间的凹陷处。主治：头痛，眩晕，失眠，颈项强痛，视物不清，目赤痛，耳鸣，惊厥，癫痫，热病，感冒等。操作：针尖向下朝鼻尖方向斜刺 0.5～0.8 寸，深部中间为延髓，必须严格掌握针刺的角度与深度；可灸。

Name of an acupoint. It belongs to the Gallbladder Meridian of Foot-Shaoyang. Location：On the nape, below the occipital bone, on the level of Fengfu(GV16), in

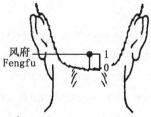

the depression between the upper ends the sternocleidomastoid and trapezius muscles. Indications：Headache, vertigo, insomnia, pain and stiffness of the neck, blurred vision, red and painful eyes, tinnitus, convulsion, epilepsy, febrile diseases, common cold, etc. Method：Puncture obliquely towards the nasal apex 0. 5-0. 8 cun, the angle and depth of acupuncture must be controlled precisely because the deeper part of the point is the medulla oblongata. Moxibustion is applicable.

风府 Fengfu(GV16)

经穴名。属督脉。定位：在项部,当后发际正中直上 1 寸,枕外隆凸直下,两侧斜方肌之间凹陷中。主治：头痛项强,视物不清,鼻衄,咽喉肿痛,中风不语,偏瘫,癫狂等。操作：向下颌方向缓慢刺入 0. 5 寸,不可深刺或向上斜刺,以免误伤延髓。

Name of an acupoint. It belongs to the Governor Vessel. Location：On the nape, 1 cun directly above the midpoint of the posterior hairline, directly below the external occipital protuberance, in the depression between the trapezius muscle of both sides. Indications：Headache, neck rigidity, blurred vision, epistaxis, sore throat, aphasia from apoplexy, hemiplegia, mental disorder, etc. Method：Puncture slowly obliquely towards the lower jaw 0. 5 cun, deep or upward puncture is prohibited, otherwise the medulla oblongata may be injured.

风关 Fengguan

小儿按摩用穴,示指掌面第一、二、三节总称三关。其本节称风关,中节称气关,末节称命关。主要用于诊察和按摩。又指示指根横纹中,称风关穴,针刺见血治小儿惊风。

Name of an infantile massage point. The three palmar phalanges of the index finger are collectively called sanguan, the proximal one called fengguan, the intermediate one called qiguan and the distal one called mingguan. All these are used for diagnosis and massage. It also refers to the extra point fengguan located at the midpoint of the index finger radical crease, curing the infantile convulsion by pricking and letting out blood.

风寒湿痹 arthralgia due to wind-cold-damp evil

即风寒湿邪相合侵袭机体,阻闭肢体经络而引起的关节疼痛、运动障碍的一种疾病。治宜散寒除湿、通络止痛。取穴：足三里、商丘、阴陵泉、膝阳关。

A disease marked by arthralgia and limitation of joint movement, caused by wind-cold-damp evils attacking the body and blocking the meridians of the limbs.

Treatment principle: Dispel cold and remove dampness, remove obstructions in the meridians and collaterals to relieve pain. Point selection: Zusanli (ST36), Shangqiu(SP5), Yinlingquan (SP9), Xiyangguan(GB33).

风门 Fengmen(BL12)

经穴名。属足太阳膀胱经。定位:在背部,当第二胸椎棘突下,后正中线旁开 1.5 寸。主治:伤风感冒,咳嗽,发热头痛,项强背痛等。操作:向内斜刺 0.5～0.8 寸;可灸。

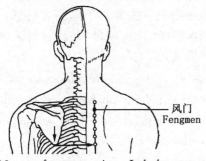

风门
Fengmen

Name of an acupoint. It belongs to the Bladder Meridian of Foot-Taiyang. Location: On the back, below the spinous process of the 2nd thoracic vertebra, 1.5 cun lateral to the posterior midline. Indications: Common cold, cough, fever and headache, neck rigidity, back pain, etc. Method: Puncture obliquely 0.5-0.8 cun towards the interspace of the spines. Moxibustion is applicable.

风热 wind-heat

即风邪和热邪相结合的致病因素,致病时可引起发热重、恶寒轻,并有咳嗽、口渴、咽喉疼痛、舌质红、舌苔微黄及脉浮数等症状。治宜祛风、除湿、清热。取穴:风池、风市、阴陵泉、行间、膈俞。

The pathogenic factor blended with wind-evil and heat-evil, which may cause symptoms as high fever, mild aversion to cold, cough, thirst, sore throat, red tongue with yellowish fur, floating and rapid pulse, etc. Treatment principle: Dispel the wind, clear the dampness and the heat. Point selection: Fengchi(GB20), Fengshi (GB31), Yinlingquan (SP9), Xingjian(LR2), Geshu(BL17).

风湿 rheumatism

风和湿两种病邪结合所引起的病证。多表现为各种痹证。

A syndrome caused by the attack of wind and dampness-evils; usually manifested as all kinds of bi syndromes.

风市 Fengshi(GB31)

经穴名。属足少阳胆经。定位:在大腿外侧部的中线上,当腘横纹上 7寸,或直立垂手时中指尖处。主治:腰腿酸痛,下肢偏瘫,脚气,全身瘙痒等。操作:直刺 1～2寸;可灸。

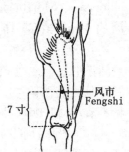

风市
Fengshi

7寸

Name of an acupoint. It belongs to the Gallbladder Meridian of Foot-Shaoyang. Location: On the lateral midline of the thigh, 7cun above the popliteal crease, or at the place touching the tip of the middle finger when the patient stands upright with the arms hanging down freely. Indications: Pain and soreness in the thigh and lumbar region, paralysis of the lower limbs, beriberi, general pruritus, etc.

Method: Puncture perpendicularly 1-2 cun. Moxibustion is applicable.

风溪 Fengxi

耳穴名。又称过敏区、荨麻疹点、结节内。在指、腕两穴之间。主治：荨麻疹，皮肤瘙痒症，过敏性鼻炎。

Name of an ear point. It is also called allergic zone, urticaria point, interior tubercle, located at the midpoint between Zhi and Wan. Indications: Urticaria, itching of the skin, allergic rhinitis.

锋针 sharp needle

古代九针之一。即现代用的三棱针。针体圆，针尖呈三棱状，有刃。主要用于刺破皮下静脉及小血管，治疗痈肿、热病、急性胃肠炎等。

One of the nine needles of the ancient times. Namely, the modern three-edged needles. Its body is round and its tip is triangular with sharp edges. It is mainly used to prick subcutaneous veins and small vessels for treating abscess and carbuncle, febrile diseases, acute gastroenteritis, etc.

凤凰展翅 the phoenix spreads its wings

针刺手法名。同"飞法"。

Name of acupuncture manipulations, i. e. , the need-handle twisting.

跗 instep

指足背部。

Dorsum of foot.

跗阳 Fuyang (BL59)

经穴名。属足太阳膀胱经。定位：在小腿后侧，外踝后，昆仑穴直上3寸。主治：头重头痛，腰背痛，外踝红肿，下肢瘫痪

等。操作：直刺0.5～1寸；可灸。

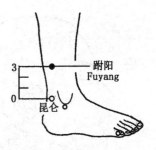

Name of an acupoint. It belongs to the Bladder Meridian of Foot-Taiyang. Location: On the posterior side of the leg, po-sterior to the lateral malleolus, 3 cun directly above Kunlun(BL60). Indications: Heavy sensation of the head, headache, low back pain, redness and swelling of the external malleolus, paralysis of the lower extremities, etc. Method: Puncture perpendicularly 0. 5-1 cun. Moxibustion is applicable.

敷 topical application of herb

把新鲜的植物药捣烂，或用干药末加一定量的溶液调和，敷在身体表面的某一部位，定期换药。适用于局部的疮疡、肿痛及外伤等。

Local application of pounded fresh medicinal herbs or moisturized medicinal powder on the affected part, which needs to be changed at regular intervals, applicable to local sore and ulcer, swelling, pain and trauma.

浮白 Fubai (GB10)

经穴名。属足少阳胆经。定位：在头部，当耳后乳突的后上方，天冲与完骨的弧线连线的中1/3与上1/3交点处。主治：头痛，耳鸣，耳聋等。操作：平刺0.3～0.8寸；可灸。

Name of an acupoint. It belongs to the

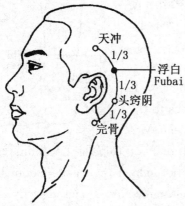

Gallbladder Meridian of Foot-Shaoyang. Location: On the head, posterior and superior to the mastoid process behind the ear, at the junction of the middle third and upper third of the curved line connecting Tianchong (GB9) and Wangu (GB12). Indications: Headache, tinnitus, deafness, etc. Method: Puncture horizontally 0. 3-0. 8 cun. Moxibustion is applicable.

浮刺 superficial needling

十二刺法之一。用于治疗寒性肌肉痉挛。方法是从患处的侧旁进行浅刺。

One of the twelve needling techniques for treating muscle spasm of cold nature. It is to administer a shallow puncture on the sides of the affected part.

浮络 floating collateral

指位于皮下浅表的络脉。

The collaterals located superficially in the skin.

浮脉 floating pulse

脉浮浅,轻按即得的一种脉象。主病在表,浮而有力为表实,浮而无力为表虚。

A pulse condition in which the beats are superficial and palpable by light pressure, indicating that the disease is on the surface of the body. The floating and strong pulse indicates a superficial sthenia syndrome, while the floating and weak pulse indicates a superficial asthenia syndrome.

浮郄 Fuxi (BL38)

经穴名。属足太阳膀胱经。定位:在腘横纹外侧端,委阳上 1 寸,股二头肌肌腱的内侧。主治:臀股麻木,腘挛筋急等。操作:直刺0. 8～1. 5 寸;可灸。

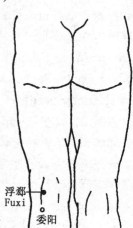

Name of an acupoint. It belongs to the Bladder Meridian of Foot-Taiyang. Location: At the lateral end of the popliteal crease, 1 cun above Weiyang(BL39), medial to the tendon of the biceps femoris of the thigh. Indications: Numbness of the gluteal and femoral regions, contracture of the tendons in the popliteal fossa, etc. Method: Puncture perpendicularly 0. 8-1. 5 cun. Moxibustion is applicable.

伏冲 deep part of the Thoroughfare Vessel

冲脉循行进入脊椎骨内的部分。

The part of Thoroughfare Vessel running through the spinal column of the body.

伏兔 Futu(ST32)

经穴名。属足阳明胃经。定位：在大腿前面，当髂前上棘与髌底外侧端的连线上，髌底上6寸。主治：腰胯疼痛，腿膝冷痛，下肢麻痹，脚气等。操作：直刺1～2寸；可灸。

Name of an acupoint. It belongs to the Stomach Meridian of Foot-Yangming. Location：On the anterior side of the thigh and on the line connecting the anterior superior iliac spine and the superior lateral corner of

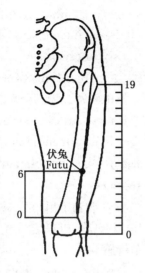

the patella, 6 cun above this corner. Indications：Pain in the lumbar and hip, coldness and pain of the knee and leg, paralysis of the lower extremities, beriberi, etc. Method：Puncture perpendicularly 1-2 cun. Moxibustion is applicable.

伏羲 Fuxi

传说中中华民族的祖先，选草药并制九针。

Ancestor of Chinese nation in the legend. It is said that he selected the medicinal herbs and invented the nine kind of needles.

伏针、伏灸 acupuncture and moxibustion in hot summer days

指在盛夏三伏天进行针灸。因此时天气炎热，阳气升发，针灸对一些慢性病及秋冬易发病具有良好的防治作用。

Acupuncture and moxibustion in hot summer days can give excellent preventing and curing effect on some chronic diseases and other dieases easily contracted in autumn and winter because of the rising and opening of yang-qi during this kind of weather.

扶突 Futu(LI18)

经穴名。属手阳明大肠经。定位：在颈外侧部，结喉旁，当胸锁乳突肌的前后缘之间。主治：咳嗽气喘，咽喉肿痛，暴喑，瘰疬，瘿气等。操作：直刺0.5～0.8寸；可灸。

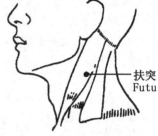

Name of an acupoint. It belongs to the Large Intestine Meridian of Hand-Yangming. Location：On the lateral side of the neck, beside the laryngeal prominence, between the anterior and posterior borders of the sternocleidomastoid muscle. Indications：Cough, asthma, sore throat, sudden loss of voice, scrofula, goiter, etc. Method：Puncture perpendicularly 0.5-0.8 cun. Moxibustion is applicable.

扶正固本 supporting the healthy qi

使用调补阴阳气血的药物，以增强人体抗病能力的治法。

A treatment for strengthening the

body's resistance by the application of drugs for the invigoration of yin, yang, qi and blood.

扶正祛邪 supporting healthy qi to e-liminate evils

治疗原则名。扶正指扶助正气,增强机体抗病能力;祛邪指祛除病邪,使邪去正安。

Name of therapeutic principle. To support vital qi is to strengthen body's resistance to pathogen; to eliminate evils means getting rid of pathogenic factors to facilitate restoration of healthy qi.

府舍 Fushe (SP13)

经穴名。属足太阴脾经。定位:在下腹部,脐下 4 寸,冲门上方 0.7 寸,距前正中线 4 寸。主治:下腹痛,疝气等。操作:直刺 0.5～1 寸;可灸。

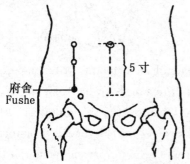

Name of an acupoint. It belongs to the Spleen Meridian of Foot-Taiyin. Location: On the lower abdomen, 4 cun below the center of the umbilicus, 0.7 cun above Chongmen(SP12), 4 cun lateral to the anterior midline. Indications: Lower abdominal pain, hernia, etc. Method: Puncture perpendicularly 0.5-1 cun. Moxibustion is applicable.

府俞 Fu shu

指六腑诸阳经的井、荥、输、原、经、合各穴。

It refers to the Jing-Well points, Ying-Spring points, Shu-Stream points, Yuan-Primary points, Jing-River points and He-Sea points of all the yang meridians of the six fu-organs.

腑会 influential point of Fu-organs

指中脘穴。为八会穴之一。

It refers to Zhongwan (CV12), one of the eight influential points.

辅助手法 supplementary manipulations

指针刺过程中的一些配合手法,如按压、拨动等,以确定穴位,帮助进出针,调节针感等。

Some supplementary manipulations during acupuncture, such as pressing, stirring, etc. , to help to locate the points, insert or withdraw the needle, and regulate the needling sensations, etc.

复溜 Fuliu (KI7)

经穴名。属足少阴肾经,本经经穴。定位:在 小 腿 内 侧,太溪上

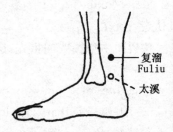

2 寸,跟腱的前方。主治:水肿,腹胀,泄泻,肠鸣,下肢痿痹,盗汗,热病无汗等。操作:直刺 0.5～1 寸;可灸。

The name of the acupoint, Jing-River point of the Kidney Meridian of Foot-Shaoyin. Location: On the medial side of the leg, 2 cun directly above Taixi(KI3), anterior to the Achilles tendon. Indications: Edema, abdominal distension, diarrhea, borborygmus, muscular atrophy of the leg, night sweating, febrile disease without sweating, etc. Method: Puncture perpendicularly 0. 5-1 cun. Moxibustion is applicable.

附分 Fufen (BL41)

经穴名。属足太阳膀胱经。定位：在背部，当第二胸椎棘突下，旁开3寸。主治：肩背颈项强痛，肘臂麻木等。操作：斜刺0.5～0.8寸；可灸。

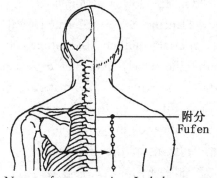

Name of an acupoint. It belongs to the Bladder Meridian of Foot-Taiyang. Location: On the back, below the spinous process of the 2nd thoracic vertebra, 3 cun lateral to the posterior midline. Indications: Stiffness and pain of the shoulder, back, neck, numbness of the elbow and arm, etc. Method: Puncture obliquely 0. 5-0. 8 cun. Moxibustion is applicable.

附子饼灸 aconite-cake moxibustion

间接灸的一种。取中药附子切碎、研细末，加入黄酒调和制成2～3 cm厚的薄饼，中间透刺数孔，置于施灸的腧穴上，将艾炷置薄饼上点燃灸之。多用于阴性疮疡久不收口等病症。

A form of indirect moxibustion. Cut aconite into small pieces and grind it into powder, then mix it with yellow wine to make thin cakes about 2-3 cm, prick several holes in the center of the cake, place it on an acupoint, and put the moxa cone on it for moxibustion, primarily used for chronic ulcers, carbuncles, etc.

腹 abdomen；Fu

①位于胸部与骨盆之间的身体部分。②耳穴名。在腰骶椎前侧耳腔缘。主治：腹痛，腹胀，腹泻，急性腰扭伤。

①The portion of the body which lies between the thorax and pelvis. ②Name of an ear point. It is in front of Yaozhui, on the margin of the ear cavity. Indications: Abdominal pain and distention, diarrhea, acute lumbar muscle sprain.

腹哀 Fuai(SP16)

经穴名。属足太阴脾经。定位：在上腹部，当脐中上3寸，距前正中线4寸。主治：腹痛，消化不良，便秘，痢疾等。操作：直刺0.8～1.5寸；可灸。

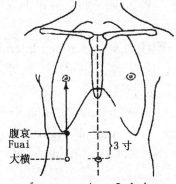

Name of an acupoint. It belongs to the Spleen Meridian of Foot-Taiyin. Location：On the upper abdomen，3 cun above the center of the umbilicus and 4 cun lateral to the anterior midline. Indications：Abdominal pain，indigestion，constipation，dysentery，etc. Method：Puncture perpendicularly 0. 8-1. 5 cun. Moxibustion is applicable.

腹第二侧线 second abdominal lateral line

经穴定位线,距腹正中线 2 寸,为足阳明胃经循行处。

Meridians and points locating line，2 cun lateral to the abdominal midline，where the Stomach Meridian of Foot-Yangming passes.

腹第三侧线 third abdominal lateral line

经穴定位线,距腹正中线 3. 5 寸,为足太阴脾经、足厥阴肝经和足少阳胆经循行处。

Meridians and points locating line，3. 5 cun lateral to the abdominal midline，where the Spleen Meridian of Foot-Taiyin，the Liver Meridian of Foot-Jueyin and the Gallbladder Meridian of Foot-Shaoyang pass.

腹第一侧线 first abdominal lateral line

经穴定位线,距腹正中线 0. 5 寸,为足少阴肾经循行处。

Meridians and points locating line，0. 5 cun lateral to the abdominal midline，where the Kidney Meridian of Foot-Shaoyin passes.

腹结 Fujie (SP14)

经穴名。属足太阴脾经。定位:在下腹部,大横下 1. 3 寸,距前正中线 4 寸。主治:脐周痛,腹胀,疝气,泄泻,便秘等。操作:直刺1～1. 5 寸;可灸。

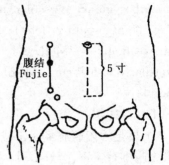

Name of an acupoint. It belongs to the Spleen Meridian of Foot-Taiyin. Location：On the lower abdomen，1. 3 cun below Daheng（SP15），4 cun lateral to the anterior midline. Indications：Pain around the navel，abdomial distension，hernia，diarrhea，constipation，etc. Method：Puncture perpendicularly 1-1. 5 cun. Moxibustion is applicable.

腹满 fullness of the abdomen

指腹部胀满的症状。有虚实之分。虚证多因脾阳失运所致,喜按喜暖;实证多因热结胃肠所致,腹满痛拒按,大便秘结。治宜调畅三焦气机。取穴:三焦俞、偏历、气海、水分、足三里。

A disorder classified into asthenia syndrome and sthenia syndrome. The former is usually caused by the dysfunction of spleen-yang，characterized by prefering to local pressure and heat；while the latter is usually caused by the retention of heat-evil in the gastric intestinal tract，characterized by abdominal pain refusing to pressure and constipation，etc. Treatment principle：Regulate the movement of qi in sanjiao. Point selection：Sanjiaoshu (BL22)，Pianli（LI6），Qihai（CV6），Shuifen(CV9)，Zusanli(ST36).

腹通谷 Futonggu（KI20）

经穴名。属足少阴肾经。定位：在上腹部，当脐中上5寸，距前正中线0.5寸。主治：腹痛，腹胀，呕吐，消化不良等。操作：直刺1～1.5寸；可灸。

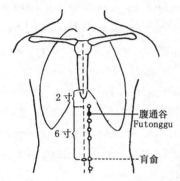

Name of an acupoint. It belongs to the Kidney Meridian of Foot-Shaoyin. Location：On the upper abdomen，5 cun above the center of the umbilicus and 0.5 cun lateral to the anterior midline. Indications：Abdominal pain and distension，vomiting，indigestion，etc. Method：Puncture perpendicularly 1-1.5 cun. Moxibustion is applicable.

腹痛 abdominal pain

指因外感六淫、饮食不节、七情所伤、气机郁滞、血脉瘀阻及虫积等因素引起的腹部疼痛。治宜补脾温肾、调畅气机。取穴：脾俞、肾俞、章门、关元、太冲。

A symptom caused by the attack of six external pathogens，immoderate diet，emotional upsets，stagnation of qi，obstruction of blood circulation and parasitic infestation，etc. Treatment principle：Reinforce the spleen and warm the kidney，regulate the movement of qi. Point selection：Pishu（BL20），Shenshu（(BL23)，Zhangmen（LR13），Guanyuan（CV4），Taichong(LR3).

腹正中线 abdominal midline

经穴定位线，为任脉循行处。

Meridians and points locating line where the Conception Vessel passes.

G

干脚气 dry beriberi

没有浮肿的脚气病。因体质素有阴虚内热,湿热、风毒之邪从热化,伤及营血,筋脉失养所致。临床表现为下肢无力、麻木、酸痛挛急,脚不肿而日见枯瘦,饮食减少,小便赤热,舌红,脉弦数等。治宜养血滋阴。取穴:解溪、阴市、血海、复溜、照海、悬钟。

A type of beriberi occurring in the patient suffering from yin deficiency and internal heat syndrome due to attack of damp-heat and wind-evils which transform to heat-evil and damages the nutrient-blood, leading to the malnutrition of tendons and vessels; manifested as weakness, numbness, soreness and spasm of the lower limbs, foot muscle loss without edema, loss of appetite, hot and deep-colored urine, red tongue, wiry and rapid pulse, etc. Treatment principle: Replenish the blood and nourish the yin. Point selection: Jiexi (ST41), Yinshi (ST33), Xuehai (SP10), Fuliu (KI7), Zhaohai (KI6), Xuanzhong (GB39).

干咳 dry cough

由于火郁、伤燥或肺阴不足所致的病症。以咳嗽无痰为特征。治宜滋阴润肺、清热止咳。取穴:太溪、肺俞、列缺、照海。

A disorder due to retention of fire-evil, impairment of lung caused by dryness-evil or insufficiency lung-yin characterized by non-productive cough. Treatment principle: Nourish yin and moisten the lung, clear heat to relieve cough. Point selection: Taixi(KI3), Feishu(BL13), Lieque (LU7), Zhaohai(KI6).

干呕 retching

即患者作呕吐之态,但有声而无物吐出,胃虚气逆或胃寒、胃热均可引起本症。治宜疏肝和胃。取穴:上脘、阳陵泉、太冲、梁丘、神门。

It refers to vomiting with sound but without vomitus, mainly caused by stomach asthenia with adverse rising of qi, stomach-cold or stomach-heat. Treatment principle: Dispersing stagnated liver-qi for regulating stomach. Point selection: Shangwan(CV13), Yanglingquan (GB34), Taichong (LR3), LiangQiu (ST34), Shenmen(HT7).

干针 simple acupuncture

指单纯的针刺,在针刺麻醉中与电针、水针相对而言。

In acupuncture anesthesia, simple acupuncture is named in comparison with electroacupuncture and hydroacupuncture.

干支 stems-branches

即十天干与十二地支,它们相互配合以志时序。针灸按时配穴法也以此为依据。

The ten heavenly stems and the twelve earthly branches which can be combined together to record time and order. In acupuncture the point-combinating methods according to time is based on this.

肝 liver;Gan

①五脏之一。主要功能是贮藏和调节

血液,维持筋腱关节的运动功能及调节脾胃的消化吸收功能。此外,与精神活动也有密切关系。②耳穴名。在胃和十二指肠穴的后方。主治:胁痛,眩晕,月经不调,眼病,高血压,肝炎,肋间神经痛等。

① One of the five zang organs. It's main functions are to store and regulate the blood, to control the movement of the joints and tendons, and to adjust the digestive function of the spleen and stomach. Furthermore, it is closely related to the mental activities. ② Name of an ear point. On the posterior side of Wei and Shierzhichang. Indications: Hypochondriac pain, vertigo, irregular menstruation, eye diseases, hypertension, hepatitis, intercostal neuralgia, etc.

肝合胆 liver is connected with gallbladder

指肝和胆之间相互关联、相互影响。它们通过经络的联系互为表里,在生理上互相协调,在病理上互相影响。

The paired relationship between the liver and the gallbladder, which are connected with each other by the network of meridians to form an exterior-interior relationship. They cooperate in functioning and involving each other when diseased.

肝火上炎 liver-fire flaring up

指肝经气火上逆的证候,症见头痛眩晕、耳聋耳鸣、急躁易怒、面红目赤、胁肋疼痛、溲赤便秘、苔黄、脉弦数等。治宜平肝降火。取穴:太冲、行间、肝俞、水泉。

It refers to qi and fire rising adversely from liver, manifested as headache, dizzines, deafness, tinnitus, irritability, flushed face and red eyes, pain in the lateral thorax, red urine, constipation, yellow coating on the tongue, wiry and rapid pulse, etc. Treatment principle: Calm the liver and relieve the fire. Point selection: Taichong (LR3), Xingjian (LR2), Ganshu (BL18), Shuiquan (KI5).

肝经 Liver Meridian

足厥阴肝经的简称。

Abbreviation for the Liver Meridian of Foot-Jueyin.

肝脾不和 disharmony between liver and spleen

由于肝气郁结、肝脾两脏制约关系失调致消化功能长期紊乱的病理。症见胁胀或胁痛、嗳气、厌食、腹胀痛、泄泻、性情急躁、脉弦缓等。治宜平肝调中、抑木扶土。取穴:中脘、天枢、足三里、太冲、阴陵泉、期门。

A morbid condition of prolonged digestive disorder caused by the stagnation of liver-qi and the failure of mutual restraint between liver and spleen; manifested as hypochondriac distention or pain, eructation, anorexia, abdominal distending pain, diarrhea, irritability, wiry and slow pulse, etc. Treatment principle: Calm the liver and regulate the function of the spleen, suppress hyperfunction of the liver and strengthen the spleen. Point selection: Zhongwan (CV12), Tianshu (ST25), Zusanli (ST36), Taichong (LR3), Yinlingquan (SP9), Qimen (LR14).

肝气 liver-qi

①肝脏的精气。②指肝脏的功能,包括神经系统、消化系统和内分泌系统的部分功能。

①The essence of the liver. ②Referring to the functions of the liver, including some functions of nervous, digestive and endocrine systems.

肝肾同源 liver and kidney coming from the same origin

①指肝和肾互相滋养的关系。②肝藏血,肾藏精,精和血可以互相转化。

①The mutual supply of nutrients between the liver and the kidney. ②The liver stores blood and the kidney stores essence, the essence and blood are able to transform into each other.

肝肾阴虚 yin deficiency of liver and kidney

肝肾阴液亏虚,阴不制阳,虚热内扰的病理。症见眩晕、头汗、耳鸣、视物不明、咽干口燥、五心烦热、遗精、失眠、腰膝酸痛、舌红少津等。治宜滋补肝肾。取穴:肝俞、肾俞、命门、阴谷、太溪。

A morbid condition due to yin-fluid deficiency of liver and kidney failing to control yang resulting in internal deficient heat; manifested as dizziness, head sweating, tinnitus, poor vision, dry mouth and throat, five center heat, nocturnal emission, insomnia, soreness of waist and knees, red and dry tongue, etc. Treatment principle: Nourish the liver and kidney. Point selection: Ganshu (BL18), Shenshu (BL23), Mingmen (GV4), Yingu(KI10), Taixi(KI3).

肝俞 Ganshu (BL18)

经穴名。属足太阳膀胱经,肝的背俞穴。定位:在背部,当第九胸椎棘突下,旁开1.5寸。主治:黄疸,胁痛,目赤,视物不清,夜盲,精神失常,痫证,背痛,吐衄等。操作:向内斜刺0.5～0.8寸;可灸。

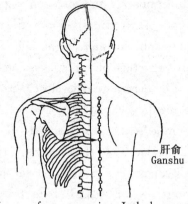

肝俞
Ganshu

Name of an acupoint. It belongs to the Bladder Meridian of Foot-Taiyang. Back-shu point of liver. Location: On the back, below the spinous process of the 9th thoracic vertebra, 1.5 cun lateral to the posterior midline. Indications: Jaundice, pain in the hypochondriac region, redness of the eye, blurred vision, night blindness, mental disorders, epileptic syndrome, back pain, hematemesis and epistaxis, etc. Method: Puncture obliquely 0.5-0.8 cun towards the interspace of the spines. Moxibustion is applicable.

肝阳 liver yang

肝的阳气,与肝阴相对而言。主升发疏泄,促进脾胃运化,调畅气机。肝阳升发太过则易阳亢动风。

It refers to the yang-qi of the liver, contrast with the liver-yin. It governs the functions of ascending, smoothing and regulating the flow of qi, promotes the functions of the spleen and stomach in transportation and transformation. Excessive ascending of liver yang will lead to hyperactivity of yang and endogenous wind.

肝阳上亢 hyperactivity of liver yang

由于肝肾阴虚导致肝阳偏亢的病理。症见头晕、目眩、头痛、面赤、口苦、舌红、脉弦细或弦数等。治宜平肝潜阳。取穴太冲、行间、肝俞、水泉。

A morbid condition dues to deficiency of liver-yin and kidney-yin; manifested as dizziness, headache, flushed cheeks, bitter taste, red tongue, stringy and thin or stringy and rapid pulse, etc. Treatment principle: Calm the liver and subdue yang. Point selection: Taichong (LR3), Xingjian (LR2), Ganshu (BL18), Shuiquan (KI5).

肝郁 stagnation of liver-qi

由于情志不遂或其他病因使肝气疏泄受阻而引起的一类病症。其表现为两胁胀痛、嗳气、脉弦等。治宜疏肝理气。取穴：膻中、内关、太冲、阳陵泉。

A morbid state dues to emotional upsets or other factors; manifested as bilateral hypochondriac distending pain, eructation, wiry pulse, etc. Treatment principle: Dispersing the stagnated liver-qi and regulate the flowing of qi. Point selection: Danzhong (CV17), Neiguan (PC6), Taichong (LR3), Yanglingquan (GB34).

肝主筋 liver governing tendons

五脏分主五体，肝主全身之筋膜，与肢体运动有关。肝之气血充盛，筋膜得养，则筋力强健，运动灵活。

Five zang-organs govern five parts of the body. Liver governs the tendons all over the body, and is related with body movements. If the blood and qi of liver is sufficient, the tendons will be nourished naturally, and the body movement will be agile.

感觉区 sensory zone

位于运动区向后平移 1.5cm 处。该区上 1/5 主治对侧腰腿疼痛、麻木、感觉异常，后头部疼痛，头晕；中 2/5 处主治对侧上肢麻木、疼痛、感觉异常；下 2/5 处主治对侧偏头痛和面部麻木。

It is the zone parallel to and 1.5 cm backwards from the motor zone. Indications: On the upper 1/5, it is used for treating pain, numbness and paresthesia of the waist and the lower limb on the opposite side, occipital headache, and dizziness; at the middle 2/5, it is used for treating numbness, pain and paresthesia of the upper limb on the opposite side; on the lower 2/5, it is used for treating migraine and numbness of face on the opposite side.

感冒 common cold

指由风邪侵袭人体所致的一种疾病。临床上以发热、头痛、鼻塞、流涕、恶风、脉浮为特征。分风寒和风热两种类型。治宜疏风解表。取穴：风门、风池、列缺、大椎、外关。

A disease caused by the attack of wind-evil, characterized by fever, headache, stuffy nose, nasal discharge, aversion to wind, floating pulse, etc.,; classified as wind-cold and wind-heat types. Treatment principle: Expel wind and relieve superficial evils. Point selection: Fengmen (BL12), Fengchi (GB20), Lieque (LU7), Dazhui (GV14), Waiguan (TE5).

肛裂 anal fissure

因血热肠燥,大便干结,排便用力,引起肛管齿线以下皮肤破裂。症见便时肛门灼痛,出少量鲜血。治宜清热利湿、和营止血。取穴:长强、次髎、上巨虚、承山。

A fissure at the margin of the anus, caused by blood-heat and dryness of intestines leading to dry and hard stools, and forcible strain during defecation; manifested as burning pain of the anus during defecation with small amount of fresh blood. Treatment principle: Clear heat and drain dampness, regulate nutrient qi to stop bleeding. Point selection: Changqiang (GV1), Ciliao (BL32), Shangjuxu(ST37),Chengshan(BL57).

肛门 anus

又名魄门、后阴。为消化道最末端,能控制和排泄粪便。

Also named as pomen, posterior yin. It is the terminal opening of the digestive tract which can control and discharge the feces.

高武 Gao Wu

明代针灸学家,编有《针灸聚英》,并制针灸铜人三具(男、女、童子各一具)。

An expert in acupuncture and moxibustion in the Ming Dynasty, the author of *Collection of Gems in Acupuncture and Moxibustion*. He designed and made three bronze figures (a man, a woman and a child) with points and meridians marked on them.

膏肓 Gaohuang (BL43)

①经穴名。属足太阳膀胱经。定位:在背部,当第四胸椎棘突下,旁开 3 寸。主治:肺痨,咳嗽,气喘,吐血,盗汗,健忘,遗精等。②原指心下膈上的部位,后将发病部位较深、治疗很困难者,称为"病入膏肓"。

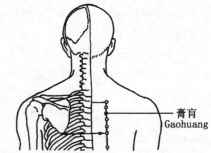

膏肓 Gaohuang

① Name of an acupoint. It belongs to the Bladder Meridian of Foot-Taiyang. Location: On the back, below the spinous process of the 4th thoracic vertebra, 3 cun lateral to the posterior midline. Indications: Pulmonary tuberculosis, cough, asthma, hematemesis, night sweating, poor memory, nocturnal emission, etc. ② Originally, it is the area below the heart and above the diaphragm. Later on, it is used to describe a deeply seated and incurable disease as "the diseases invaded Gaohuang".

膏淋 chyluria

指以小便混浊如米泔或如脂膏、排尿不畅为主症的一种淋证。常有虚实之分。虚证多因脾肾虚弱，不能制约脂液引起；实证多因湿热蕴结下焦，气化不利，清浊相混，脂液失约所致。治宜健脾利湿、益肾固涩。取穴：肾俞、脾俞、膀胱俞、气海俞、百会、足三里、关元。

A disease characterized by dysuria and the presence of chyle in the urine, giving it a milky appearance. The condition is caused by the inability to control the chyle fluid resulting from the asthenia of spleen and kidney in the asthenic type, and from the accumulation of damp-heat in the lower jiao in the sthenic type. Treatment principle: Invigorate the spleen and remove dampness by diuresis, tonify the kidney and induce astringency. Point selection: Shenshu (BL23), Pishu (BL20), Pangguangshu (BL28), Qihaishu (BL24), Baihui (GV20), Zusanli (ST36), Guanyuan (CV4).

割治疗法 cutting therapy

指在患者身上一定部位，用手术刀切开皮肤进行机械性刺激，并摘除少量脂肪以进行治疗的疗法。

The therapeutic technique is to mechanically stimulate a certain location of the body by cutting through the skin with a scalpel and removing a little fatty tissue.

革脉 hollow pulse

弦大中空，如按鼓皮的一种脉象。多因精血亡失所致。

A pulse condition with a feeling like pressing over a drum, mostly caused by the loss of blood and essence.

阁门 Gemen

经外奇穴名。位于阴茎根部中点旁开3寸处。直刺或灸治疝气、阴囊红肿等。

Name of an extra point. Located 3 cun lateral to the midpoint of the penial root, perpendicular acupuncture or moxibustion is used to cure hernia, red and swelling scrotum, etc.

隔饼灸 moxibustion on herbal cake

指隔着有孔的药饼施灸的方法。

Mosibustion with a thin layer of porous herbal cake between skin and moxa cone.

隔葱灸 moxibustion on scallion

间接灸的一种。有两法：①将葱捣烂置于腹部穴位或脐中，在其上施灸。主治虚脱、腹胀、腹寒痛、小便不利等。②取葱白一束捆扎，长约2寸，直立于穴位上施灸，治疮痈、风湿痹痛等。

A kind of indirect moxibustion, there are two methods. ①The pounded scallion is applied to the navel or other points on the abdomen and moxibustion is performed on it to cure collapse, abdominal distension, cold and pain, dysuria, etc. ②A bundle of 2 cun long scallion stems are put vertically on the points and moxibustion is performed on them to cure sores, suppurative inflammations, rheumatic arthritis, etc.

隔姜灸 moxibustion on ginger

间接灸的一种。取厚约2 cm的生姜片，在中心处用针穿刺数孔，上置艾炷放在穴位上施灸。适用于虚寒病症。

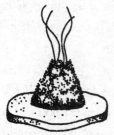

A kind of indirect moxibusion. Take a slice of fresh ginger about 2 cm thick and prick several holes in the center of the ginger with a needle before putting it on the selected point. Then place a moxa cone on top of the ginger and ignite it for moxibustion. Indications: Deficiency and cold diseases.

隔酱灸 moxibustion on thick sauce

间接灸的一种。以酱一匙涂百会穴,灸之,治脱肛。

A kind of indirect moxibustion, i. e., put a spoonful of thick soya sauce on Baihui(GV20), and perform moxibustion on it to cure anal prolapse.

隔韭灸 moxibustion on chives

间接灸的一种。把韭菜捣烂做饼,置于穴位上施灸,治风寒疮毒。

A kind of indirect moxibustion, i. e., pound the chives to pieces and make cakes, moxibustion is performed on those cakes to cure wind-cold, sores.

隔蒜灸 moxibustion on garlic

间接灸的一种。用独头大蒜切成厚度约0.1寸的薄片,用针穿刺数孔,上置艾炷放在穴位上施灸。适用于痈、疽、疮、疖、蛇蝎毒虫所伤、腹中积块及肺痨等。

A form of indirect moxibustion. Select fresh single-clove garlic, cut it into slices about 0.1 cun thick, prick holes in the center of the slice with a needle before placing it on the selected point, then put a moxa cone on the garlic slice and burn it for moxibustion. Indications: Carbuncle, deep rooted carbuncle, sore, boils, bites of snake, scorpion and toxin insect, abdominal masses, pulmonary tuberculosis, etc.

隔盐灸 moxibustion on salt

间接灸的一种。取纯净干燥的食盐适量研细或炒热,填平脐孔,上置艾炷施灸。也有于盐上放置姜片施灸的。常用于急性腹泻、呕吐、脱证等。

A form of indirect moxibustion. Take a proper amount of pure, dry salt, grind it into powder or parch it warm, then fill the salt in the umbilicus until it is at the level of the skin. Place a moxa cone on the salt and burn it for moxibuston. Another method is to put a ginger slice between the salt and moxa cone. Indications: Acute diarrhea, vomiting, collapse syndrome, etc.

膈 diaphragm

即横膈膜。此膜将体腔分为腹腔和胸腔。

Musculomembranous partition separating the coelom into thoracic and abdominal cavities.

膈关 Geguan (BL46)

经穴名。属足太阳膀胱经。定位:在背部,当第七胸椎棘突下,旁开3寸。主治:饮食不下,呃逆,呕吐,嗳气,脊背强痛等。

Name of an acupoint. It belongs to the Bladder Meridian of Foot-Taiyang. Loca-

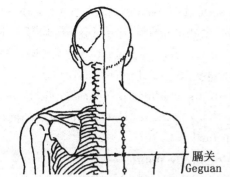

膈关
Geguan

tion: On the back, below the spinous process of 7th thoracic vertebra, 3 cun lateral to the posterior midline. Indications: Dysphagia, hiccup, vomiting, belching, pain and stiffness of the back, etc.

膈俞 Geshu (BL17)

经穴名。属足太阳膀胱经,八会穴之一,血会膈俞。定位:在背部,当第七胸椎棘突下,旁开1.5寸。主治:呕吐,呃逆,咳嗽,气喘,吐血,潮热,盗汗等。操作:向内斜刺0.5~0.8寸;可灸。

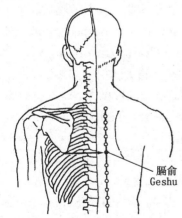

膈俞
Geshu

Name of an acupoint. It belongs to the Bladder Meridian of Foot-Taiyang. Influential point of blood. Location: On the back, below the spinous process of 7th thoracic vertebra, 1.5 cun lateral to the posterior midline. Indications: Vomiting, hiccup, cough, asthma, hematemesis, tidal fever, night sweating, etc. Method: Puncture obliquely 0.5-0.8 cun towards the interspace of the spines. Moxibustion is applicable.

葛洪 Ge Hong

东晋著名医药学家,道家人士(281—341),自号抱朴子,其《抱朴子》一书主要记述炼丹、饮食等,并著有《肘后备急方》。

A noted physician, pharmacologist and Taoist (281-341) of the Eastern Jin Dynasty who called himself Baopuzi. He is the author of *Handbook of Prescription for Emergencies* and *Bao Puzi's Inner Treatise*, the latter deals mainly with alchemy and dietetics.

根结 roots and terminals

指经气的所起与所归。根即根本,指四肢末端的井穴;结指归结,即头、胸、腹部。

It refers to the position of starting and ending of the meridian qi. Roots mean the starting position, i. e., the Jing-Well points in the extremities. Terminals mean the ending, i. e., the head, the thorax and the abdomen.

根穴 root points

十二经脉在四肢末端的井穴,为经脉之根,故名。

The Jing-Well points of the 12 regular meridians in the extremities which are considered to be the roots of those meridians.

跟 Gen

耳穴名。在对耳轮上脚的前上角。主治足跟痛。

Name of an ear point. Located at the superior and anterior angle of superior antihelix crus. It is used for treating heel pain.

公孙 Gongsun (SP4)

经穴名。属足太阴脾经,本经络穴,八脉交会穴之一,通于冲脉。定位:在足内侧缘,当第一跖骨基底的前下方。主治:胃痛,呕吐,腹痛腹胀,泄泻,痢疾,肠鸣等。操作:直刺 0.6～1.2 寸;可灸。

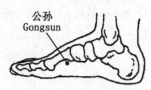

公孙
Gongsun

Name of an acupoint, Luo-Connecting point of the Spleen Meridian of Foot-Taiyin. One of the eight confluence points, communicates with the Thoroughfare Vessel. Location:On the medial border of the foot,anterior and inferior to the proximal end of the 1st metatarsal bone. Indications: Gastric pain, vomiting, abdominal pain and distension, diarrhea, dysentery, borborygmus, etc. Method: Puncture perpendicularly 0.6-1.2 cun. Moxibustion is applicable.

攻补兼施 Reinforcement and elimination in combination

攻法和补法同时使用,以达到邪去而正气不伤的目的。适用于邪气实而正气虚的患者。在这种情况下,单用攻法则正气不支,单用补法则又使邪实,只能攻补两法兼而施之。

A treatment applicable to the case with sthenia of the evil and deficiency of the vital qi. For such case, if only the therapy for elimination of evil is used, the vital qi may be exhausted, and if only the therapy for reinforcement of vital qi is used, the evil may become more sthenic, so, both therapies should be used simultaneously.

孤穴 single point

指位于身体正中线的单穴。

The single points on the midlines.

箍围药 encircling herbal treatment

外治法的一种。在初起的肿疡周围敷以一圈湿润的药泥,起消肿散结止痛或促使脓肿溃破的作用。

One of the external treatments. Circular application of moist herbal paste around an abscess of early stage to reduce swelling, relieve pain and accelerate its diabrosis.

谷气 food (nourishment) qi

指从食物中吸收的营养物质。

The nutrients absorbed from food.

股阴 medial aspect of thigh

部位名。指大腿内侧部。

Name of the body part, i. e., the medial side of the thigh.

骨 bone

为奇恒六腑之一。为人身支架,由肾所主,赖精髓以滋养。

One of the six extraordinary fu-organs, forming the framework of the body, closely related to the function of the kidney and nourished by the marrow and essence.

骨度 bone measurement

古代以骨节为主要标志测量全身各部位的长度和宽度，并以此为基础确定经穴的位置。如前发际至后发际为 12 寸，膝至外踝为 16 寸。此骨度法沿用至今。

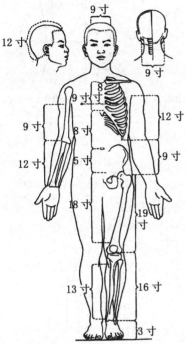

In ancient China, the lengths and widths of the body parts were measured mainly by the bones and joints as the principal landmarks, and the location of meridians as well as acupoints were based on this. For example, the distance between the anterior hairline and the posterior hairline is 12 cun while the length from the knee to the exterior ankle is 16 cun, etc. This bone measurement method has been handed down and used till now.

骨会 influential point of bone

即大杼穴，八会穴之一。

It refers to Dazhu(BL11), one of the eight influential points.

骨针 bone needle

古代以兽骨制成的医用针具，在北京周口店曾有发现，距今约 10 万年。

Medical needles made of animal bones in ancient China, some were found in Zhoukoudian near Beijing, about one hundred thousands years ago.

刮法 needle-scraping technique

针刺辅助手法之一。针刺进入一定深度后，用拇指抵住针尾，以示指或中指的指甲轻刮针柄；或示、中指抵住针尾，以拇指的指甲轻刮针柄，以加强针感。

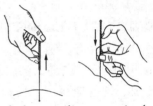

One of the anxiliary manipulations in acupuncture. After inserting the needle into an acupoint to a certain depth, press the needle tail with the thumb and scrape the handle of the needle slightly with the nail of the index or middle finger, or resist the needle tail with the index or middle finger and scrape the handle of the needle gently with the nail of the thumb to strengthen the needle sensation.

关冲 Guanchong(TE1)

经穴名。属手少阳三焦经，本经井穴。定位：在手环指末节尺侧，距指甲角 0.1 寸。主治：头痛，目赤，咽喉肿痛，舌强，热病，心烦等。操作：浅刺 0.1 寸，或三棱针点刺出血；可灸。

The acupoint, Jing-Well point, belongs to the Sanjiao Meridian of Hand-Shaoyang. Location：On the ulnar side of the distal segment of the ring finger, 0.1 cun from the corner of the nail. Indications：Headache, eye

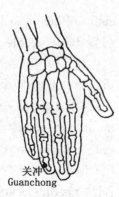

关冲 Guanchong

redness, sore throat, stiffness of the tongue, febrile diseases, irritability, etc. Method：Puncture shallowly 0.1 cun or prick with the three-edged needle to cause bleeding. Moxibustion is applicable.

关刺(渊刺、岂刺) Joint needling

五刺法之一。用于治疗筋痹。刺法是直接针刺四肢关节周围筋肉的附着部,但应防止出血。这是应用于治疗肝病的一种古代刺法。

One of the five needling techniques for treating muscular rheumatism. Method：Directly puncture the attachment of the muscles around the joints of the limbs but avoid bleeding. It is an ancient method to treat hepatic diseases.

关陵(关阳) Guanling(Guanyang)

膝阳关别名。

The other name of Xiyangguan(GB33).

关门 Guanmen (ST22)

经穴名。属足阳明胃经。定位:在上腹部,当脐中上 3 寸,距前正中线 2 寸。主治:腹胀腹痛,食欲不振,肠鸣泄泻等。操作:直刺 1～1.5 寸;可灸。

Name of an acupoint. It belongs to the Stomach Meridian of Foot-Yangming.

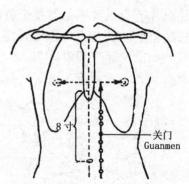

关门 Guanmen

Location：On the upper abdomen,3 cun above the center of the umbilicus and 2 cun lateral to the anterior midline. Indications：Abdominal distension and pain, anorexia, borborygmus, diarrhea, etc. Method：Puncture perpendicularly 1-1.5 cun. Moxibustion is applicable.

关仪 Guanyi

经外奇穴名。位于膝外侧中线,腘横纹上 1 寸处。直刺或艾灸,治女阴痛、小腹绞痛、腹中积寒。

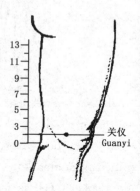

关仪 Guanyi

Name of an extra point. Location：At the lateral midline of the knee, 1 cun above the popliteal crease. Perpendicular acupuncture or moxibustion is used to cure vaginal pain, lower abdominal colic, cold accumulation in abdomen.

关元 Guanyuan (CV4)

经穴名。属任脉,小肠的募穴。定位:在下腹部,前正中线上,当脐下 3 寸。主治:遗尿,遗精,尿频,小便不利,疝气,月经不调,白带,痛经,崩漏,产后出血,下腹痛,泄泻,脱肛等。操作:直刺 0.5～1 寸;可灸。

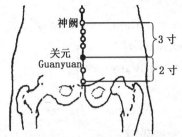

Name of an acupoint. It belongs to the Conception Vessel. Front-Mu point of the Small Intestine. Location: On the lower abdomen, on the anterior midline, 3 cun below the center of the umbilicus. Indications: Enuresis, nocturnal emission, frequent urination, dysuria, hernia, irregular menstruation, leukorrhea disease, dysmenorrhea, metrorrhagia and metrostaxis, postpartum hemorrhage, lower abdominal pain, diarrhea, anal prolapse, etc. Method: Puncture perpendicularly 0. 5-1 cun. Moxibustion is applicable.

关元俞 Guanyuanshu (BL26)

经穴名。属足太阳膀胱经。定位:在腰部,当第五腰椎棘突下,旁开1.5寸。主治:腰痛,腹胀,泄泻,遗尿,尿频等。操作:直刺0.8～1.5寸;可灸。

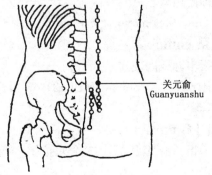

Name of an acupoint. It belongs to the Bladder Meridian of Foot-Taiyang. Location: On the low back, below the spinous process of the 5th lumber vertebra, 1. 5 cun lateral to the posterior midline. Indications: Low back pain, abdominal distension, diarrhea, enuresis, frequent urination, etc. Method: Puncture perpendicularly 0. 8-1. 5 cun. Moxibustion is applicable.

光剥苔 peeled tongue

原有舌苔突然消失。此属胃阴枯竭,胃气大伤的征象。

A sudden disappearance of fur on the tongue, the sign indicates the exhaustion of stomach-yin and serious damage of stomach-qi.

光明 Guangming (GB37)

经穴名。属足少阳胆经,本经络穴。定位:在小腿外侧,当外踝尖上5寸,腓骨前缘。主治:膝痛,下肢痿痹,视物不清,目痛,夜盲,乳胀痛等。操作:直刺0.5～0.8寸;可灸。

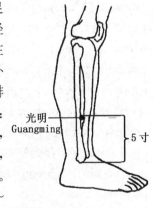

The acupoint, Luo-Connecting point, belongs to the Gallbladder Meridian of Foot-Shaoyang. Location: On the lateral side of the leg, 5 cun above the tip of the external malleolus, on the anterior border of the fibula. Indications: Pain in the knee, muscular atrophy, motor impairment and pain of the lower extremities, blurred vision, pain of eyes, night blindness, distending pain of the breast, etc. Method:Puncture perpendicularly 0. 5-0. 8 cun. Moxibustion is applicable.

归来 Guilai(ST29)

经穴名。属足阳明胃经。定位:在下腹部,当脐中下 4 寸,距前正中线 2 寸。主治:腹痛,疝气,痛经,月经不调,经闭,白带,阴挺等。操作:直刺 1~1. 5 寸;可灸。

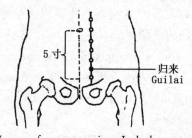

5寸

归来
Guilai

Name of an acupoint. It belongs to the Stomach Meridian of Foot-Yangming. Location:On the lower abdomen, 4 cun below the center of the umbilicus and 2 cun lateral to the anterior midline. Indications:Abdominal pain, hernia, dysmeno-rrhea, irregular menstruation, amenorrhea, leukorrhea disease, uterine or vaginal prolapse, etc. Method:Puncture perpendicularly 1-1. 5 cun. Moxibustion is applicable.

鬼藏 guicang

男指会阴穴,女指奇穴玉门头。

It refers to Huiyin(CV1) in male and extra point Yumentou in female.

鬼臣 Guichen

即曲池穴。

The other name of Quchi(LI11).

鬼城 Guicheng

经外奇穴名。即十宣穴。

Name of the extra points, i. e. , Shixuan(EX-UE11).

鬼床 Guichuang

即颊车穴。

The other name of Jiache(ST6).

鬼当 Guidang

经外奇穴名。在拇指甲后。

Name of an extra point. Located just behind the thumb nail.

鬼封 Guifeng

经外奇穴名。即海泉。

Name of the extra point, i. e. , Haiquan(EX-HN11).

鬼宫 Guigong

即水沟穴。

The other name of Shuigou(GV26).

鬼哭 Guiku

经外奇穴名。位于手足大指(趾)内甲根角处。灸治癫痫、精神病等。

Name of an extra point. Located at the medial nail root corners of the thumb and big toe. Moxibustion is used to cure epilepsy, mental diseases, etc.

鬼垒 Guilei

即隐白穴。

The other name of Yinbai(SP1).

鬼路 Guilu

指申脉或间使穴。

It refers to Shenmai(BL62) or Jianshi(PC5).

鬼门 Guimen

①指治疗癫狂的十三个穴位。②指风府穴。

① The 13 acupoints which are used

specifically to cure epilepsy and mania. ②The other name of Fengfu(GV16).

鬼受 Guishou

即尺泽穴。

The other name of Chize(LU5).

鬼堂 Guitang

指上星或尺泽穴。

The other name of Shangxing(GV23) or Chize(LU5).

鬼邪 Guixie

即足三里穴。

The other name of Zusanli (ST36).

鬼信 Guixin

即少商穴。

The other name of Shaoshang(LU11).

鬼眼 Guiyan

①经外奇穴名。即鬼哭。②腰眼别名。③膝眼别名。

①Name of the extra point, i. e., Guiku. ②The other name of Yaoyan(EX-B7). ③The other name of Xiyan(EX-LE5).

鬼营 Guiying

指间使或劳宫穴。

The other name of Jianshi(PC5) or Laogong(PC8).

鬼枕 Guizhen

即风府穴。

The other name of Fengfu(GV16).

滚筒刺 rolling acupuncture

刺法的一种,使用的针具由柄和滚筒组成,筒壁密布短针,用于较大面积的浅刺。

A kind of acupuncture method using an instrument made of a handle and a roller on which a lot of short needles are densely fixed to perform the shallow rolling acupuncture on a large area.

腘 fossa

部位名。指膝关节的后方,即腘窝。

Name of the body part, i. e., the back of the knee joint,named popliteal fossa.

过梁针 guoliangzhen

指治疗癫狂等精神疾病的十四个经外奇穴。这些奇穴都在四肢部位。

The 14 extra points located in the extremities which are used to treat the mental diseases such as epilepsy and mania.

H

海底 Haidi

会阴别名。

The other name of Huiyin(CV1).

海泉 Haiquan

经外奇穴名。位于舌系带中点处。直刺或三棱针点刺出血,主治呕吐、呃逆、舌肿痛、喉痛、腹泻、消渴等。

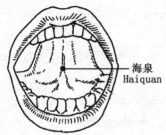

海泉
Haiquan

Name of an extra point. Located at the midpoint of the lingual frenum. Vertical acupuncture or blood-letting with a three-edged needle is used to cure vomiting, hiccup, swelling and sore tongue, sore throat, diarrhea, consumptive thirst, etc.

寒 cold

寒邪,六淫之一。属阴邪,易伤阳气而影响气血的活动。人体受寒邪侵袭而致病时表现为恶寒、发热、头痛、身痛或腹痛腹泻等症状。

Referring to the cold-evil, one of the six evils, which pertains to yin in nature, usually damages yang-qi and affects the activity of qi and blood. It may cause the symptoms such as aversion to cold, fever, headache, general aching, or abdominal pain, diarrhea, etc.

寒府 Hanfu

膝阳关别名。

The other name of Xiyangguan(GB33).

寒热往来 alternate chill and fever

指不规则的恶寒与发热交替出现的症状。本症多因外感病邪居半表半里、正邪交争所致。治宜和解表里、温阳达邪。取穴:陶道、曲池、间使、中渚、丘墟。

A symptom that chill and fever appear alternately, commonly seen in the struggle between healthy qi and pathogen, when the latter invades the half-superficies and half-interior of the body. Treatment principle: Harmonize superficies and interior, warm yang to dispel pathogenic factors. Point selection: Taodao(GV13), Quchi(LI11), Jianshi(PC5), Zhongzhu(TE3), Qiuxu(GB40).

寒则留之 retaining needles for cold syndrome

针刺治疗原则之一。指治疗寒性疾病可留针使其热为补。与"热则疾之"相对。

One of the acupuncture principles, i. e., needles can be retained to cure the cold syndrome by warming reinforcing, as contrasted with the principle of "quick needling for the heat syndrome".

寒者热之 treat cold syndrome with warm herb

属寒性的疾病,一般宜用温热的方药治疗。寒证临床上一般分表寒证、里寒证,分别采用辛温解表和温中祛寒的方法进行治疗。

A therapeutic principle for treating the cold syndrome, i. e., therapy of expelling superficial evils with herb that are acrid in taste and warm in nature is applied for cold syndrome of the superficies, and expelling cold by warming the middle jiao is applied for cold syndrome of the interior.

寒证 cold syndrome

感受寒邪或因阳气不足而产生的证候。表现为面色苍白,恶寒肢冷,腹中雷鸣,腹部疼痛,得热则减,口不渴,或渴喜热饮,大便稀薄,小便清长,舌淡苔白润,脉迟或紧等。治宜温胃健脾。取穴:脾俞、胃俞、足三里、中脘、关元。

A syndrome caused by the attack of cold-evil or the deficiency of yang-qi; manifested as pale complexion, aversion to cold, cold limbs, increased borborygmus, abdominal pain which can be relieved by heat, absence of thirst, or thirst with a desire for hot drink, loose stools, polyuria with light-colored urine, pale tongue with moist and white fur, slow or tense pulse, etc. Treatment principle: Warm the stomach and tonify the spleen. Point selection: Pishu(BL20), Weishu(BL21), Zusanli(ST36), Zhongwan(CV12), Guanyuan(CV4).

汗 sweat

五液之一,是津液代谢的产物。汗为心之液,汗液的分泌与心脏的功能有关。

One of the five kinds of body fluids. It is a product formed during the process of body fluid metabolism. Sweat comes from heart-blood, so it's secretion is related to the function of the heart.

颔厌 Hanyan(GB4)

经穴名。属足少阳胆经。定位:在头部鬓发上,当头维与曲鬓弧形连线的上 1/4 与下 3/4 交点处。主治:偏头痛,眩晕,耳鸣,目外眦痛,齿痛,癫痫等。操作:向后平刺 0.5~0.8 寸;可灸。

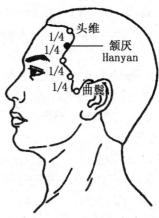

Name of an acupoint. It belongs to the Gallbladder Meridian of Foot-Shaoyang. Location: On the head, in the hair above the temples, at the junction of the upper one fourth and lower three fourths of the curved line connecting Touwei(ST8) and Qubin(GB7). Indications: Migraine, vertigo, tinnitus, pain in the outer canthus, toothache, epilepsy, etc. Method: Puncture horizontally backward 0.3-0.5 cun. Moxibustion is applicable.

颃颡 nasopharynx

指上腭与鼻相通的部位,是人体与外界进行气体交换的必经之道路。

It refers to the part where the palate meets the nasal carity, through which qi exchange between the human body and the external environment takes place.

毫针 filiform needle

古代九针之一,也是现代最常用的一种针具。针身细小如毫毛,根据针的粗细和长短,分各种不同的规格。

One of the nine needles in ancient times, also the most commonly used needle in modern times. Its body is very fine. It varies in different specifications according to the diameter and length.

禾髎 Heliao(LI19)

经穴名。属手阳明大肠经。别名长频、长髎、长颊。主治:口㖞,口噤,鼻塞,鼻衄,鼻息肉,急、慢性鼻炎等。操作:直刺0.3～0.5寸;可灸。

Name of an acupoint. It belongs to the Large Intestine Meridian of Hand-Yangming. It is also known as Chang pin, Chang liao and Chang jia. Indications: Deviation of the mouth, trismus, stuffy nose, epistaxis, nasal polyp, acute and chronic rhinitis, etc. Method: Puncture perpendicularly 0.3-0.5 cun. Moxibustion is applicable.

合谷 Hegu(LI4)

经穴名。属手阳明大肠经,本经原穴。定位:在手背,第一、第二掌骨间,当第二掌骨桡侧的中点处。主治:头颈痛,目赤肿痛,鼻衄,齿痛面肿,耳聋,咽喉肿痛,热病无汗或多汗,面瘫,腹痛,痢疾,经闭,滞产等。操作:直刺0.5～1寸;可灸。

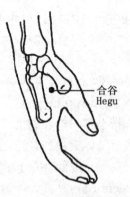

合谷 Hegu

The acupoint, Yuan-Primary point, belongs to the Large Intestine Meridian of Hand-Yangming. Location: On the dorsum of the hand, between the 1st and 2nd metacarpal bones, and at the midpoint of the radial side of the 2nd metacarpal bone. Indications: Headache, pain in the neck, redness, swelling and pain of the eyes, epistaxis, toothache, swelling of the face, deafness, sore throat, febrile disease with or without sweating, facial paralysis, abdominal pain, dysentery, amenorrhea, delayed labour, etc. Method: Puncture perpendicularly 0.5-1 cun. Moxibustion is applicable.

合谷刺 hegu puncture

五刺法之一。用于治疗肌痹。方法是在患病局部向左、右两侧斜刺,直接刺在肌肉部位,像鸡爪的形状。这是应用于脾病的一种古代针法。

One of the five needling techniques for treating painful muscles. It is to puncture the muscles of the affected region obliquely right and left just like chicken feet. It is an ancient way for treating splenic diseases.

合穴 He-Sea points

五输穴之一。位于肘关节、膝关节附近,十二经各有一个。如各处的经气像江河汇合流入大海一样,故名。

One of the five Shu points. They are located at the vicinity of the elbow and knee, one for each of the twelve regular meridians, analogous to rivers from various places flowing together and entering the sea.

合阳 Heyang(BL55)

经穴名。属足太阳膀胱经。定位:在小腿后面,当委中与承山的连线上,委中下 2 寸。主治:腰痛,下肢酸痛、麻痹等。操作:直刺1～2 寸;可灸。

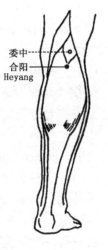

Name of an acupoint. It belongs to the Bladder Meridian of Foot-Taiyang. Location: On the posterior side of the leg, on the line connecting Weizhong (BL40)and Chengshan(BL57),2 cun below Weizhong(BL40). Indications:Low back pain, soreness and paralysis of the lower extremities, etc. Method:Puncture perpendicularly 1-2 cun. Moxibustion is applicable.

和髎 Heliao(TE22)

经穴名。属手少阳三焦经,为手足少阳、手太阳之会。主治:头痛,耳鸣,牙关拘急,口㖞等。操作:斜刺0.2～0.5 寸;可灸。

Name of an point. It belongs to San jiao Meridian of Hand-Shaoyang. It is also the crossing point of Hand-Shaoyang, Foot-Shaoyang and Hand-Taiyang Meridians. Indications:Headache, tinnitus, lockjaw, deviation of the mouth, etc. Method: Puncture obliquely 0.2-0.5 cun. Moxibustion is applicable.

核骨 walnut-like bone

第一跖趾关节内侧部呈核状突起处。

Nodular process on the medial aspect of the first metatarsophalangeal joint.

颌 He;jaw

①耳穴名。在耳垂 3 区的中央。主治:牙痛,颞颌关节紊乱症等。②下颌角的体表部位。

①Name of an ear point. It is in the center of the 3rd section of the earlobe. Indications:Toothache, disorders of temporomandibular joint, etc. ②Corresponding to the region of the submandibular angle.

鹤顶 Heding(EX-LE2)

经外奇穴名。在髌骨上缘中点凹陷处。主治:膝痛,足胫无力,瘫痪等。操作:直刺1～1.5 寸;可灸。

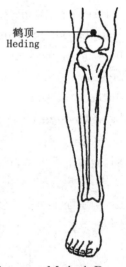

Name of an extra point. It is in the depression of the midpoint of the superior patellar border. Indications:Knee pain, weakness of foot and leg, paralysis, etc. Method:Puncture perpendicularly 1-1.5 cun. Moxibustion is applicable.

鹤膝风 crane-knee arthrosis

以膝关节肿大疼痛、股胫肌肉消瘦为特征的一种疾病。多由三阴亏损、风邪外袭、阴寒凝滞而成。治宜疏通经络、祛邪止痛。取穴:足三里、犊鼻、梁丘、阳陵泉、膝阳关。

Arthritis of the knee joint characterized by local swelling and pain with muscular emaciation of the thigh and leg; caused by the consumption of three yin and the attack of wind-evil leading to the stagnation of yin-cold. Treatment principle: Dredge the meridians and collaterals and eliminate the pathogenic factors to alleviate pain. Point selection: Zusanli (ST36), Dubi (ST35), Liangqiu (ST34), Yanglingquan (GB34), Xiyangguan (GB33).

横刺 horizontal puncture

使针身与皮肤表面成 15°～25°角刺入。适用于皮肉浅薄处的穴位或透刺。

Inserting the needle horizontally or along the skin to form an angle of 15°-25°. It is often used in the areas where the muscles is thin or used for piercing through the skin.

横骨 Henggu (KI11)

经穴名。属足少阴肾经。定位:在下腹部,当脐中下 5 寸,前正中线旁开 0.5 寸。主治:少腹胀痛,小便不利,遗尿,遗精,阳痿,阴痛等。操作:直刺 1～1.5 寸;可灸。

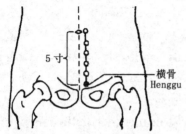

Name of an acupoint. It belongs to the Kidney Meridian of Foot-Shaoyin. Location: On the lower abdomen, 5 cun below the center of the umbilicus and 0.5 cun lateral to the anterior midline. Indications: Fullness and pain of the lateral lower abdomen, dysuria, enuresis, nocturnal emission, impotence, vaginal pain, etc. Method: Puncture perpendicularly about 1-1.5 cun. Moxibustion is applicable.

横纹 transverse crease

皮肤上的皱纹,可以作为取穴的体表标志。

The creases on the skin which are often used as landmarks for locating points.

横指寸 transverse finger cun

同身寸的一种,又名"一夫法",即患者将示指、中指、环指、小指并拢,以中指中节背侧横纹处为准,四指横为 3 寸。

A kind of proportional unit of body, also named "4-finger-breadth measurement", i.e., close the four fingers (index, middle, ring and little finger) together, the width of them at the level of the dorsal transverse crease of the middle segment of the middle finger is taken as 3 cun.

洪脉 surging pulse

脉象名。脉体宽大,充实有力,滔滔满指,如波涛汹涌,来盛去衰。以轻取即得,按之势不减为特点。多见于里热炽盛的病症。

A pulse condition with a large volume that feels full and forceful, like dashing waves coming vigorously and going gently. It is palpable on gentle pressure, remaining forceful on pressing, usually indicating interior excessive heat syndrome.

后顶 Houding (GV19)

经穴名。属督脉。定位：在头部，当后发际正中之上 5.5 寸。主治：头痛眩晕，癫狂，痫证。操作：平刺 0.5～0.8 寸；可灸。

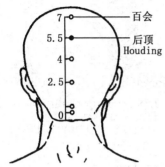

Name of an acupoint. It blongs to the Governor Vessel. Location：On the head, 5.5 cun directly above the midpoint of the posterior hairline. Indications：Headache, vertigo, mania, epilepsy, etc. Method：Puncture horizontally 0.5-0.8 cun. Moxibustion is applicable.

后发际 Houfaji

经外奇穴名。位于后发际正中。灸治鼻衄。

Name of an extra point. Located at the midpoint of the posterior hairline. Moxibustion is used to cure epistaxis.

后关 Houguan

听会穴别名。

The other name of Tinghui (GB2).

后曲 Houqu

瞳子髎穴别名。

The other name of Tongziliao (GB1).

后溪 Houxi(SI3)

经穴名。属手太阳小肠经，本经输穴，八脉交会穴之一，通于督脉。定位：在手掌尺侧，微握拳，当小指本节后的远侧掌

横纹头赤白肉际。主治：头痛，项强，耳鸣耳聋，咽喉肿痛，癫狂，疟疾，急性腰扭伤，盗汗，热病，手指、肘肩挛痛等。操作：直刺 0.5～1 寸；可灸。

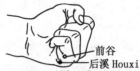

The acupoint, Shu-Stream point, belongs to the Small Intestine Meridian of Hand-Taiyang. One of the eight confluence points, communicate with the Governor Vessel. Location：On the dorsoventral boundary of the hand, along the ulnar border of the hand, at the ulnar end of the distal palmar crease, proximal to the 5th metacarpophalangeal joint when a hollow fist is made. Indications：Headache, rigidity of neck, tinnitus, deafness, sore throat, mania, malaria, acute lumbar sprain, night sweating, febrile diseases, contracture and numbness of fingers, pain in shoulder and elbow, etc. Method：Puncture perpendicularly 0.5-1 cun. Moxibustion is applicable.

后阴 houyin

指肛门，与前阴（外生殖器）相对。

The anus, as contrasted with qianyin (the external genital organ).

候气 waiting for qi

针刺入穴位后，采用一定的方法来促使得气的过程。

After the needle is inserted into the point, use certain methods to induce the arrival of qi.

候时 waiting for the proper time

《黄帝内经》刺法理论。即针灸需结合日月天时的运行,为子午流注法所本。

Theory of acupuncture manipulations stated in *Huangdi's Canon of Medicine*, i. e., the acupuncture must be performed in accordance with the time of the solar and lunar movements, on which the midnight-noon and ebb-flow point selection based.

呼吸补泻 reinforcing-reducing method by respiration

患者吸气时进针,呼气时出针属"泻"法;呼气时进针,吸气时出针属"补"法。

When the needle is inserted as the patient inhales and withdrawn as the patient exhales, it is "reinforcing". When the needle is inserted as the patient exhales and withdrawn as the patient inhales, it is "reducing".

虎口 Hukou

①合谷穴别名。②经外奇穴名。位于合谷穴前方赤白肉际处。灸刺治疗头痛、眩晕、失眠、牙痛、扁桃体炎等。

① The other name of Hegu(LI4). ②Name of an extra point. Located at the thenar just in front of Hegu(LI4). Acupuncture or moxibustion is adopted to cure headache, dizziness, insomnia, toothache, tonsillitis, etc.

华盖 Huagai (CV20)

经穴名。属任脉。定位:在胸部,前正中线上,平第一肋间。主治:咳嗽,气喘,胸胁胀痛等。

Name of an acupoint. It belongs to the Conception Vessel. Location: On the

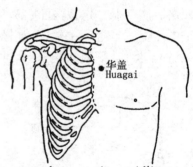

chest, on the anterior midline and the level of the 1st intercostal space. Indications: Cough, asthma, distending pain in the chest and hypochondrium, etc.

华佗 Hua Tuo

东汉末年杰出的医学家。倡导用体育疗法,创编五禽戏,尤以应用麻醉药物进行腹部手术而闻名。

An outstanding medical scientist in the last years of the Eastern Han Dynasty, the first exponent of sports therapy who introduced the Frolics of Five Animals for physical training. His fame rests mainly on his using of anesthetics and success in performing abdominal operations.

华佗夹脊穴 Hua Tuo jiaji points

在脊柱区,第一胸椎至第五腰椎棘突下两侧,后正中线旁开0.5寸,一侧17穴,共34穴。

A group of 34 points on both sides of the spinal column, 0.5 cun lateral to the lower border of each spinous process from the 1st thoracic vertebra to the 5th lumbar vertebra.

滑精 spermatorrhea

指无梦而遗精者,甚至清醒时精液流出

者。多因肾元亏损，精关不固所致，少数则因下焦湿热而引起。治宜补益精气、固涩精关。取穴：气海、三阴交、志室、肾俞。

Involuntary and frequent discharge of semen without dream or even at awaking state, mostly caused by the inability to control ejaculation resulting from the consumption of primordial energy of the kidney, or by the attack of damp-heat evil to the lower jiao in a few cases. Treatment principle: Tonify the kidney-qi so as to control the gate of essence. Point selection: Qihai(CV6), Sanyinjiao(SP6), Zhishi(BL52), Shenshu(BL23).

滑脉 slippery pulse

脉搏流利、指感圆滑的一种脉象。一般主痰饮、食滞。滑数无力者则属虚热。

A kind of pulse condition with fluent and smooth pulsation, indicates phlegm retention and indigestion. Slippery rapid weak pulse suggests asthenia heat syndrome.

滑肉门 Huaroumen (ST24)

经穴名。属足阳明胃经。定位：在上腹部，当脐上 1 寸，距前正中线 2 寸。主治：胃痛，呕吐，癫狂等。操作：直刺 1～1.5 寸；可灸。

Name of an acupoint. It belongs to the Stomach Meridian of Foot-Yangming. Location: On the upper abdomen, 1 cun above the center of the umbilicus and 2 cun lateral to the anterior midline. Indications: Gastric pain, vomiting, mania, etc. Method: Puncture perpendicularly 1-1.5 cun. Moxibustion is applicable.

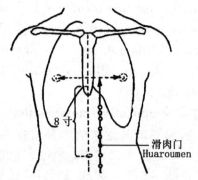

滑寿 Hua Shou

元代著名医家，撰有《十四经发挥》等书。

A distinguished physician of the Yuan Dynasty, the author of *Elucidation of the Fourteen Meridians*.

滑胎 habitual abortion

指连续发生 3 次以上的自然流产者，即习惯性流产。多因气虚、肾虚、血热、外伤等所致。

The spontaneous expulsion of a nonviable fetus on three or more consecutive occasions, mostly due to qi deficiency, kidney deficiency, blood-heat, external injury, etc.

滑泄 lingering diarrhea

以泄泻不禁，常伴有四肢厥冷或肿胀、形寒气短、消瘦等为主要临床表现的一种病症。多因久泻气陷下脱所致。治宜健脾益气、升阳止泻。取穴：中脘、章门、胃俞、脾俞、足三里。

Diarrhea with involuntary control of fecal discharge; often accompanied with edema or coldness of limbs, chills, shortness of breath and emaciation; usually due to collapse of qi resulting from chronic diarrhea. Treatment principle:

Strengthen the spleen and replenish qi，elevate the yang to arrest diarrhea. Point selection：Zhongwan（CV12），Zhangmen（LR13），Weishu（BL21），Pishu（BL20），Zusanli（ST36）.

化脓灸 suppurative moxibustion

引起局部皮肤化脓的一种直接灸法。将艾炷直接置于穴位上，灸至皮肤起疱，继而化脓。适用于哮喘、肺结核、瘰疬等慢性疾病。

A kind of direct moxibustion method by burning a moxa cone directly on the acupoint to produce local vesiculation and then suppuration；applicable to chronic diseases such as asthma, pulmonary tuberculosis, scrofula, etc.

化痰开窍 dissipating phlegm for resuscitation

又称豁痰醒脑，是治疗因痰浊之邪阻闭心窍致神志昏迷的方法。临床上常分为清热化痰开窍和逐寒开窍两种。

It has the same meaning with "eliminate phlegm for arousing the brain". It is a treatment for coma due to phlegm-evil blocking the heart orifice, clinically applied for the purpose of waking up the patient from unconsciousness either by clearing away the heat-evil and dissipating phlegm or by dispelling the cold-evil.

踝 Huai

耳穴名。在跟、膝穴之间。主治踝扭伤及相应部位的疼痛。

Name of an ear point. Location：Between Gen and Xi. It is used for treating ankle sprain and pain in the affected area.

环谷 huangu

即脐中。

The center of the umbilicus.

环跳 Huantiao（GB30）

穴位名。属足少阳胆经。定位：侧卧屈股，当股骨大转子最高点与骶管裂孔连线的外 1/3 与内 2/3 交点处。主治：腰腿痛，下肢痿痹，半身不遂等。操作：直刺 2～3 寸；可灸。

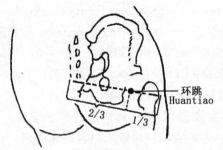

Name of an acupoint. It belongs to the Gallbladder Meridian of Foot-Shaoyang. Location：On the lateral side of the junction of the lateral one third and medial two thirds of the line connecting the prominence of the greater trochanter of femur and the sacral hiatus when the patient is in a lateral recumbent position with the thigh flexed. Indications：Pain of the lumbar and thigh, muscular atrophy of the lower limbs, hemiplegia, etc. Method：Puncture perpendicularly 2-3 cun. Moxibustion is applicable.

环中 Huanzhong

经外奇穴名。在环跳与腰俞穴连线的中点。主治腰腿痛。

Name of an extra point. It is on the midpoint of the line between Huantiao

(GB30) and Yaoshu(GV2). It is used for treating lumbar and thigh pain.

缓脉 moderate pulse

脉率正常,来去和缓的一种脉象。若和缓、均匀,则为正常脉象;缓而无力、弛缓,常见于湿邪致病和脾胃虚弱。

A pulse condition characterized by coming and going gently with normal rate. Pulse beating gently and regularly is considered as normal, while pulse with weak and slow beats indicates the syndrome caused by dampness-evil and the deficiency of spleen and stomach.

缓则治本 relieving the primary symptom in a chronic disease

在病情较轻、病势和缓的情况下,应针对疾病的根本原因进行治疗。

A principle of treatment applied when the disease is neither acute nor severe and temporary secondary symptom has been relieved.

患门 Huanmen

经外奇穴名。位于第五胸椎棘突旁开1.5寸处。主治:五劳七伤,面黄肌瘦,饮食无味,困倦乏力,咳嗽痰喘,盗汗遗精,胸背引痛等。宜施灸治。

Name of an extra point. Located 1.5 cun lateral to the process of the 5th thoracic vertebra. Moxibustion is adopted to cure the five kinds of overdoings and seven kinds of injury, yellow face and emaciation, short appetite, over fatigue, cough and asthma with phlegm, nocturnal sweating and emission, thoracic and back pains, etc.

肓门 Huangmen(BL51)

经穴名。属足太阳膀胱经。定位:在第一腰椎棘突下,后正中线旁开3寸。主治:腹痛,便秘,痞块等。操作:斜刺0.5～0.8寸;可灸。

Name of an acupoint. It belongs to the Bladder Meridian of Foot-Taiyang. Location: On the lower back, below the spi-

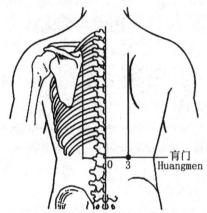

nous process of the 1st lumbar vertebra, 3 cun lateral to the posterior midline. Indications: Abdominal pain, constipation, abdominal mass, etc. Method: Puncture obliquely 0.5-0.8 cun. Moxibustion is applicable.

肓募 Huangmu

经外奇穴名。以乳头至脐距离的一半,从乳头直下度量,终点为穴。灸治腹中积块、疼痛,黄疸,虚弱等。

Name of an extra point. Located at the end of the line equal to half of the distance between the nipple and the navel, and the line start from the nipple directly go downwards. Moxibustion is used to cure abdominal mass and pain, jaundice, weakness, etc.

肓俞 Huangshu(KI16)

经穴名。属足少阴肾经。定位：在中腹部,当脐中旁开 0.5 寸。主治：腹痛、腹胀,呕吐,便秘,泄泻等。操作：直刺 1～1.5 寸;可灸。

Name of an acupoint. It belongs to the Kidney Meridian of Foot-Shaoyin. Location: On the middle abdomen, 0. 5 cun

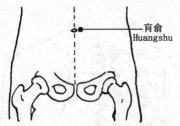

肓俞
Huangshu

lateral to the center of the umbilicus. Indications: Abdominal pain and distension, vomiting, constipation, diarrhea, etc. Method: Puncture perpendicularly 1-1. 5 cun. Moxibustion is applicable.

皇甫谧 Huangfu Mi

晋代文学家、医学家。编有《针灸甲乙经》,对古代针灸知识系统化做出了贡献。

A literati and physician of Jin Dynasty, the author of the book *A-B Classic of Acupuncture and Moxibustion*. He made contribution to the systematization of the knowledge of acupuncture.

黄疸 jaundice

以身黄、目黄、小便黄为主症的疾病。一般分为阴黄和阳黄两大类。治宜清热除湿、疏肝利胆。取穴：至阳、腕骨、阳陵泉、太冲。

A disease characterized by yellow appearance of skin, sclerae and urine, classified into two types, i. e. , yang jaundice and yin jaundice. Treatment principle: Clear heat, eliminate dampness and smooth the liver and gallbladder. Point selection: Zhiyang(GV9), Wangu(SI4), Yanglingquan(GB34), Taichong(LR3).

《黄帝内经》 *Huangdi's Canon of Medicine*

简称《内经》,中国现存最早的医学著作,成书于战国时期,作者不详。其内容包括《素问》《灵枢》两部分。前者主要为医学理论,后者主要论述针灸等理论。

Canon of Medicine for short, the earliest medical classic extant in China, which appeared in the Warring States Period with the authorship unknown. It consists of two parts: *Plain Questions* and *Miraculous Pivot*. The former deals mainly with basic theories of medicine, while the latter acupuncture.

黄苔 yellowish fur

舌苔呈黄色。一般是里热证的表现。其厚薄、干湿度及颜色的深浅反映不同的病理变化。如微黄薄苔,常为外感风热之邪。

A sign generally indicates interior heat syndrome. Different pathological changes are indicated and vary with the thickness and moisture of the fur, and the degree of its colouration, e. g. , a thin, light yellowish fur usually suggests an exposure to wind-heat evil.

灰苔 greyish fur

舌苔色灰白。若灰白而滑润,为三阴寒证;若灰黄而干燥,为里热实证。

The tongue coating is grayish white. A

grey and moist fur on the tongue signifies cold syndrome of three yin; while a grey yellowish and dry fur signifies sthenia heat syndrome of the interior.

恢刺 relaxing puncture

十二刺法之一。用于治疗筋痹（肌肉痉挛、疼痛等）。方法是将针直刺在病痛部位的一侧，并上下、前后、左右摇动针体，以促使肌肉弛缓。

One of the twelve needling techniques for treating muscle aching and spasm, etc. It is to puncture one side of the painful muscle, and shake the needle upward and downward, anteriorly and posteriorly, right and left to relax the muscle.

回肠 ileum

指小肠下段，上接空肠，下连大肠。

The distal portion of the small intestine, extending from the jejunum to the cecum.

回发五处 Huifawuchu

经外奇穴名。即当头顶旋毛正中及其前后左右共5穴。灸治头风眩晕。

Name of extra points. Located at the center of the hair whorl on the head and four others at the anterior, posterior, left and right around the center. Moxibustion can be used to treat recurrent headache, dizziness and vertigo.

回气 Huiqi

经外奇穴名。位于骶骨尖端。灸治大便失禁、便血、痔疮等。

Name of an extra point. Located at the sacral tip. Moxibustion is used to cure fecal incontinence, bloody stool and hemorrhoids, etc.

回旋灸 circling moxibustion

指将点燃的艾条对着穴位处反复回旋移动施灸的一种灸法。

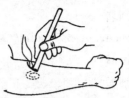

Administering the ignited moxa stick in a circular movement over the point.

回阳九针穴 nine emergency points

指具有回阳救逆作用的九个急救穴，即哑门、劳宫、三阴交、涌泉、太溪、中脘、环跳、足三里、合谷。临床用于阳虚欲脱之晕厥肢冷、口噤不开、不能言语等症。

The nine emergency points which are used to revive yang and recover conscious are Yamen (GV15), Laogong (PC8), San-yinjiao (SP6), Yongquan (KI1), Taixi (KI3), Zhongwan (CV12), Huantiao (GB30), Zusanli (ST36) and Hegu (LI4). These points are clinically used to cure syncope and cold extremities, trismus, aphasia, etc.

回阳救逆 restoring yang from collapse

将温肾祛寒药与益气固脱药合用治疗阳气衰微将脱、阴寒内盛的方法。此法适用于汗出不止、四肢厥冷、呼吸衰弱、脉微欲绝等症。

A treatment for exhaustion of yang-qi and over abundance of yin-cold in the interior by using both herb warming kidney and expelling cold-evil and those supplementing qi and relieving collapse, this therapy is applicable to cases manifested as profuse perspiration, cold limbs, faint respiration and impalpable pulse, etc.

会额 Huie

脑户穴别名。

The other name of Naohu(GV17).

会维 Huiwei

地仓穴别名。

The other name of Dicang(ST4).

会穴 hui(meeting) points

①两条或两条以上经脉相交会的部位。②八会穴的简称。

①The site where two or more meridians converse;②An abbreviation for the eight influential points.

会厌 epiglottis

七冲门之一。呼吸时会厌开启,吞咽或呕吐时则关闭,中医认为会厌是声音之户。

One of the seven important openings. It opens during respiration and closes during swallowing and vomiting. It is considered as the aperture of voice.

会阳 Huiyang (BL35)

经穴名。属足太阳膀胱经。定位:在骶部,尾骨端旁开 0.5 寸。主治:痢疾,便血,泄泻,痔疾,阳痿,白带等。操作:直刺 1~1.5 寸;可灸。

Name of an acupoint. It belongs to of the Bladder Meridian of Foot-Taiyang. Location:On the sacrum, 0.5 cun lateral to the tip of the coccyx. Indications:Dysentery, bloody stools, diarrhea, hemorrhoids, impotence, leukorrhea disease, etc. Method:Puncture perpendicularly 1-1.5 cun. Moxibustion is applicable.

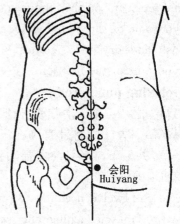

会阴 Huiyin (CV1)

经穴名。属任脉。定位:在会阴部,男性当阴囊根部与肛门连线的中点,女性当大阴唇后联合与肛门连线的中点。主治:阴道炎,小便不利,痔疾,遗精,遗尿,月经不调,癫狂等。操作:直刺 0.5~1 寸,可灸。

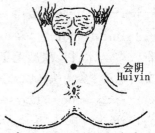

Name of an acupoint. It belongs to of the Conception Vessel. Location:On the perineum, at the midpoint between the root of the scrotum and anus in men and between the posterior commissure of the large labia and anus in women. Indications:Vaginitis, retention of urine, hemorrhoids, nocturnal emission, enuresis, irregular menstruation, mental disorder, etc. Method:Puncture perpendicularly 0.5-1 cun. Moxibustion is applicable.

会原 Huiyuan

冲阳穴别名。

The other name of Chongyang(ST42).

会宗 Huizong (TE7)

经穴名。属手少阳三焦经,本经郄穴。定位:在前臂背侧,当腕背横纹上3寸,支沟尺侧尺骨的桡侧缘,距离支沟一指宽。主治:耳聋,耳痛,痫证,臂痛等。操作:直刺0.5~1寸;可灸。

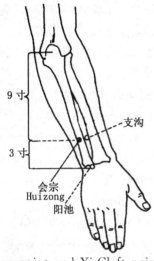

9寸

支沟

3寸

会宗
Huizong
阳池

The acupoint and Xi-Cleft point of the Sanjiao Meridian of Hand-Shaoyang. Location:On the dorsal side of the forearm, 3 cun above the transverse crease of the dorsum of the wrist, at the level of Zhigou(TE6), about one finger breadth away from Zhigou(TE6), on the radial side of the ulna. Indications:Deafness, earache, epilepsy, pain of the arm, etc. Method:Puncture perpendicularly 0. 5-1 cun. Moxibustion is applicable.

昏厥 syncope

指突然仆倒、四肢厥冷、短暂的意识丧失状态。治宜泻热救阴、平肝熄风。取穴:风府、大椎、曲池、涌泉、太冲、十二井穴。

Temporary loss of consciousness accompany with cold extremities after a sudden fall. Treatment principle:Purge heat to rescue yin, calm liver to stop wind. Point selection:Fengfu(GV16), Dazhui(GV14), Quchi(LI11), Yongquan(KI1), Taichong(LR3) and the twelve Jing-Well points.

昏聩 mental confusion

指神识昏乱、不明事理的症状。治宜醒脑开窍。取穴:水沟、十二井穴、太冲、丰隆、劳宫。

A state of mental derangement and confused mind. Treatment principle:Activate the brain and regain consciousness. Point selection:Shuigou (GV26), the twelve Jing-Well points,Taichong (LR3), Fenglong (ST40), Laogong (PC8).

昏迷 coma

指各种原因引起的重度意识丧失,患者对任何刺激均不反应。多为邪阻清窍,神明被蒙所致。治宜熄风开窍、清心豁痰。取穴:水沟、十二井穴、太冲、丰隆、劳宫。

A state of severe unconsciousness from which the patient cannot be wakened, even by powerful stimulation; caused by the attack of evils to the upper orifices resulting in deterioration of the mind. Treatment principle:Calm the endopathic wind and regain consciousness, remove heat from the heart and eliminate phlegm. Point selection:Shuigou (CV26), the twelve Jing-Well points, Taichong (LR3), Fenglong (ST40), Laogong (PC8).

昏睡 lethargic sleep

指沉睡,可以唤醒,但一般不能准确回答问题的一种意识障碍。通常是病情危重的反映。治则同"昏瞆"。

A critical condition manifested as partial consciousness with a lethargic condition which can be wakened but the patient is unable to answer questions accurately. Treatment principle: Same to "mental confusion".

魂门 Hunmen (BL47)

经穴名。属足太阳膀胱经。定位:在背部,第九胸椎棘突下,旁开3寸。主治:胸胁疼痛,背痛,呕吐,泄泻等。操作:直刺0.5～0.8寸;可灸。

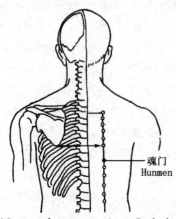

魂门
Hunmen

Name of an acupoint. It belongs to the Bladder Meridian of Foot-Taiyang. Location: On the back, below the spinous process of the 9th thoracic vertebra, 3 cun lateral to the posterior midline. Indications: Pain in the chest and hypochondriac region, back pain, vomiting, diarrhea, etc. Method: Puncture perpendicularly 0.5-0.8 cun. Moxibustion is appli-

cable.

魂舍 Hunshe

奇穴名。位于脐两边各1寸处。直刺或灸治泻痢。

Name of extra points. Located 1 cun lateral to the navel, perpendicular acupuncture or moxibustion is used to cure diarrhea and dysentery.

火 fire

①六淫之一,温热、暑热均属火邪。其性属阳,致病时表现为热证、功能亢进。②五行之一。指一类阳性、热性的事物或亢进的状态。③生理性的火,为阳气所化,生命的动力,如命门之火等。

①One of the six evils which is yang in nature, including the warm-heat and summer-heat evils, and may cause heat syndrome and hyperactivity state. ②One of the five phases which represents the substances with yang and hot nature or the state of hyperactivity. ③Physiologically, referring to the motive force of life which is transformed from yang-qi, such as the fire of the life-gate.

火罐法 fire cupping method

拔罐法的一种,系利用点火燃烧法排出罐内空气,形成负压,以吸附在体表上。

One kind of cupping method refers to expelling the air in the jar by fire to form negative pressure, so the jar can be adsorbed onto the surface of the human body.

火针 fire needle

针刺疗法中用的一种金属针,长10～13 cm,针体粗圆,针尖锐利,针柄用角质或竹木包裹，用时先将针尖烧红再入针。

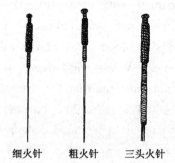

细火针　　粗火针　　三头火针

A metallic needle used for acupuncture therapy，10-13 cm in length，with round body and sharp tip. The handle of the needle is made of horn or bamboo，and the tip needs to burnt to red before inserted into the skin.

火针疗法 fire needle acupuncture

古代针刺法，指将针烧红迅速刺入病痛部位并迅速拔出的针刺法。此法多用于治疗某些外科疾病及风湿性关节炎。

An ancient acupuncture technique refers to inserting a red-hot needle into the affected area and withdraw it swiftly. It is mainly used in treating some external diseases and rheumatic arthritis.

活血化瘀 activating blood circulation to dissipate blood stasis

畅旺血流、消散瘀滞的一种治疗方法。适用于血液瘀滞所致的瘀血证。

A treatment for promoting blood circulation and accelerating the absorption of extravasated blood，applicable to the blood-stasis syndrome.

机关 Jiguan

颊车穴别名。

The other name of Jiache(ST6).

肌腠 muscular striae

即肌肉的纹理。肌肉的组织间隙以及其中的结缔组织。

The spaces and the connective tissues between the strips of muscles.

肌肉不仁 numbness

指肌肉麻木，不知痛痒冷热，常见于痿痹、中风、麻风等病。治宜通经活络、补脾益气。取穴：合谷、足三里、肾俞、气海、三阴交。

Lack or diminution of sensation of the skin, commonly seen in case of flaccidity syndrome, apoplexy and leprosy, etc. Treatment principle: Clear and activate the meridians and collaterals, invigorate the spleen and replenish qi. Point selection: Hegu(LI4), Zusanli(ST36), Shenshu(BL23), Qihai(CV6), Sanyinjiao(SP6).

积聚 abdominal mass

指腹内结块，或胀或痛的病患。结块固定不移，痛有定处，病在血分者，为积证；积块时聚时散，痛无定处，病在气分者，为聚证。因情志郁结、饮食所伤、寒邪外袭、肝脾受损、气机阻滞、瘀血或痰湿内停所致。治宜疏肝理气、活血化瘀。取穴：气海、太冲、三阴交、阳陵泉、血海、足三里、关元。

Formation of mass in the abdomen accompanied with distention or pain. Fixed mass and pain indicates that the disease is in blood phase and is called Ji syndrome. Wandering mass without fixed pain indicates that the disease is in qi phase and is called Ju syndrome. It is mostly caused by emotional depression, impairment by improper diet, invasion of exopathogenic cold, impairment of the liver and spleen, obstruction of qi movement, blood stasis or phlegm retention. Treatment principle: Relieve the depressed liver and regulate the flow of qi, promote blood circulation to remove blood stasis. Point selection: Qihai (CV6), Taichong (LR3), Sanyinjiao (SP6), Yanglingquan (GB34), Xuehai (SP10), Zusanli (ST36), Guanyuan (CV4).

箕门 Jimen(SP11)

经穴名。属足太阴脾经。定位：在大腿内侧，当血海与冲门连线上，血海上6寸。主治：小便不通，遗溺，腹股沟肿痛等。操作：直刺1～1.5寸；可灸。

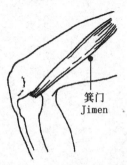

箕门
Jimen

Name of an acupoint. It belongs to the Spleen Meridian of Foot-Taiyin. Location: On the inner thigh and on the line connecting Xuehai(SP10) and Chongmen(SP12), 6 cun above Xuehai (SP10). Indications：Dysuria, enuresis, pain and swelling in the inguinal region, etc. Method：Puncture perpendicularly 1-1.5 cun. Moxibustion is applicable.

极泉 Jiquan(HT1)

经穴名。属手少阴心经。定位：在腋窝顶点,腋动脉搏动处。主治：胸胁疼痛,瘰疬,肘臂冷痛,咽干等。操作：直刺 0.3～0.5 寸。

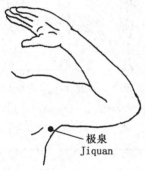

极泉
Jiquan

Name of an acupoint. It belongs to the Heart Meridian of Hand-Shaoyin. Location：At the apex of the axillary fossa, where the pulsation of the axillary artery is palpable. Indications：Pain in the chest and hypochondrium, scrofula, cold pain of the elbow and arm, dryness of the throat, etc. Method：Puncture perpendicularly 0.3-0.5 cun.

急惊风 acute infantile convulsion

多因邪热炽盛、热极生风所致。发病急,突然高热烦躁、牙关紧闭、气促痰壅,继而四肢抽搐,神志昏迷,头项强硬,甚则角弓反张。治宜清热驱邪、开窍熄风。取穴：大椎、合谷、太冲、阳陵泉、十二井穴。

A disease caused by the hyperactivity of pathogenic heat leading to the production of wind-evil; characterized by sudden onset of high fever, irritability, lockjaw, dys-pnea, abundant sputum, and followed by convulsion, coma, stiff neck, or even opisthotonos. Treatment principle：Clear heat and eliminate evils, cause resuscitation and calm the endopathic wind. Point selection：Dazhui (GV14), Hegu (LI4), Taichong (LR3), Yanglingquan(GB34), the twelve Jing-Well points.

急脉 Jimai(LR12)

经穴名。属足厥阴肝经。定位：在耻骨结节的外侧,当气冲下方,腹股沟股动脉搏动处,前正中线旁开 2.5 寸。主治：少腹痛,疝气,外阴痛等。操作：直刺 0.5～1 寸;可灸。

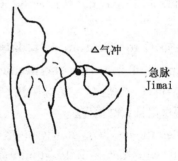

△气冲

急脉
Jimai

'Name of an acupoint. It belongs to the Liver Meridian of Foot-Jueyin. Location：Lateral to pubic tubercle, inferior to Qichong (ST30), in the inguinal groove where the pulsation of the femoral artery is palpable, 2.5 cun lateral to the anterior midline. Indications：Lower abdominal pain, hernia, pain in the external genitalia, etc. Method：Puncture perpendicularly 0. 5-1 cun. Moxibustion is applicable.

急者治标 relieving the secondary symptom in an acute case

在临床上，有的症状虽属于标证，但由于它起病急、发展快，给患者造成痛苦甚至危险，应先予治疗。

A principle of treatment applied when the secondary symptom occurs abruptly with a rapid progress and is harmful to the patient.

疾而徐则虚 fast insertion and slow withdrawal to reduce

针刺泻法要领。意为迅速进针、缓慢出针则可泻邪气，与"徐而疾则实"相对。

An important principle of reducing acupuncture, i. e. , the fast insertion and slow withdrawal of the needle will expel the evils, as contrasted with the principle of "slow insertion and fast withdrawal to reinforce."

疾徐补泻 tonification or sedation by the speed of inserting the needle

缓慢进针，疾速出针，属"补"法；疾速进针，缓慢出针，属"泻"法。

When the needle is slowly inserted and swiftly withdrawn, it is "tonification". When the needle is swiftly inserted and slowly withdrawn, it is "sedation".

脊 spine

即脊椎骨。共 21 节：胸椎 12 节，腰椎 5 节，骶椎 4 节。

Vertebrae in traditional Chinese medicine, twenty one in total (12 thoracic vertebrae, 5 lumbar vertebrae, and 4 sacral vertebrae).

脊中 Jizhong(GV6)

经穴名。属督脉。定位：在背部，后正中线上，第十一胸椎棘突下凹陷中。主治：腹痛，泄泻，黄疸，癫痫，背脊痛等。操作：稍向上斜刺 0.5～1 寸；可灸。

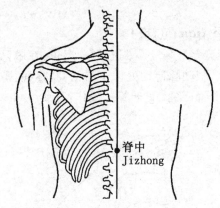

脊中
Jizhong

Name of an acupoint. It belongs to the Governor Vessel. Location：On the back and on the posterior midline, in the depression below the spinous process of the 11th thoracic vertebra. Indications：Abdominal pain, diarrhea, jaundice, epilepsy, stiffness and pain of the back, etc. Method：Puncture obliquely upward 0. 5-1 cun. Moxibustion is applicable.

脊椎 vertebral column

椎骨的总称。成年人的椎骨一般包括颈椎 7 块、胸椎 12 块、腰椎 5 块、骶椎 1 块、尾椎 1 块，共 26 块。

The collective name of the spinal vertebra. In adult, there are seven in the neck, twelve in the thorax, five in the lumbar, 1 in the sacrum, and 1 in the coccyx, 26 vertebrae in all.

季胁 jixie

①季胁部。②章门穴别名。

① The hypochondrium. ② The other name of Zhangmen (LR13).

季胁痛 hypochondriac pain

多因肝虚所致。兼见胆怯善惊、视物模糊、耳鸣者,属肝气虚;兼见烦热口干、头眩眼花者,属肝血不足。治宜疏肝利胆、通络止痛。取穴:期门、支沟、阳陵泉、太冲、膈俞。

A symptom due to asthenia of liver; if accompanied with timidness, blurred vision and tinnitus, it is due to the deficiency of liver-qi; if accompanied by dysphoria with feverish sensation, dry mouth and dizziness, it is due to the insufficiency of liver-blood. Treatment principle:Sooth the liver and promote bile secretion, remove obstruction in the meridians and collaterals to relieve pain. Point selection:Qimen (LR14), Zhigou (TE6), Yanglingquan (GB34), Taichong (LR3), Geshu(BL17).

夹承浆 Jiachengjiang

经外奇穴名。在承浆穴旁1寸处。主治:口眼歪斜,面肌挛痛。

Name of an extra point. It is 1 cun lateral to Chengjiang (CV24). Indications: Deviation of eyes and mouth, spasm of facial muscle.

夹持进针法 gripping insertion

进针法之一。即用左手拇、示指夹住针身下段,露出针尖,对准穴位,右手持针柄,两手同时配合用力,将针快速刺入穴位的方法。适用于长针直刺。

One of the needle-inserting methods, i. e. , the lower part of the needle is

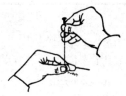

tightly gripped between the thumb and index finger of the left hand exposing the needle tip which aims at the acupoint, and the upper part of the needle is held by the right hand. The needle will be quickly inserted into the point by the combined force of the two hands. This method is often adopted in the perpendicular acupuncture with long needles.

夹脊 Jiaji (EX-B2)

经外奇穴名。在第一胸椎至第五腰椎各椎棘突下旁开0.5寸处。主治病症见下表。

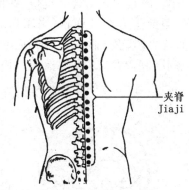

Name of extra points. They are 0. 5 cun lateral to the lower border of each spinous process from the first thoracic vertebra to the fifth lumbar vertebra. Indications are in the following table.

夹脊穴 Jiaji points		主治 Indications
T.	1 2 3	T1～T3　上肢疾患 diseases in the upper limbs
	4 5 6	T1～T8　胸部疾患 diseases in the chest region
	7 8	T6～L5　腹部疾患 diseases in the abdominal region
L.	1 2 3 4 5	L1～L5　下肢疾患 diseases in the lower limbs

颊车 Jiache(ST6)

经穴名。属足阳明胃经。定位:在面颊部,下颌角前上方约一横指,当咀嚼时咬肌隆起,按之凹陷处即是。主治:面瘫,齿痛,面颊肿,腮腺炎,口噤不语等。操作:直刺0.3～0.5寸,或向地仓穴斜刺0.5～1寸;可灸。

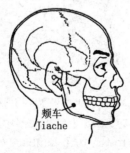

颊车
Jiache

Name of an acupoint. It belongs to the Stomach Meridian of Foot-Yangming. Location: On the cheek, one finger breadth anterior and superior to the mandibular angle, in the depression where the mas-seter muscle is prominent when chewing. Indications: Facial paralysis, toothache, swelling of the cheek and face, mumps, trismus, etc. Method: Puncture perpendicularly 0.3-0.5 cun, or obliquely 0.5-1 cun towards Dicang(ST4). Moxibustion is applicable.

甲根 Jiagen

经外奇穴名。位于蹞趾甲内、外根角处,共4穴。此穴针刺1分(0.1寸),主治疝气。

Name of extra points. Located at the medial and lateral corners of the big toe nail root, 4 points in all, acupuncture 0.1 cun to treat hernia.

肩 Jian;shoulder

①耳穴名。在肘、锁骨穴之间。主治肩部疼痛。②上臂和躯干连接的部位。

① Name of an ear point. Location: Midway between Zhou and Suogu. It is used for treating pain in shoulder region. ② The junction between the upper limb and the trunk.

肩背痛 pain of shoulder and back

肩背部疼痛。因劳伤,或风寒、风湿等外邪侵袭膀胱经或肺经所致。治宜调气活血、舒筋散寒。取穴:大椎、膈俞、风池、天柱、后溪、悬钟。

A condition due to overload, or attack of wind-cold evil or wind-damp evil to the Bladder Meridian or to the Lung Meridian. Treatment principle: Promote the flow of qi and blood circulation, relax muscles and dispel cold. Point selection: Dazhui(GV14), Geshu(BL17), Fengchi

(GB20)，Tianzhu(BL10)，Houxi(SI3)，Xuanzhong(GB39).

肩胛 scapula

①肩胛骨的部位。②即肩胛骨。

①Scapular region. ②Shoulder blade.

肩井 Jianjing (GB21)

经穴名。属足少阳胆经。定位：在肩上，乳头直上，当大椎与肩峰连线的中点上。主治：颈项强痛，肩胛背痛，手臂不举，乳汁少，乳痈，瘰疬，难产，中风。操作：直刺 0.5～0.8 寸，内有肺尖，不可深刺；可灸。

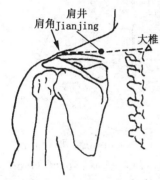

Name of an acupoint. It belongs to the Gallbladder Meridian of Foot-Shaoyang. Location：On the shouder, directly above the nipple, at the midpoint of the line connecting Dazhui(GV14) and the acromion. Indications：Pain and rigidity of the neck, pain in the shoulder and back, motor impairment of the arm, insufficient lactation, acute mastitis, scrofula, difficult labour, apoplexy, etc. Method：Puncture perpendicularly 0. 5-0. 8 cun. Deep puncture is prohibited, because the deeper area of the point is the apex of the lung. Moxibustion is applicable.

肩髎 Jianliao(TE14)

经穴名。属手少阳三焦经。定位：在肩部，肩髃后方，当臂外展时肩峰后下方呈现的凹陷处。主治：肩、上臂痛不能举等。操作：直刺 0.5～1 寸；可灸。

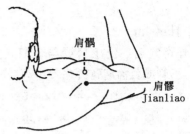

Name of an acupoint. It belongs to the Sanjiao Meridian of Hand-Shaoyang. Location：On the shouder, posterior to Jianyu(LI15), in the depression inferior and posterior to the acromion when the arm is abducted. Indications：Pain and motor impairment of the shoulder and upper arm, etc. Method：Puncture perpendicularly 0. 5-1 cun. Moxibustion is applicable.

肩内俞 Jianneishu

经外奇穴名。位于肩髃与云门穴连线中点下 1 寸。直刺或灸治肩臂疼痛不举等。

Name of an extra point. Located 1 cun below the midpoint of the line between Jianyu(LI15) and Yunmen(LU2). Perpendicular acupuncture or moxibustion is used to cure shoulder and arm pain and inability to raise hands, etc.

肩前 Jianqian

经外奇穴名。在腋前皱襞顶端与肩髃穴连线的中点。主治：肩臂痛，上肢瘫痪等。

Name of an extra point. Located at the

midpoint of the line connecting Jianyu (LI15) and the tip of the front axillary crease. Indications: Pain in the shoulder and arm, paralysis of the upper limbs, etc.

肩俞 Jianshu

经外奇穴名。位于肩髃与云门穴连线中点,直刺或灸治肩臂疼痛不举等。

Name of an extra point. Located at the midpoint of the line between Jianyu (LI15) and Yunmen(LU2). Perpendicular acupuncture or moxibustion is used to cure shoulder and arm pain and inability to raise hands, etc.

肩外俞 Jianwaishu(SI14)

经穴名。属手太阳小肠经。定位:在背部,当第一胸椎棘突下,旁开 3 寸。主治:肩背疼痛,颈项强急等。操作:斜刺 0.5～0.8 寸,不宜深刺,以免刺伤肺脏,引起气胸;可灸。

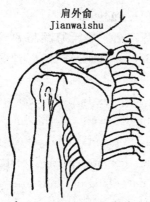

肩外俞
Jianwaishu

Name of an acupoint. It belongs to the Small Intestine Meridian of Hand-Tai-yang. Location: On the back, below the spinous process of the 1st thoracic vertebra, 3 cun lateral to the posterior midline. Indications: Pain of the shoulder and back, pain and rigidity of the neck, etc. Method: Puncture obliquely 0.5-0.8 cun. Avoid to puncture deeply, otherwise the lung may be injured and the pneumothorax may occur. Moxibustion is applicable.

肩髃 Jianyu(LI15)

经穴名。属手阳明大肠经。定位:在肩部,三角肌上,臂外展或向前平伸时,当肩峰前下方凹陷处。主治:肩臂挛痛不遂,瘾疹,瘰疬等。操作:直刺或向下斜刺 0.8～1.5 寸;可灸。

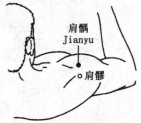

肩髃
Jianyu

肩髎

Name of an acupoint. It belongs to the Large Intestine Meridian of Hand-Yang-ming. Location: On the the deltoid muscle of the shoulder, in the depression anterior and inferior to the acromion when the arm is abducted or stretched forward. Indications: Pain in the shoulder and arm, motor impairment of the upper limbs, urticaria, scrofula, etc. Method: Puncture perpendicularly or obliquely downward 0.8-1.5 cun. Moxibustion is applicable.

肩贞 Jianzhen(SI9)

经穴名。属手太阳小肠经。定位:在肩关节后下方,臂内收时,腋后纹头上 1 寸。主治:肩胛痛,手臂不举等。操作:直刺0.5～1 寸,不宜向胸侧深刺;可灸。

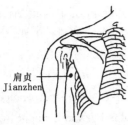

Name of an acupoint. It belongs to the Small Intestine Meridian of Hand-Taiyang. Location: Posterior and inferior to the shoulder joint, 1 cun above the posterior end of the axillary fold when the arm abducted. Indications: Pain in the scapular region, motor impairment of the arm, etc. Method: Puncture perpendicularly 0.5-1 cun. Avoid to puncture deeply towards the chest. Moxibustion is applicable.

肩中俞 Jianzhongshu(SI15)

经穴名。属手太阳小肠经。定位:在背部,当第七颈椎棘突下,后正中线旁开 2 寸。主治:咳嗽,气喘,咯血,肩背痛等。操作:直刺或斜刺 0.5～0.8 寸;可灸。

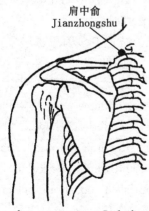

Name of an acupoint. It belongs to the Small Intestine Meridian of Hand-Taiyang. Location: On the back, below the spinous process of the 7th cervical vertebra, 2 cun lateral to the posterior midline. Indications: Cough, asthma, hemoptysis, pain in the shoulder and back, etc. Method: Puncture perpendicularly or obliquely 0.5-0.8 cun. Moxibustion is applicable.

间谷 Jiangu

二间穴别名。

The other name of Erjian(LI2).

间使 Jianshi(PC5)

经穴名。属手厥阴心包经,本经经穴。定位:在前臂掌侧,当曲泽与大陵的连线上,腕横纹上 3 寸,掌长肌腱与桡侧腕屈肌腱之间。主治:心痛,心悸,胃痛,呕吐,热病,烦躁,疟疾,癫、狂、痫,腋肿,肘臂挛痛等。操作:直刺 0.5～1 寸;可灸。

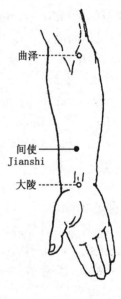

The acupoint and Jing-River point belongs to the Pericardium Meridian of Hand-Jueyin. Location: On the palmar side of the forearm, on the line connecting Quze(PC3) and Daling(PC7), 3 cun above the transverse crease of the wrist, between the tendons of palmaris longus and flexor carpi radialis. Indications: Cardiac pain, palpitation, stomachache, vomiting, febrile diseases, irritability, malaria, mental disorders, epilepsy, swelling of the axilla, contracture and pain of the elbow and arm, etc. Method: Puncture perpendicularly 0. 5-1 cun. Moxibustion is applicable.

兼证 associated symptom and sign

指疾病的伴发症状和体征,与主证相对而言,可作为诊断时的参考。

The symptoms and signs accompanying with the primary ones, serving as reference for diagnosis.

间接灸 indirect moxibustion

又称间隔灸。指将艾炷隔着一层东西(如姜片、蒜片、食盐、药饼等)进行灸治的方法。

Also called partition moxibustion. It refers to administer moxibustion with a burning moxa cone on a slice of ginger or garlic, a thick layer of salt, or a thin paste of herbs, etc. , over an acupoint.

建里 Jianli (CV11)

经穴名。属任脉。定位:在上腹部,前正中线上,当脐中上3寸。主治:胃痛,呕吐,腹胀,肠鸣,水肿等。操作:直刺0.8~1.2寸;可灸。

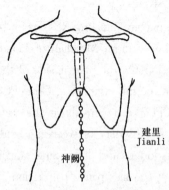

Name of an acupoint. It belongs to the Conception Vessel. Location: On the upper abdomen and on the anterior midline, 3 cun above the center of the umbilicus. Indications: Stomachache, vomiting, abdominal distension, borborygmus, edema, etc. Method: Puncture perpendicularly 0. 8-1. 2 cun. Moxibustion is applicable.

健脾疏肝 invigorating the spleen and soothing the liver

治疗肝气郁结引起的脾运化功能障碍的方法。常用于肝郁脾虚。症见两胁胀痛、不思饮食、腹胀肠鸣、大便稀薄、苔白腻、脉弦。

A treatment for the disturbance of digestive function of the spleen due to stagnation of liver-qi, applicable to the case with stagnation of liver-qi and spleen deficiengcy, manifested as distending pain over the hypochondrium, anorexia, abdominal distention, borborygmus, discharge of loose stools, whitish and greasy fur on the tongue, wiry pulse.

健忘 forgetfulness

指记忆力减退。多因思虑过度,心肾不足所致。治宜健脾补肾、益气养血。取穴:足三里、关元、心俞、百会、脾俞。

Decline of memory, usually dues to over anxiety and deficiency of the heart and kidney. Treatment principle: Strengthen the spleen and tonify the kidney, reforce qi and nourish blood. Point selection: Zusanli(ST36), Guanyuan(CV4), Xinshu(BL15), Baihui(GV20), Pishu(BL20).

降压沟 Jiangyagou

耳穴名。主治:高血压。

Name of an ear point. Indications: hypertension.

交叉取穴 selection of contralateral points

取穴方法之一。即：①左右交叉取穴。②左右上下双向交叉取穴。

One of the point-selecting methods，i. e.，①Left-right side symmetrical point selection. ② Symmetrical point selection in the two opposite directions of left-right side and upper-lower part.

交冲 Jiaochong

后顶穴别名。

The other name of Houding(GV19).

交感 Jiaogan

耳穴名。在对耳轮下脚的末端与耳轮内缘交界处。主治：内脏痛，心悸，盗汗，自主神经功能紊乱。

Name of an ear point. It is at the junction of the terminal of inferior antihelix crus and medial border of helix. Indications：Pain of internal organs，palpitation，night sweating，functional disorders of autonomous nerve system.

交会穴 crossing point

指两经或两条以上经脉所交会的腧穴，多分布在头面及躯干部。

The point where two or more meridians intersect，most of which are located on the face，head and trunk.

交经八穴 eight confluence points

即八脉交会穴，是奇经八脉与十二经脉相通的八个特定穴。

The eight crossing points of the eight extra meridians with the twelve regular meridians.

交信 Jiaoxin（KI8）

经穴名。属足少阴肾经，阴跷脉郄穴。定位：在小腿内侧，当太溪之上2寸，复溜前0.5寸，胫骨内侧缘的后方。主治：月经不调，痛经，尿血，阴挺，泄泻，便秘，睾丸肿痛等。操作：直刺0.5~1寸；可灸。

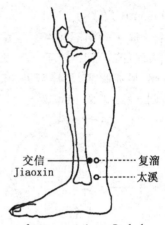

Name of an acupoint. It belongs to the Kidney Meridian of Foot-Shaoyin. It is the Xi-Cleft point of the Yin Heel Vessel. Location：On the medial side of the leg，2 cun above Taixi（KI3），and 0. 5 cun anterior to Fuliu(KI7)，poterior to the medial border of the tibia. Indications：Irregular menstruation，dysmenorrhea，urinating bleeding，prolapse of the uterus，diarrhea，constipation，pain and swelling of testis，etc. Method：Puncture perpendicularly 0. 5-1 cun. Moxibustion is applicable.

交仪 Jiaoyi

蠡沟穴别名。

The other name of Ligou(LR5).

椒饼灸 moxibustion on pepper paste

指隔着胡椒粉和水制成的药饼施灸的方法。

Moxibustion with a thin layer of herbal

cake made of pepper powder and water between skin and moxa cone.

角法 horn cupping

古代称拔罐疗法为角法。

In ancient China, the cupping therapy was called horn cupping.

角孙 Jiaosun(TE20)

经穴名。属手少阳三焦经。定位：在头部，折耳廓向前，当耳尖直上入发际处。主治：耳鸣，目赤肿痛，齿痛龈肿，痄腮等。操作：平刺 0.3～0.5 寸；可灸。

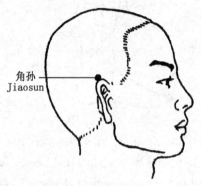

角孙 Jiaosun

Name of an acupoint. It belongs to the Sanjiao Meridian of Hand-Shaoyang. Location: On the head, above the ear apex when the auricle is folded, within the hairline. Indications: Tinnitus, redness, pain and swelling of the eyes, swelling of the gum, toothache, mumps, etc. Method: Puncture horizontally 0.3-0.5 cun. Moxibustion is applicable.

角窝上 Jiaowoshang

耳穴名。又称降压点。在三角窝前上方。主治高血压。

Name of an ear point, also known as Jiangyadian. It is anterior and superior to the triangular fossa. It is mainly used for treating hypertension.

角针 cone needle

针具名。即以塑料或金属制成的高为 0.1 寸，底面直径也为 0.1 寸的圆锥。使用时，将锥尖按于穴位上，使底面与皮肤面平，再以胶布固定。

Name of a special kind of needle made of plastics or metal with a cone shape, the height and the diameter of the bottom are both 0.1 cun, when use it, press the tip of the cone on the point so that the bottom is at the same level of the skin around and then fix it with a tape.

脚气 beriberi

以腿足软弱、行动不便为特征的疾病。本病多由湿邪壅滞，流注于脚所致。临床上分干、湿脚气两种。治宜疏通经络、清化湿热。取穴：足三里、三阴交、阳陵泉、八风。

A disease characterized by weakness and difficulty in movement of the lower limbs, due to the local retention of dampness-evil; clinically classified as dry and wet beriberi. Treatment principle: Dredge the meridians and remove heat and dampness. Point selection: Zusanli (ST36), Sanyinjiao(SP6), Yanglingquan (GB34), Bafeng(EX-LE10).

接经法 meridian-connected method

配穴法之一。指在同一条经脉上选用相近的几个穴位，使经气相互连接，以加强作用。

One of the point-combining methods, i. e., selecting several points close to each other in the same meridian to make a continuation of qi to increase the effects.

接经取穴 selecting points in the connected meridian

取穴法之一。又称同名经取穴法。十二经脉中,手足同名经上下相连。根据这种关系,对某一经脉的病变可取与其相连的手经或足经穴来进行治疗。

One of the point-selecting methods, known as "selecting points in the corresponding hand-food meridians". It is known that the corresponding hand-food meridians of the twelve meridians are connected with each other. According to this relationship, the points of the hand or foot meridians can be used to treat the disease of the corresponding foot-hand meridians.

接气通经 moving qi throughout the meridian

针刺法之一。古代对各经均规定一定长度,气的运行也有一定速度。针刺某经时应根据该经的长度和气的运行速度来决定运针的时间,以使经气相通。

One of the acupuncture methods. In ancient China, the lengths of all the meridians were determined and the moving speed of qi was also measured, so the time of acupuncture manipulations should be calculated according to the length of the punctured meridian and the moving speed of qi to ensure qi connected with each other.

节气 solar term

农历推算四季气候的单位。一般以 15 日为 1 个节气,一年共有 24 个节气,如立春、雨水等。

The unit used to calculate the climate of the four seasons according to the lunar calendar. A climatic period is approximately equivalent to 15 days. There are 24 solar terms in a year, e. g., "Beginning of Spring" "Rain Water", etc.

截疟 jienüe

经外奇穴名。位于乳头直下 4 寸处。此穴施灸治疗疟疾、胸胁痛等。

Name of an extra point. Located 4 cun below the nipples. Moxibustion is used to cure malaria, chest and hypochondrium pain, etc.

解溪 Jiexi (ST41)

经穴名。属足阳明胃经,本经经穴。定位:在足背与小腿交界处的横纹中央凹陷处,当跚长伸肌腱与趾长伸肌腱之间。主治:踝关节痛,肌萎缩,下肢痿痹,癫痫,头痛,头晕,

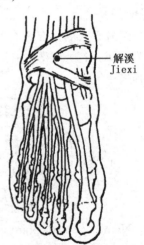

解溪 Jiexi

腹胀,便秘等。操作:直刺 0.3～0.5 寸;可灸。

The acupoint and Jing-River point of the Stomach Meridian of Foot-Yangming. Location:In the central depression of the crease between the instep of the foot and leg, between the tendons of the long extensor muscle of the great toe and the long extensor muscle of the toes. Indications: Pain of the ankle joint, muscular atrophy, pain and paralysis of the lower limbs, epilepsy, headache, vertigo, abdominal distension, constipation, etc. Method: Puncture perpendicularly 0.3-0.5 cun. Moxibustion is applicable.

巾针 scarf needle

古代针具之一,《灵枢》云其似镵针,头大而末锐。

An ancient type of needle which is described in the *Miraculous Pivot* as being similar to the arrow-head needle, having a large head and a tapered tip.

金津、玉液 Jinjin, Yuye (EX-HN12, EX-HN13)

经外奇穴名。在舌系带两侧静脉上,左为金津,右为玉液。主治:舌肿,呕吐,舌强失语等。

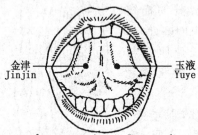

Name of extra points. Located on the veins on both sides of the frenulum of the tongue, Jinjin is on the left, and Yuye is on the right. Indications: Swelling of the tongue, vomiting, aphasia with stiffness of tongue, etc.

金门 Jinmen (BL63)

经穴名。属足太阳膀胱经,本经郄穴。定位:在足外侧,当外踝前缘直下,骰骨下缘处。主治:癫、狂、痫,小儿惊风,外踝痛,下肢痿痹等。操作:直刺 0.3～0.5 寸;可灸。

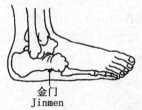

金门
Jinmen

The acupoint and Xi-Cleft point of the Bladder Meridian of Foot-Taiyang. Location: On the lateral side of the foot, below the anterior border of the external malleolus, on the lower border of the cuboid bone. Indications: Mania, epilepsy, infantile convulsion, pain in the external malleolus, motor impairment and pain of the lower extremities, etc. Method: Puncture perpendicularly 0.3-0.5 cun. Moxibustion is applicable.

金针 gold or metal needle

①黄金制成的医用针具。②泛指金属制成的针具。

①Gold medical needle. ②Needle made of metals for acupuncture.

津 thin fluid

是人体体液的组成部分,质清稀,流动性大,主要分布于皮肤、肌肉、孔窍,有营养肌肉和润泽皮肤的功能。此外,中医学认为,汗和尿液均来源于津,出汗过多和排尿过多均可伤津。

A component of body fluid, which is clear and thin with great fluidity. It distributes in the skin, muscles and orifics, with the function of nourishing the muscles and moisturizing the skin. The sweat and urine are originated from the thin fluid. Profuse sweating and polyuria may cause the consumption of thin fluid.

津液 fluid

体液的总称。其向体外流泄者为津,存于体内起滋润作用者为液。

The general name of the body fluid. The fluid excreted from the body is called Jin while the fluid nourishing in the body is called Ye.

筋 tendon

筋:组织器官名,即肌腱,附着于骨节的称筋,包于肌外的叫筋膜。筋和筋膜的功能由肝所主,因此,肝的精气盛衰与筋力的强弱有密切关系。

A terminology of tissue and organ. It refers to tendon. The one that is attached to the joints is called tendon and the one that wraps the tendons is known as fascia or aponeurosis, both of them are controlled by the liver. Therefore, the strength of the tendons is closely related to the condition of liver.

筋会 influential point of tendons

即阳陵泉穴。八会穴之一。

Yanglingquan(GB34). One of the eight influential points.

筋缩 Jinsuo(GV8)

经穴名。属督脉。定位:在背部,第九胸椎棘突下凹陷中。主治:癫痫,脊强,胃痛等。操作:稍向上斜刺 0.5～1 寸;可灸。

Name of an acupoint. It belongs to the Governor Vessel. Location: On the back, in the depression of the spinous

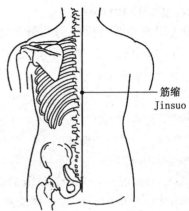

筋缩
Jinsuo

process of the 9th thoracic vertebra. Indications: Epilepsy, stiffness of the back, gastric pain, etc. Method: Puncture obliquely upward 0.5-1 cun. Moxibustion is applicable.

筋之府 residence of tendons

指膝部。

It refers to the knees.

紧按慢提 swift, vigorous thrusting and slow, gentle lifting

刺法用语。即快而重地插针和轻而缓地提针,为补法,与"紧提慢按"相对。

A term of acupuncture, i. e. , thrust the needle swiftly and vigorously and lift it slowly and gently to reinforce, as contrasted with "swift, vigorous lifting and slow, gentle thrusting".

紧脉 tight pulse

指感紧张有力的一种脉象,如牵绳转索,按之弹指,多见于寒证及痛证。

A pulse condition with tense and vigorous beats, like a stretched and twisted cord, frequently seen in cold syndrome and pain syndrome.

紧提慢按 swift, vigorous lifting and

slow, gentle thrusting

刺法用语。即慢而轻的插针和快而重的提针,为泻法。与"紧按慢提"相对。

A term of acupuncture, i. e. , lift the needle swiftly and vigorously and thrust it slowly and gently to reduce, as contrasted with "swift, vigorous thrusting and slow, gentle lifting".

禁刺 acupuncture contraindication

包括禁针部位如内脏部位禁深刺,孕妇的腹部、婴幼儿囟门部及其他禁针穴位禁刺。酒醉、过饥、过饱、过度疲劳、情绪激烈变化等情况下,不可立刻进行针刺,以免发生意外。

The locations of human body and the condition of the patient to which acupuncture is contraindicated. The former includes the abdomen of pregnant women, the fontanel of infants, certain particular points, and the parts over viscera (for deep puncture). The latter includes the patients who are drunken, over hunger, over fed, over fatigue, under emotional upsets, etc.

禁灸穴 moxibustion-prohibited points

有些穴位因接近重要器官或动脉,不宜直接灸,如五处、心俞、素髎等,但各书所列禁灸穴不尽一致,临床可根据病情选用不同的灸法。

Certain points are prohibited for moxibustion due to the important organs or arteries close to them, for example, Wuchu (BL5), Xinshu (BL15), Suliao (GV25), etc. The prohibited acupoints listed in different medical books are not always the same, so they can be clinically selected for suitable moxibustion according to the disease conditions.

禁针穴 acupuncture-prohibited acupoints

指禁用针刺的穴位。古书中所列禁针穴较多,现代除乳中及神阙两穴外,临床上均可酌情使用。

It refers to the acupoints prohibited to puncture. In ancient medical works a lot of acupoints were prohibited to puncture, but in modern times, all the points except Ruzhong(ST17) and Shenque(CV8) can be punctured according to the disease conditions.

进气法 inspiration method

针刺手法名。即先直刺,紧提慢按六数,得气后将针斜对病痛处,行气后让患者吸气五口或七口,以助运气。用于各种痛证。

Name of the acupuncture method, i. e. , insert the needle perpendicularly first, then swiftly lift and slowly thrust it six times. After having got the needling sensation, turn the needle obliquely into the direction of the disease, perform manipulations and ask the patient to inspire five or seven times to help qi move. The method can be used in all kinds of pain syndrome.

进针 insertion of the needle

针刺手法之一。即将毫针刺入体内的方法。

One of the acupuncture techniques, i. e. , the method to insert a filiform needle into the body.

进针管 insertion tube

进针时的辅助用具。用手指弹压管内的针具,使之快速刺入皮内,以减轻进针时的痛感。

A supplementary tool for insertion. Flick the needle in the tube swiftly into the skin to reduce the pain during insertion.

进针器 needle inserter

一种利用弹簧装置将针迅速刺入皮下以减轻痛感的用具。

A kind of tool with spring mechanism which is used to insert the needle quickly into the skin to reduce the pain during insertion.

近道取穴 adjacent point selection

指于病痛的局部或邻近部位取穴,与远道取穴相对。

Selecting the points in or near the diseased part, contrary to the method of distal point selection.

近节段取穴 adjacent segment point selection

取穴法之一。指在针灸或针麻时选用与疼痛或手术部位属于同一或邻近脊髓节段所支配的穴位。

One of the point-selecting methods, i. e., selecting the points innervated by the same or adjacent spinal segment corresponding to the parts of the disease or operation during the acupuncture or acupuncture anesthesia.

京骨 Jinggu (BL64)

经穴名。属足太阳膀胱经,本经原穴。定位:在足外侧,第五跖骨粗隆下方,赤白肉际处。主治:头痛,项强,腰腿痛,痫证

等。操作:直刺 0.3～0.5 寸;可灸。

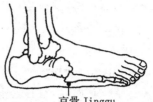

京骨 Jinggu

The acupoint and Yuan-Primary point of the Bladder Meridian of Foot-Taiyang. Location:On the lateral side of the foot, below the tuberosity of the 5th metatarsal bone, on the dorso-ventral boundary of the foot. Indications:Headache, neck rigidity, pain in the lower back and thigh, epilepsy. Method:Puncture perpendicularly 0.3-0.5 cun. Moxibustion is applicable.

京门 Jingmen (GB25)

经穴名。属足少阳胆经,肾的募穴。定位:在侧腰部,当第十二肋骨游离端的下方。主治:腹胀,肠鸣,泄泻,腰胁痛等。操作:直刺 0.5～1 寸;可灸。

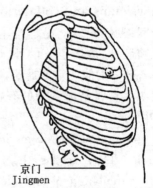

京门
Jingmen

The acupoint belongs to the Gallbladder Meridian of Foot-Shaoyang. The Front-Mu point of the kidney. Location:On the lateral side of the waist, below the free end of the 12th rib. Indications:Abdominal distension, borborygmus, diarrhea, pain in the lumbar and hypochondriac region, etc. Method: Puncture perpendicularly 0. 5-1 cun. Moxibustion is applicable.

经刺 meridian puncture

①当某一经脉有病时,在该经脉上进行针刺的方法。②九刺法之一。指针刺与患病局部同一经脉的结聚不通的部位。

① When a meridian is affected, acupuncture is manipulated along that meridian. ②One of the nine needling techniques to needle the meridian related to the affected part.

经筋 meridian muscle regions

与十二经脉相类似,全身有十二经筋,起于四肢,结于骨节,不入脏腑。

Similar to the 12 meridians, there are 12 meridian muscle regions in the human body, which originate from the extremities and converge in the joints but don't enter the viscera.

经络 meridians and collaterals

经脉和络脉的总称,是运行全身气血、联络脏腑肢节、沟通上下内外、调节脏腑及机体各部分功能的重要通路,起着把人体各组织器官联结成统一的有机整体的重要作用。

The gerneral name of meridians and collaterals. They act as the important route for circulating qi and blood, connecting viscera with extremities, communicating the upper with the lower and the interior with the exterior, regulating the activities of viscera and other parts of the body, and play an important role in joining the tissues and organs of the body to build up an organic whole.

经络电测定法 the electric measurement of a meridian

测定人体皮肤电阻的各种变化,以了解有关脏腑经络生理、病理情况的一种方法。

To measure the changes of the electric resistance of the skin so as to recognize the physiologic and pathologic conditions of the related viscera of a meridian.

经络感传现象 propagated sensations along meridians

指刺激穴位时,有酸、麻、胀、重的感觉从被刺激的穴位开始沿着经络循行路线进行传导的一种现象。

The evoked sensations of soreness, numbness, distension and heaviness with acupuncture may radiate from the stimulated acupoint along the route of the meridian.

经络敏感点、线、区 the sensitive point, line and zone of the meridian

沿着经络路线出现的某一敏感点称为经络敏感点;出现的线状感称为经络敏感线;出现的片状感称为经络敏感区。

A sensitive point on the route of a meridian is called the sensitive point; the linear sensation along a meridian is called the sensitive line; the sensitive area along a meridian is called the sensitive zone.

经络敏感人 meridian-sensitive person

针刺时较易出现经络感传现象的人。

The one who is apt to experience propagated sensation along meridians when being needled.

经络学说 theory of meridians and collaterals

研究人体经络系统的生理功能、病理变化及其与脏腑相互关系的学说。

The theory to study the physiologic functions and pathologic changes of the meridians and collaterals, and their relationship with the viscera.

经脉 meridian

联系人体各部分及运行气血的主要干线。

The main passage connecting different parts of the body in which qi and blood circulate.

经脉之海 convergence of the meridians

指冲脉。

It refers to the Thoroughfare Vessel.

经气 meridian qi

指运行于经脉中的气。它包括经脉的功能和经脉中流动着的精微。

It refers to the qi circulating in the meridians. It contains the function of the meridians and the nutrients flowing in the meridians.

经渠 Jingqu(LU8)

经穴名。属手太阴肺经,本经经穴。定位:在前臂掌面桡侧,桡骨茎突与桡动脉之间凹陷处,腕横纹上1寸处。主治:咳嗽,气喘,发热,咽喉肿痛,胸痛,腕痛等。操作:避开血管,直刺0.3~0.5寸。

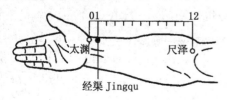

经渠 Jingqu

The acupoint and the Jing-River point belongs to the Lung Meridian of Hand-Taiyin. Location: On the radial side of the palmar side of the forearm, 1 cun above the transverse crease of the wrist, in the depression between the styloid process of the radius and radial artery. Indications: Cough, asthma, fever, sore throat, pain in the chest and wrist, etc. Method: Puncture perpendicularly 0.3-0.5 cun, avoiding the radial artery.

经隧 meridian passage

经络学术语,指潜布于体表以下运行气血的经络通道。

A terminology of meridians. It refers to the meridians which circulating the qi and blood under the surface of the body.

经外奇穴 extra points

又称奇穴,指既有一定的穴名,又有明确的位置,但尚未列入十四经系统的腧穴。

It refers to the points with certain names and clear locations but not included in the fourteen meridians system.

经穴 Jing-River points; acupoints

①五输穴之一。位于腕关节、踝关节附近,十二经各一个。因经气在此像较大的河流一样迅速流行,畅通无阻,故名。②指十四经的经穴。

①One of the five Shu points in the vicinity of the wrist and the ankle, one for each of the twelve regular meridians named as analogous to a large river flowing swiftly. ②Referring to the points of the fourteen meridians.

经穴电测定法 acupoint electrometry

测定经络穴位电位、电阻等电学特征的方法。

Measurement of the electric potential and resistance of an acupoint, etc.

经穴探测仪 acupoint detector

现代针疗仪器,用以探测皮肤电阻,经络循行、生理变化和经穴部位。

Modern acupuncture instrument used to measure skin electric resistance, detect the course and physiological changes of meridians, and locate acupoints.

经中 Jingzhong

经外奇穴名。位于气海穴旁3寸。直刺或灸治二便不能、带下、月经不调、腹泻等。

Name of an extra point. Location: 3 cun lateral to Qi hai(CV6). Perpendicular acupuncture or moxibustion is used to cure constipation, retention of urine, leukorrhea, irregular menstruation, diarrhea, etc.

惊风 infantile convulsion

突然发作四肢抽搐和意识不清的病证,1～5岁的儿童多见。治宜清热驱邪、熄风开窍。取穴:大椎、合谷、太冲、阳陵泉、十二井穴。

A disease usually seen in children aged 1-5 years, marked by sudden onset of convulsion accompanied with loss of consciousness. Treatment principle: Clear heat and eliminate evils, calm the endopathic wind for resuscitation. Point selection: Dazhui(GV14), Hegu(LI4), Taichong(LR3), Yanglingquan(GB34), the twelve Jing-Well points.

睛明 Jingming (BL1)

经穴名。属足太阳膀胱经。定位:在面部,目内眦角稍上方凹陷处。主治:目赤肿痛,内眦痒痛,流泪,夜盲,色盲,视物不清,近视等。操作:嘱患者闭目,医者左手将眼球轻轻推向外侧固定,右手将针沿眼眶边缘缓慢直刺入0.5～1寸,不捻转,不提插,出针后按压针孔片刻,以防出血。一般不留针;禁灸。

Name of an acupoint. It belongs to the Bladder Meridian of Foot-Taiyang. Location: On the face, in the depression slightly above the inner canthus. Indica-

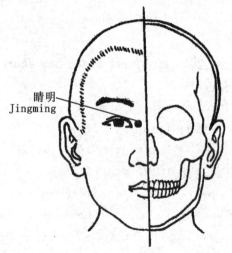

睛明
Jingming

tions: Redness, swelling and pain of the eyes, itching of the canthus, lachrymation, night blindness, colour blindness, blurred vision, myopia, etc. Method: Ask the patient to close his eyes, fix the patient's eyeballs after gently pushing it laterally with the left hand, insert the needle perpendicularly and closely to the orbital margin 0.5-1 cun with the right hand, without twirling, lifting, or thrusting. Press the needle hole for a moment after withdrawal of the needle，otherwise bleeding may be caused. Generally，it is not advisable to retain the needle，and moxibustion is prohibited.

睛中 Jingzhong

经外奇穴名。位于瞳孔正中。于角膜缘处刺，以金针治疗各种白内障。

Name of an extra point. Located on the center of the pupil，used mainly to treat various kinds of cataracts with a gold needle entering the eyeball from the corneal margin.

精 essence

指构成和维持人体生命的基本物质，包括先天之精和后天之精。

Fundamental substances constituting the body and maintaining the life，including both the congenital and acquired essences.

精灵、威灵 Jingling, Weiling

按摩用穴。位于手背四、五和二、三掌骨间隙后缘凹陷处。前者称精灵，后者称威灵。掐按此处用于急救。近来针刺用于治疗头痛、目眩、耳鸣、惊风、手痛、腰痛、腕关节炎等。

Points for massage. Jingling and Wei ling are located at the dorsal side of the posterior metacarpal depression between the fourth and fifth meta carpal bones and between the second and third meta carpal bones respectively. Press and pinch these two points mainly for emergencies. Recently，acupuncture is also used on these points to cure headache，blurred vision，tinnitus，infantile convulsion，hand pain，lumbago，wrist ar-

thritis，etc.

精明 Jingming

睛明穴别名。

The other name of Jingming(BL1).

精明之府 residence of intelligence

指头部，因脏腑经络之精气会聚于此。

The head where the essential qi of the viscera and meridians converge.

井穴 Jing-Well points

五输穴之一。位于手指或足趾末端处，十二经各一个。如水之发源地，故名。

One of the five Shu points. Located at the tips of the fingers and toes. Each of the Twelve Regular Meridians has one. They are analogous to the headwaters of a river.

颈 Jing

耳穴名。在颈椎前侧耳腔缘。主治：落枕，颈项强痛。

Name of an ear point. It is on the border of cavum conchae，anterior to the cervical vertebrae. Indications：Stiffness and pain of the neck.

颈椎 Jingzhui

耳穴名。在对耳轮体部，将轮屏切迹至对耳轮上、下脚分叉处分为五等份，下 1/5 为颈椎。主治相应部位的疼痛。

Name of an ear point. In the body of anthelix，the curved line from intertragic notch to the branching area of superior and inferior antihelix crus can be divided into 5 equal segments. The lower 1/5 is Jingzhui. It is used for treating pain in the corresponding part of the spine.

胫 tibia

骨骼名,是小腿的大骨。

Name of the big bone of the lower leg.

鸠尾 Jiuwei(CV15)

经穴名。属任脉。本经络穴。定位:在上腹部,前正中线上,当剑胸结合部下1寸。主治:胸区疼痛,恶心,癫狂,痫证等。操作:向下斜刺0.4～0.6寸;可灸。

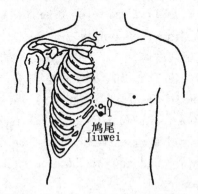

鸠尾
Jiuwei

Name of the acupoint, Luo-Connecting point, belongs to the Conception Vessel. Location: On the upper abdomen and on the anterior midline, 1 cun below the xiphosternal synchondrosis. Indications: Pain in the cardiac region and the chest, nausea, mental disorders, epilepsy, etc. Method: Punctue obliquely downward 0.4-0.6 cun. Moxibustion is applicable.

九刺 nine techniques of needling

《内经》刺法分类,出自《灵枢·官针》。指治疗九类不同性质的病变运用的九种不同的刺法,即输刺、远道刺、经刺、络刺、分刺、大泻刺、毛刺、巨刺、焠刺。

A category of acupuncture technique in *Huangdi's Canon of Medicine*, originates from *Miraculous Pivot*: *Guanzhen*, referring to the nine different needling acupuncture techniques employed for trea-

ting nine kinds of diseases, i. e. , shupoint needling, distant needling, meridian needling, collateral needling, crack needling, evacuation needling, shallow needling, opposite needling, and fire needling.

九宫 nine palaces

古代将八方及中央定为九宫,各有专名,并以一定数字来代表。九宫与季节及部位相配是古代的一种取穴法。

In ancient China, the eight directions and the center were named as nine palaces, each having a specific name and a designated number. The combination of the nine palaces, the seasons and the parts was one of the point-locating methods in ancient China.

九六补泻 nine for reinforcing and six for reducing

针刺时的补泻与数字有关,九为补,六为泻。

In acupuncture the reinforcing and the reducing are related to the numbers of nine and six. Nine is related to reinforcing while six is related to reducing.

九六数 nine-six numbers

刺法用语。古代以九为阳数,六为阴数。在后世刺法的组合中,补法的操作以九为基数,泻法的操作则以六为基数。

A term used in acupuncture. In ancient China, the number of nine was considered to be a yang number while the number of six a yin number. Since then in the prescription of acupuncture, the reinforcing manipulation has been based on the number of nine while the reducing manipulation on the number of six.

九曲中府 Jiuquzhongfu

经外奇穴名。位于腋窝正中直下,第七肋间隙下 3 寸处。主治:恶风邪气入经,内有瘀血,胸胁疼痛,腹痛等。治法常用斜刺或灸治。

Name of an extra point. Located directly downward from the middle of the armpit, 3 cun under the 7th intercostal space. Indications: Stagnation of blood, thoracic pain, hypochondriac pain, and abdominal pain caused by wind-evil invading the meridians, etc. Oblique acupuncture or moxibustion can be used.

九宜 indications of the nine needles

九针根据形状特点各有其适应的范围。

Because of the different shapes and characteristics of the nine kinds of acupuncture needles, they can be used in different cases or indications.

九针 nine needles

指古代九种不同形状和不同用法的针。其名称是镵针、圆针、锃针、锋针、铍针、圆利针、毫针、长针、大针。

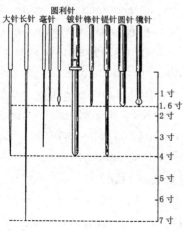

The needles of nine different varieties used by ancient acupuncturists. Their names are arrowhead needle, round needle, blunt needle, sharp needle, sword-shaped needle, round-sharp needle, filiform needle, long needle and large needle.

久泻不止 protracted diarrhea

即大便泄泻日久不止。多因脾肾阳虚而致。治宜健脾益气、升阳止泻。取穴:中脘、章门、胃俞、脾俞、足三里。

Diarrhea for a long time, due to gastrointestinal dysfunction resulting from the deficiency of spleen-yang and kidney-yang. Treatment principle: Strengthen the spleen and replenish qi, elevate the spleen to arrest diarrhea. Point selection: Zhongwan(CV12), Zhangmen(LR13), Weishu(BL21), Pishu(BL20), Zusanli(ST36).

灸瘢 moxibustion scar

因灸治而造成的瘢痕。

Scar caused by moxibustion.

灸板 moxibustion board

灸用器具。为有孔长板,上可置艾施灸。

A kind of moxibustion tool, i. e., a long board with many holes on which moxa can be placed to do moxibustion.

灸疮 post-moxibustion sore

艾火灼伤皮肤,或因灼伤护理不当感染化脓形成疮疡。

A lesion formed by burning of the skin during moxibustion or complication from local infection.

灸法 moxibustion

指利用艾绒或其他药物烧灼、熏熨体表一定部位,以温热的刺激来防治疾病的方法。

A therphy of applying ingnited moxa or other medical herbs to a certain part of the body to prevent and treat diseases with warmth.

灸痨 Jiulao

经外奇穴名。位于背部。自中趾尖经足心至腘窝横纹之长为度,自鼻尖沿正中线至背脊尽处为标点,旁开各半口寸处是穴。灸治肺痨、盗汗、咳嗽、咯血、消瘦、乏力等。

Name of extra points. Location: On the back, using the distance from the middle toe tip through the center of the sole to the popliteal crease as the set length of a line and then start the line from the nose tip along the midline to the back. The points are 0.5 mouth cun bilaterally away from the end point of the line. Moxibustion is used to cure pulmonary tuberculosis, night sweating, cough, hemoptysis, emaciation, fatigue, etc.

灸器灸 moxibustion with tools

用特制的灸器盛放点燃的艾绒,在穴位上进行熨灸或熏灸。

A kind of moxibustion with special tools in which the burning moxa can be placed to perform ironing or fuming moxibustion on the points.

灸哮 Jiuxiao

经外奇穴名。位于背部,以绳环颈下垂至鸠尾穴,环转向背,绳端着脊中处是穴。灸治哮喘、咳嗽、支气管炎等。

Name of an extra point. A cord with two ends at Jiuwei (CV15) is wrapped around the neck, swing the two ends of the cord to the back with the cord still wrapped around the neck, the point where the two ends touching the posterior midline is the location for the point. Moxibustion is used to cure asthma, cough, bronchitis, etc.

灸血病 Jiuxuebing

经外奇穴名。位于第三骶椎棘突高点处。灸治吐血、衄血、便血等血证。

Name of an extra point. Located on top of the spinous process of the 3rd sacral vertebra. Moxibustion is used to cure blood disease such as hematemesis, epistaxis, bloody stool, etc.

酒熨 alcohol press therapy

古代理疗法之一。用净布蘸热酒从胸部至腹部反复搽抹,待皮肤潮红、周身发热而止,可促使气血通畅。适用于情志不舒、气机不调、胸胁胀满等症。

An ancient physiotherapy repeatedly rubbing of the area extending from the chest to the abdomen with cloth soaked with hot wine until the skin is flushed and the patient experience a sensation of warmth. This method is used to promote the flow of qi and blood and to treat emotional distress, disturbance of functional activity of qi and fullness of the chest and hypochondriac regions.

居髎 Juliao (GB29)

经穴名。属足少阳胆经。定位:在髋部,当髂前上棘与股骨大转子最凸点连线的中点处。主治：腰腿痹痛，下肢痿痹，瘫痪等。操作：直刺或斜刺 1～2 寸；可灸。

Name of an acupoint. It belongs to the

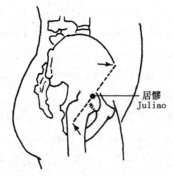

居髎
Juliao

Gallbladder Meridian of Foot-Shaoyang. Location：On the hip，at the midpoint of the line connecting the anterior superior iliac spine and the prominence of the great trochanter. Indications：Pain and numbness in the thigh and lumbar region，muscular atrophy of the lower limbs，paralysis，etc. Method：Puncture perpendicularly or obliquely 1-2 cun. Moxibustion is applicable.

局部选穴法 local point selection

选穴方法之一，在病变局部选穴治疗，如胃痛选中脘、肩痛选肩髃、腹痛选关元等。

A method of point selection，in which points at the disease site are needled. For example，for gastralgia，Zhongwan(CV12) is selected；for shoulder pain，Jianyu (LI15) is chosen；for abdominal pain，Guanyuan(CV4) is needled.

巨刺 opposing needling

九刺法之一。身体一侧（左或右侧）有病时，针刺对侧（右或左侧）穴位的一种方法。主要应用于：①身体一侧疼痛而对侧的脉象出现异常者。②经脉有病者。

One of the nine needling techniques. When a disease occurs at one side(left or right) of the body，the acupoints on the opposite side（right or left）are punctured. It is mainly used for：①Unilateral pain of the body with abnormal pulse on the opposite side. ②Meridian disease.

巨骨 Jugu (LI16)

经穴名。属手阳明大肠经。定位：在肩上部，当锁骨肩峰端与肩胛冈之间凹陷处。主治：上肢疼痛不遂，肩背痛等。操作：直刺 0.5～0.8 寸；可灸。

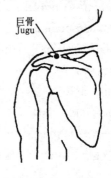

巨骨
Jugu

Name of an acupoint. It belongs to the Large Intestine Meridian of Hand-Yangming. Location：On the shoulder，in the depression between the acromial end of the clavicle and scapular spine. Indications：Pain and motor impairment of the upper extremities，pain in the shoulder and back，etc. Method：Puncture perpendicularly 0.5-0.8 cun. Moxibustion is applicable.

巨髎 Juliao (ST3)

经穴名。属足阳明胃经。定位：在面部，瞳孔直下，平鼻翼下缘处，当鼻唇沟外侧。主治：面瘫，眼球瞷动，鼻衄，齿痛，唇颊肿痛等。操作：直刺 0.2～0.5 寸；可灸。

Name of an acupoint. It belongs to of the Stomach Meridian of Foot-Yang-

ming. Location:
On the face,
directly below
the pupil, on
the level of the
lower border of
the nasal ala,
beside the naso-
labial groove.

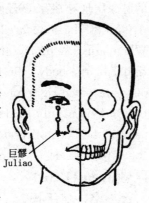

巨髎
Juliao

Indications: Facial paralysis, twitching of eyelids, epistaxis, toothache, pain and swelling of lips and cheek, etc. Method: Puncture perpendicularly 0.2-0.5 cun. Moxibustion is applicable.

巨阙 Juque (CV14)

经穴名。属任脉,心的募穴。定位:在上腹部,前正中线上,当脐中上 6 寸。主治:心区疼痛,恶心,吞酸,吞咽困难,呕吐,癫狂,痫证,心悸等。操作:向下斜刺0.8~1.2寸;可灸。

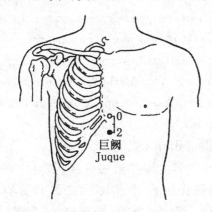

巨阙
Juque

Name of an acupoint. It belongs to the Conception Vessel. Front-Mu point of the heart. Location: On the upper abdomen and on the anterior midline, 6 cun above the center of the umbilicus. Indications: Pain in the cardiac region and chest, nausea, acid regurgitation, difficulty in swallowing, vomiting, mental disorders, epilepsy, palpitation, etc. Method: Puncture obliquely downward 0.8-1.2 cun. Moxibustion is applicable.

巨阙俞 Juqueshu

经外奇穴名。位于后正中线第四、五胸椎棘突之间。主治:咳嗽、喘息、支气管炎、神经衰弱等。治疗常用艾炷灸或温灸。

Name of an extra point. Located between the spinous process of the 4th and 5th thoracic vertebrae on the posterior midline. Indications: Cough, asthma, bronchitis, neurasthenia, etc., by moxa cone moxibustion or warm moxibustion.

巨虚上廉 Juxushanglian

上巨虚别名。

The other name of Shangjuxu(ST37).

巨虚下廉 Juxuxialian

下巨虚别名。

The other name of Xiajuxu(ST39).

巨阳 juyang

①太阳经的别名。②指申脉穴。

①The other name of Taiyang Meridian.
②The other name of Shenmai(BL62).

巨针 great needle

针具名。原指九针中的大针。近代有以不锈钢制成的巨针,直径 0.5~1 mm,长 10~35 cm,用于皮下横刺和肌腱部刺,以治疗瘫痪和肌肉挛缩等症。

Name of an acupuncture needle. It originally refers to the big needle of the nine kinds of ancient needles. In modern times, big needles made of stainless steel have been developed with diameters of 0.5-1 mm and lengths of 10-35 cm, and have been used to puncture subcutaneously or in the tendon-muscular regions to cure paralysis, muscular contracture, etc.

聚泉 Juquan (EX-HN10)

经外奇穴名。位于舌面正中。直刺或三棱针点刺出血。主治：哮喘、咳嗽、消渴、舌强、舌肌麻痹等。

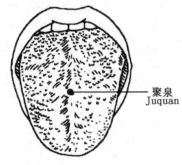

聚泉
Juquan

Name of an extra point. Located at the center of the tongue. Perpendicular acupuncture or blood letting with a three-edged needle is used to cure asthma, cough, consumptive thirst, stiff tongue, lingual paresis, etc.

绝骨 juegu

①部位名。指外踝上方凹陷处。②悬钟穴别名。③阳辅穴别名。

①Name of the body part, i. e. , the depression above the lateral malleolous. ② The other name of Xuanzhong(GB39). ③The other name of Yangfu(GB38).

绝阳 Jueyang

商阳穴别名。

The other name of Shangyang(LI1).

厥逆 syncope syndrome

①四肢厥冷。②指胸腹剧痛、两足暴冷、脉涩的一种疾病。③因寒邪犯脑所致的慢性头痛。症见头痛连齿痛，日久不愈。治宜回阳救逆。针百会、气海，灸神阙。

①Coldness of limbs. ②A disease characterized by excruciating pain of the chest and abdomen, extreme coldness of the limbs and choppy pulse. ③Prolonged headache radiating to the teeth, due to cold-evil attacking the brain. Treatment principle：Recuperate depleted yang and rescue the patient from collapse. Puncture Baihui(GV20),Qihai(CV6) and do moxibustion on Shenque(CV8).

厥阳 jueyang

①飞扬穴别名。②证候名。即肾阴衰，阳气独盛，表现为手足热等。

①The other name of Feiyang(BL58). ②Name of signs and symptoms, i. e. , the deficiency of kidney-yin and the excess of yang manifested as the heat of hands and feet, etc.

厥阴 jueyin

经脉名称之一，是阴气发展的最后阶段。

One of the Meridian names. It means that the yin-qi is at the final stage of development.

厥阴经 Jueyin Meridians

手厥阴心包经与足厥阴肝经之总称。

A joint name of the Pericardium Meridian of Hand-Jueyin and the Liver Meridian of Foot-Jueyin.

厥阴俞 Jueyinshu（BL14）

经穴名。属足太阳膀胱经，心包背俞穴。定位：在背部，当第四胸椎棘突下，旁开1.5寸。主治：咳嗽，心痛，心悸，胸闷，呕吐等。操作：向内斜刺0.5～1寸；可灸。

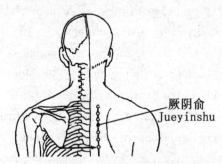

厥阴俞
Jueyinshu

Name of an acupoint. It belongs to the Bladder Meridian of Foot-Taiyang. It is the Back-Shu point of the pericardium. Location: On the back, below the spinous process of the 4th thoracic vertebra, 1.5 cun lateral to the posterior midline. Indications: Cough, cardiac pain, palpitation, stuffy chest, vomiting, etc. Method: Puncture obliquely inward 0.5-1 cun. Moxibustion is applicable.

厥阴为阖 the Jueyin Meridians are a-nalogous to the inner closed door

指厥阴经位于身体三阴经的最里部位。

The Jueyin Meridians are in the inner-most part of the three Yin Meridians.

腘 muscular prominence

肌肉的突起部分。如肱二头肌、腓肠肌等。

Prominent appearance of muscles, such as the biceps brachii, gastrocnemius, etc.

K

咯血 hemoptysis

咳嗽时血块或鲜血从气道经口排出的症状。多因阴虚火旺或肺有燥热,血络受伤所致。治宜益阴养肺、清热止血。取穴:尺泽、鱼际、孔最、颈百劳、然谷。

The expectoration of blood or blood-stained sputum, usually due to damage of blood vessels resulting from yin deficiency with hyperactivity of sthenia fire or from the retention of dryness-heat evil in the lungs. Treatment principle: Supplement yin and nourish the lungs, clear heat to stop bleeding. Point selection: Chize (LU5), Yuji (LU10), Kongzui (LU6), Jingbailao (EX-HN15), Rangu (KI2)

开、阖、枢 opening, closing, and switching (pivoting)

指经脉的开放、闭合、枢纽三种不同作用。如太阳经主开,阳明经主阖,少阳经主枢;太阴经主开,厥阴经主阖,少阴经主枢。

The three different actions of the meridians. For example, the Taiyang and Taiyin Meridian have the opening action; the Yangming and Jueyin Meridian, the closing action; the Shaoyang and Shaoyin Meridian, the switching (pivoting) action.

开阖补泻 tonification or purgation by opening or closing the needle hole

出针后用手揉按针孔,使针孔闭塞,属"补"法;出针时摇大针孔,不加揉按,属"泻"法。

After withdrawal of the needle, massage the hole to close it. This is "tonification". While the hole is enlarged by shaking the needle and not to be massaged. This is "purgation".

开窍通神 open the orifices and regain consciousness

治疗邪阻心窍神志昏迷的方法。适用于邪盛气实的闭证。通常有凉开、温开之别。

A treatment for coma due to obstruction of the heart-orifice by the evils, applicable to the sthenia syndrome of coma when the evil is hyperactive and qi is hyper-functioning, usually treated by using drugs of cool nature or of warm nature.

尻 sacrococcygeal region

骶尾部的通称。

The region overlying the sacrum and coccyx.

颏 chin

下颌的前中部凹陷处。

The anterior middle depression of the lower jaw.

咳血 hemoptysis

指血随咳嗽而出。多因外感风邪不解,化热化烦,损伤脉络,或肝火犯肺所致。治宜泻肝清肺、和络止血。取肺俞、鱼际、劳宫、行间。

Bleeding from the respiratory tract, due to the damage of pulmonary collaterals resulting from the attack of wind-evil with production of heat and dryness e-vils, or due to attack of the lungs by li-ver-fire. Treatment principle: Clear fire from the liver and remove heat from the lungs, regulate collaterals and stop bleeding. Point selection: Feishu(BL13), Yuji(LU10), Laogong (PC8), Xingjian (LR2).

孔最 Kongzui (LU6)

经穴名。属手太阴肺经，本经郄穴。定位：在前臂掌面桡侧，当尺泽与太渊连线上，腕横纹上7寸。主治：胸痛，气喘，咳血，咽喉肿痛，肘臂挛痛等。操作：直刺0.5~1寸；可灸。

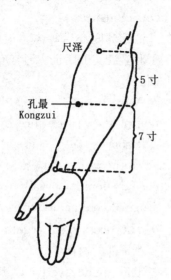

The acupoint, Xi-Cleft point of the Lung Meridian of Hand-Taiyin. Loca-tion: On the radial side of the palmar side of the forearm, and on the line connect-ing Chize(LU5) and Taiyuan(LU9), 7 cun above the transverse crease of the wrist. Indications: Pain in the chest, asthma, hemoptysis, sore throat, spas-modic pain of the elbow and arm, etc. Method: Puncture perpendicularly 0.5-1 cun. Moxibustion is applicable.

芤脉 hollow pulse

脉浅表、大而柔软，按之有空虚感的一种脉象，多见于大量失血后的患者。

A pulse condition which is superficial, large and soft, with a hollow feeling while pressing; commonly seen in pa-tients after massive haemorrhage.

口 Kou; oral cavity

①耳穴名。在外耳道开口的后上方。主治：面瘫，胃炎等。②七窍之一，包括唇、舌、齿、腭等部分，通过咽部与食管相连，与脾有密切关系。大肠经、胃经、脾经、心包经、肾经、三焦经、胆经、督脉、任脉、冲脉等经脉都循行于此。

①Name of an ear point. It is close to the posterior and superior border of the orifice of the external auditory meatus. Indications: Facial paralysis, stomatitis, etc. ②One of the seven orifices, inclu-ding the lips, tongue, teeth and palate, etc. It connects with the esophagus through the pharynx and is closely relat-ed to the function of the spleen. The Me-ridians of the Large Intestine, Stomach, Spleen, Pericardium, Kidney, Sanjiao, Gallbladder, and the Governor Vessel, the Conception Vessel, the Throughfare Vessel all pass through the mouth.

口疮 aphtha

由脾胃积热或虚火上炎引起的口腔黏膜小溃疡。治宜清胃泻热。取穴：内庭、陷谷、合谷、太溪。

Small ulcer in the mouth caused by re-tention of heat evil in the spleen and stomach and flaming-up of the asthenic fire. Treatment principle: Clear the heat of the stomach. Point selection: Neiting (ST44), Xiangu (ST43), Hegu (LI4), Taixi(KI3).

口寸 mouth-cun

经外奇穴取穴比量法之一。系以患者本人两口角之间的距离为1寸。

Measuring unit for locating the extra points. The length between the two corners of the patient's mouth is considered to be 1 cun.

口禾髎 Kouheliao(LI19)

经穴名。属手阳明大肠经。定位:在上唇部,鼻孔外缘直下,平水沟穴。主治:鼻塞,鼻衄,口㖞等。操作:直刺0.3～0.5寸;可灸。

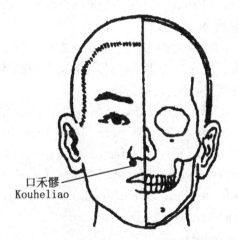

口禾髎
Kouheliao

Name of an acupoint. It belongs to the Large Intestine Meridian of Hand-Yangming. Location: On the upper lip, directly below the lateral border of the nostril, on the level of Shuigou (GV26). Indications: Nasal obstruction, epistaxis, deviation of the mouth, etc. Method: Puncture perpendicularly 0.3-0.5 cun. Moxibustion is applicable.

口苦 bitter taste in the mouth

口中常常有苦味,多属于实热证的表现。治宜清肺泻热、生津。取穴:肺俞、鱼际、太渊、少府。

A condition usually referring the bitter taste in the mouth, mostly belongs to the sthenia heat syndrome. Treatment principle: Clear lung-heat, promote the production of fluid. Point selection: Feishu (BL13), Yuji (LU10), Taiyuan (LU9), Shaofu(HT8).

口苦咽干 bitter taste and dry throat

指口中有苦味,咽喉干燥。多由肝胆积热,胆火上炎,灼伤津液所致。常见于少阳实热证患者。治宜清肝利胆。取穴:合谷、腕骨、阳陵泉、太冲。

A symptom manifested as the bitter taste in the mouth and dry feeling in the throat usually due to consumption of body fluid resulting from the accumulation of heat-evil in the liver and gallbladder and flaring-up of the gallbladder-fire, mostly seen in the patients suffering from Shaoyang sthenia heat syndrome. Treatment principle: Clear heat, eliminate dampness and smooth the liver and gallbladder. Point selection: Hegu (LI4), Wangu (SI4), Yanglingquan (GB34), Taichong(LR3).

口眼歪斜 deviation of mouth and eyes

由于风痰阻于经络所致的面部外形特征性改变。表现为口角下垂及眼裂增宽而不能闭合,常见于面神经麻痹。治宜祛风通络。取穴:风池、颊车、合谷、翳风、地仓、太冲。

Characteristic changes of the face due

to obstruction of meridians by wind-phlegm evil, manifested as dropping of the corner of the mouth and widening of the palpebral fissure with inability of eye closure; often seen in facial paralysis. Treatment principle: Dispel wind, dredge the meridians and collaterals. Point selection: Fengchi (GB20), Jiache (ST6), Hegu (LI4), Yifeng (TE17), Dicang (ST4), Taichong(LR3).

叩刺 tapping

用皮肤针（梅花针或七星针）在穴位皮肤上轻敲。

A manipulation of acupuncture by tapping around an acupoint with dermal needle (plum-blossom needle or seven-star needle) on the skin.

叩击法 tapping technique

轻轻叩击肢体的治疗方法。

Tapping the body and extremities as a therapeutic method.

库房 Kufang(ST14)

经穴名。属足阳明胃经。定位：在胸部，当第一肋间隙，距前正中线 4 寸。主治：胸胀痛，咳嗽等。操作：斜刺 0.5～0.8 寸；可灸。

Name of an acupoint. It belongs to the Stomach Meridian of Foot-Yangming. Location: On the chest, in the 1st intercostal space, 4 cun lateral to the anterior midline. Indications: Distending pain in the chest, cough, etc. Method: Puncture obliquely 0.5-0.8 cun. Moxibustion is applicable.

髋 Kuan

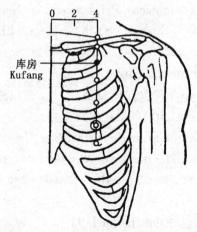

耳穴名。在对耳轮上脚的下 1/3 处。主治：髋关节疼痛，坐骨神经痛。

Name of an ear point. It is at inferior 1/3 of the superior antihelix crus. Indications: Pain in the hip joint, sciatica.

髋骨 Kuangu

①环跳穴别名。②经外奇穴名。位于梁丘穴外开 1 寸。斜刺、直刺或灸治脚膝肿痛，风湿性关节炎等。

①The other name of Huantiao(GB30). ②Name of an extra point, 1 cun lateral to Liangqiu(ST34). Oblique or perpendicular acupuncture or moxibustion is used to cure swelling and pain of the foot and knee, rheumatic arthritis, etc.

狂 mania

因七情郁结，五志化火，痰蒙心窍所致的精神病。症见过度兴奋，狂妄自大，甚至怒骂号叫、胡言乱语等。治宜清肝泻火、清心豁痰。取穴：劳宫、水沟、丰隆、大钟、内庭、行间。

A phase of mental disorder due to emotional depression causing formation of fire-evil and obstruction of the heart orifice by phlegm; manifested as hyperirritability, megalomania, irrational rage and shouting, raving. Treatment principle: Clear the liver fire, remove heat from the heart and eliminate phlegm for resuscitation. Point selection: Laogong(PC8), Shuigou（GV26）, Fenglong（ST40）, Dazhong(KI4), Neiting(ST44), Xingjian (LR2).

昆仑 Kunlun (BL60)

经穴名。属足太阳膀胱经,本经经穴。定位:在足部,外踝后方,当外踝与跟腱之间的凹陷中。主治:头痛,目眩,项强,鼻衄,肩背臂痛,足跟肿痛,难产等。操作:直刺0.5～1寸;可灸。

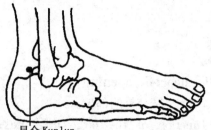

昆仑 Kunlun

The acupoint and the Jing-River point of the Bladder Meridian of Foot-Taiyang. Location: Posterior to the lateral malleolus, in the depression between the tip of the external malleolus and achilles tendon. Indications: Headache, dizziness, neck rigidity, epistaxis, pain in the shoulder, back and arm, swelling and pain of the heel, difficult labour, etc. Method: Puncture perpendicularly 0. 5-1 cun. Moxibustion is applicable.

L

阑门 ileocolic opening

指大、小肠交界的部位。

Junction of the large intestine and small intestine.

阑尾 Lanwei

耳穴名。位于大肠穴与小肠穴之间。主治:阑尾炎,腹泻等。

Name of an ear point. Location: Between Dachang and Xiaochang. Indications: Appendicitis, diarrhea, etc.

阑尾 Lanwei(EX-LE7)

经外奇穴名。在足三里穴下约 2 寸的压痛明显处。主治:急慢性阑尾炎,消化不良,下肢瘫痪等。操作:直刺1.5～2寸;可灸。

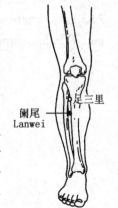

阑尾 Lanwei / 足三里

Name of an extra point. It is the tender point about 2 cun below Zusanli(ST36). Indications: Acute and chronic appendicitis, indigestion, paralysis of the lower extremities, etc. Method: Puncture perpendicularly 1.5-2 cun. Moxibustion is applicable.

劳宫 Laogong(PC8)

经穴名。属手厥阴心包经,本经荥穴。定位:在手掌心,当第二、三掌骨之间,偏于第三掌骨,握拳屈指时中指尖处。主治:心痛,癫狂,痫证,胃痛,口臭,恶心,呕吐。操作:直刺 0.3～0.5 寸;可灸。

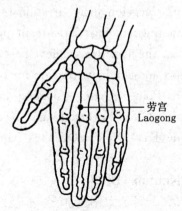

劳宫 Laogong

The acupoint, Xing-Spring point, belongs to the Pericardium Meridian of Hand-Jueyin. Location: At the center of the palm, between the 2nd and 3rd metacarpal bones but close to the latter, at the tip of the middle finger when a fist is made. Indications: Cardiac pain, mental disorders, epilepsy, stomachache, foul breath, nausea, vomiting, etc. Method: Puncture perpendicularly 0.3-0.5 cun. Moxibustion is applicable.

烙法 cautery

指将针烧红快速地点烙一定穴位的方法。

To rapidly dot the acupoint with a red-hot needle.

落枕 Laozhen

经外奇穴名。在手背第二、三掌骨间,指掌关节后约 0.5 寸处。主治:落枕,肩臂痛等。

Name of an extra point. It is located on the dorsum of the hand, between the second and third metacarpal bones, about 0.5 cun posterior to metacarpophalangeal joint. Indications: Stiff neck, pain in the shoulder and arm，etc.

雷公 Lei Gong

传说中上古的名医。相传为黄帝之臣，精于针灸，曾与黄帝论医药。《内经》中有七篇内容为黄帝与雷公论医药。

A legendary famous physician in ancient times，believed to be a minister of Huangdi and proficient in acupuncture and moxibustion，who discussed medical problems with the Emperor. Seven treatises in *Huangdi's Canon of Medicine* were written in the form of a dialogue between the Emperor and Lei Gong.

雷火神针 thunder-fire miraculous moxa stick

以多味中药制成艾条，施灸时隔纸十层按灸于患处，使热气直入病所。

Place a moxa stick made of various Chinese traditional herbs on the points covered with ten sheets of paper so the heat can directly reach the diseased part.

肋头 Leitou

经外奇穴名。位于胸骨两侧缘，平第三及第二肋骨头上缘处，共 4 穴。主治：瘕癖、咳嗽、哮喘、呃逆、支气管炎、肋间神经痛等。治疗常用斜刺及灸治。

Name of extra points. Location：At the bilateral border of sternum and levelled with the upper margins of the 2nd and 3rd rib head（4 points in total）. Indications：Mass and pain，cough，asthma，hiccup，bronchitis，intercostals neuralgia，etc.，using oblique acupuncture or moxibustion.

肋罅 Leixia

经外奇穴名。位于乳头外 4 寸肋间隙处。常用灸治腹痛、胁肋痛等。

Name of extra points. Location：4 cun lateral to the nipple，in the intereostal space. Moxibustion is used to treat abdominal pain，hypochondriac pain，costalgia，etc.

泪孔 Lei kong

睛明穴别称。

The other name of Jingming(BL1).

类经 *Classified Canon*

明代张介宾编，1624 年成书。该书对《内经》进行类编，是学习和研究《内经》的重要参考书。

A rearrangement of the contents of *Huangdi's Canon of Medicine*，an important reference book in the study of this classic，compiled by Zhang Jiebin in the Ming Dynasty and finished in 1624.

类经图翼 *Illustrated Supplementary to The Classified Canon*

明代张介宾撰，本书用图解补充《类经》的不足。

A supplementary to *Classified Canon* with illustration compiled by Zhang Jiebin in the Ming Dynasty.

冷灸 cold moxibustion

又称天灸、自灸。指将可以引起皮肤发疱的草药贴敷在一定的穴位上，使皮肤发疱的治疗方法。

Also called heavenly moxibustion or crude herb moxibustion. Irritating medicinal herbs are crushed and applied to a point to cause blisters of the skin.

冷针 cold acupuncture

即单纯的针刺，与"温针"相对。

Simple acupuncture, contrary to warm acupuncture.

厘正按摩要术 *Revised Synopsis of Massage*

清代张振鋆辑。本书在明代周于蕃《小儿推拿秘诀》的基础上，进一步校辑而成。包括辨证立法、各种按摩手法、取穴法，以及 24 种疾病的推拿方法。

An amendment and supplementary to Zhou Yufan's *Secret Principles of Pediatric Massage* written in the Ming Dynasty, which includes methods of diagnosis, massage manipulation, point locating and methods of massage for 24 kinds of illness, compiled by Zhang Zhenjun in the Qing Dynasty.

蠡沟 Ligou(LR5)

经穴名。属足厥阴肝经，本经络穴。定位：在内踝尖上 5 寸，胫骨内侧面的中央。主治：小便不利，遗尿，疝气，月经不调，带下，阴痒，下肢痿痹等。操作：直刺 0.5～0.8 寸；可灸。

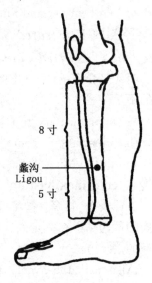

The acupoint, Luo-Connecting point, belongs to the Liver Meridian of Foot-Jueyin. Location: 5 cun above the tip of the medial malleolus, at the center of the medial aspect of the tibia. Indications: Retention of urine, enuresis, hernia, irregular menstruation, leukorrhea, pruritus vulvae, weakness and atrophy of the leg, etc. Method: Puncture perpendicularly 0.5-0.8 cun. Moxibustion is applicable.

李杲 Li Gao

金代著名医家。著有《脾胃论》《内外伤辨惑论》《医学发明》等书。为补土派的创始人。

A famous physician in the Jin Dynasty, author of *The Treatise on Spleen and Stomach*, *Differentiation on Endogenous and Exogenous Diseases* and *Elucidation of Medicine*. He is the founder of the school of strengthening the earth, i. e., the spleen and stomach.

李时珍 Li Shizhen

明代伟大的医学家、科学家（1518—1593 年）。曾于太医院任职，著有本草巨著《本草纲目》及《濒湖脉学》《奇经八脉考》等。

A great physician and scientist(1518-1593) in the Ming Dynasty, once a member of the College of Imperial Physicians, compiler of the monumental work *Compendium of Materia Medical*, author of *Binhu's Sphygmology* and *A Study on the Eight Extra Vessels*.

里急后重 tenesmus

阵发性腹痛、时时欲泻、肛门重坠、便出不爽的症状。多因湿热气滞所致。多见于痢疾。治宜清热利湿、调理肠胃。取穴：合谷、天枢、上巨虚、曲池、内庭。

A symptom refers to sudden onset of

abdominal pain with frequent desire for defecation, heavy sensation of anus and unsmooth defecation, which is commonly caused by qi obstruction in the intestines due to damp-heat stagnation and mostly seen in dysentery. Treatment principle: Clear heat and eliminate dampness, regulate the intestines and stomach. Point selection: Hegu (LI4), Tianshu (ST25), Shangjuxu(ST37), Quchi(LI11), Neiting(ST44).

里内庭 Lineiting

经外奇穴名。位于足掌面,与内庭穴相对。直刺或灸治小儿惊风、癫痫、足趾痛。

Name of an extra point. Located at the point just opposite Neiting(ST44) on the sole. Perpendicular acupuncture or moxibustion is used to cure infantile convulsion, epilepsy, toe pain.

理气 regulating qi

调理气机的方法,通常使用行气、降气的方法或药物使气机恢复正常。适用于治疗气滞、气逆所产生的证候。

A treatment for stagnation and adverse rising of qi with the medicines or methods of activating qi and keeping the adverse qi downwards.

理瀹骈文 Rhymed Discourses on External Therapy

书名。清代吴尚先撰。以骈文体记述以膏药为主的常见病外治疗法专著,具有简、便、廉、验的特点。

A book in rhythmical prose dealing with the application mainly of sticking plaster to cure common diseases, in which most of the methods and remedies recorded are simple, convenient, cheap and effective, compiled by Wu Shangxian in the Qing Dynasty.

厉兑 Lidui(ST45)

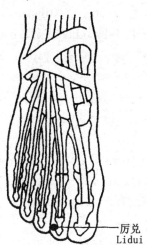

经穴名。属足阳明胃经,本经井穴。定位:在第二趾外侧,趾甲角旁约 0.1 寸处。主治:面肿口㖞,鼻衄,牙痛,咽喉肿痛,声音嘶哑,腹胀,热病等。操作:浅刺 0.1 寸;可灸。

The acupoint and the Jing-Well point belongs to the Stomach Meridian of Foot-Yangming. Location: On the lateral side of the 2nd toe, 0.1 cun posterior to the corner of the nail. Indications: Facial swelling, deviation of the mouth, epistaxis, toothache, sore throat, hoarse voice, abdominal distension, febrile disease, etc. Method: Puncture shallowly 0.1 cun. Moxibustion is applicable.

利湿 eliminate dampness-evil

用利水渗湿药物,使湿邪从小便排出的方法。

A treatment for eliminating the dampness-evil from the urine by the application of diuretics.

痢疾 dysentery

以腹痛、里急后重、大便次数增加、黏液及脓血样便为特征的一种急性肠道传染病。多因外受湿热疫毒之气，内伤饮食生冷，积滞于肠中所致。治宜清热解毒、利湿导滞。取穴：合谷、天枢、上巨虚。

An acute intestinal infectious disease marked by abdominal pain, tenesmus, and frequent defecation of bloody and mucous stools; due to attack of pestilent damp-heat evil and impairment of the intestine by cold and raw food. Treatment principle: Clear heat and toxic material, eliminate dampness and remove stagnancy. Point selection: Hegu(LI4), Tianshu (ST25), Shangjuxu(ST37).

廉 side

古代中医解剖学术语。即侧或面的意思，如上廉即上侧（上面），外廉即外侧（外面）。

An ancient anatomical term in traditional Chinese medicine meaning side or aspect. For example, Shanglian refers to the superior surface and Wailian, the lateral aspect or side.

廉泉 Lianquan(CV23)

经穴名。属任脉。定位：在喉结上方，舌骨体下缘凹陷处。主治：舌下肿痛，舌纵涎出，中风后舌强失语，暴喑，食不下等。操作：向舌根方向刺入0.5～1寸；可灸。

Name of an acupoint. It belong to the Conception Vessel. Location: Above the Adam's apple, in the depression of the lower border of the hyoid bone. Indications: Swelling and pain of the subglossal region, salivation with glossoptosis, apha-

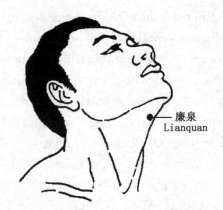

廉泉 Lianquan

sia with stiffness of tongue after apoplexy, sudden hoarseness of the voice, difficulty in swallowing, etc. Method: Puncture obliquely 0.5-1 cun towards the root of the tongue. Moxibustion is applicable.

廉洗法 pricking-rinsing therapy

用三棱针或毫针轻刺患处，然后以生理盐水冲洗，常用于结膜滤泡症。

Treatment of conjunctival folliculosis by pricking the follicles with a three-edged needle or a filiform needle, and then rinsing the wounds with physiological saline.

臁疮 ecthyma

多由湿热下注，瘀血凝滞经络所致。常继发于轻微外伤或湿疹等疾病。治宜清热利湿、活血化瘀。取穴：太渊、足三里、承山、三阴交。

A ulcerative impetigo commonly occurring on the shins, usually secondary to minor trauma or eczema; due to stagnation of blood in the meridians resulting from the attack of damp-heat evil. Treatment principle: Clear heat and eliminate dampness, promote blood circulation to remove blood stasis. Point selection: Taiyuan(LU9), Zusanli(ST36), Chengshan(BL57)，Sanyinjiao(SP6).

梁门 Liangmen(ST21)

经穴名。属足阳明胃经。定位：在脐上4寸，前正中线旁开2寸处。主治：胃痛，呕吐，食欲不振，腹胀，泄泻等。操作：直刺1～1.5寸；可灸。

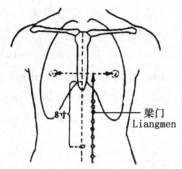

Name of an acupoint. It belongs to the Stomach Meridian of Foot-Yangming. Location：4 cun above the umbilicus，2 cun lateral to the anterior midline. Indications：Gastric pain，vomiting，anorexia，abdominal distension，diarrhea，etc. Method：Puncture perpendicularly 1-1.5 cun. Moxibustion is applicable.

梁丘 Liangqiu (ST34)

经穴名。属足阳明胃经，本经郄穴。定位：在髂前上棘与髌骨外侧缘连线上，髌骨外上缘2寸处。主治：膝痛，胃痛，乳痛，下肢不遂。操作：直刺1～1.5寸；可灸。

The acupoint and the Xi-Cleft point of the Stomach Meridian of Foot-Yangming. Location：On the line connecting anterior superior iliac spine and lateral border of the patella，2 cun above the lateral superior border of the patella. Indications：Pain of the knee，gastric pain，a-

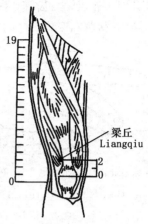

cute mastitis，motor impairment of the lower extremities，etc. Method：Puncture perpendicularly 1-1.5 cun. Moxibustion is applicable.

两衡 liangheng

指两眉之间的部位，为色诊的主要部位。

The part between the two eyebrows which is an important part for color diagnosis.

髎髎 Liaoliao

经外奇穴名。位于阴陵泉穴直下3寸处。灸治崩漏、月经不调、腿内侧风疮痒痛等。

Name of an extra point. Location：3 cun below Yinlingquan(SP9). Moxibustion is used to cure metrorrhagia and metrostaxis， irregular menstruation， itching and pains caused by wind sore on medial side of the leg，etc.

列缺 Lieque (LU7)

经穴名。属手太阴肺经，本经络穴，八脉交会穴之一，通于任脉。定位：在桡骨茎突上方，腕横纹上1.5寸。两手虎口交叉，一手示指按在另一手桡骨茎突上，指尖下凹陷处是穴。主治：头痛项强，咳嗽气喘,咽喉肿痛,面瘫,齿痛,手腕疼痛无力等。操作:斜刺 0.5～0.8 寸;可灸。

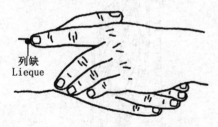

列缺
Lieque

The acupoint and the Luo-Connecting point of the Lung Meridian of Hand-Taiyin. One of the eight confluence points, communicate with the Conception Vessel. Location: Superior to the styloid process of the radius, 1.5 cun above the transverse crease of the wrist. When the index fingers and thumbs of both hands are across with the index finger of one hand placed on the styloid process of the radius of the other, it is in the depression just under the tip of the index finger. Indications: Headache, neck rigidity, cough, asthma, sore throat, facial paralysis, toothache, pain and weakness of the wrist, etc. Method: Puncture obliquely 0.5-0.8 cun. Moxibustion is applicable.

邻近选穴法 nearby point selection

于疾病所在部位附近选穴治疗。

Selecting points near the diseased area for acupuncture.

临泣 Linqi

经穴名。有二,一在头,一在足。同属胆经,为便于区分,一称头临泣,一称足临泣。

Name of acupoints. There are two of them, one is on the head, the other is on the foot, and both belong to the Gallbladder Meridian. In order to distinguish, the former is named Toulinqi (GB15) and the latter is named Zulinqi (GB41).

淋泉 Linquan

经外奇穴名。位于尾骨端尖上一口寸及左右旁开 0.5 口寸。共 3 穴,灸治淋证。

Name of extra points. Located 1 mouth-cun above the coccyx tip and 0.5 mouth-cun lateral to it. Three points in all. Moxibustion is used to cure strangury.

淋证 strangury

指以尿急、尿频、尿痛及排尿障碍淋沥不断为主症的一类病症。多因膀胱湿热或中气下陷、肾虚气化无力所致。治宜清热利湿、健脾。取穴:膀胱俞、阴陵泉、中极、行间、太溪。

A disorder characterized by frequent, difficult and painful discharge of urine, dues to accumulation of damp-heat evil in the bladder, or collapse of middle qi, or deficiency of the kidney. Treatment principle: Clear heat, eliminate dampness and strengthen the spleen. Point selection: Pangguangshu (BL28), Yinlingquan (ST9), Zhongji(CV3), Xingjian(LR2), Taixi(KI3).

灵道 Lingdao(HT4)

经穴名。属手少阴心经,本经经穴。定位:在腕横纹上 1.5 寸,尺侧腕屈肌腱的桡侧。主治:心痛,肘臂挛痛,暴喑等。操作:直刺 0.5～0.8 寸;可灸。

The acupoint and the Jing-River point

of the Heart Meridian of Hand-Shaoyin. Location: On the radial side of the tendon of the ulnar flexor muscle of the wrist, 1.5 cun above the transverse crease of the wrist.

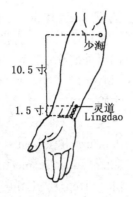

Indications: Heart pain, spasmodic pain of the elbow and arm, sudden loss of voice, etc. Method: Puncture perpendicularly 0.5-0.8 cun. Moxibustion is applicable.

灵龟八法 eight methods of the intelligent turtle

中国古代用于针灸取穴的一种学说,是以奇经八脉中的 8 个穴位配合日、时的天干、地支来决定取穴的理论。

One of the ancient theories used for selecting points in acupuncture. According to the theory, eight acupoints of the Eight Extra Vessels which are related to the day and the hour in terms of the Henvenly Stems and Earthly Branches in order to select the appropriate points.

灵枢 *Miraculous Pivot*

书名。为《黄帝内经》两大部分之一。又称《针经》,分为 24 卷、81 篇,论及九针、经络、腧穴、刺法、治疗等,是针灸学的经典著作,是研究我国战国时期医学理论和针灸学的重要文献。

A medical book also known as *Acupuncture Classic*. One of the two parts of *Huangdi's Canon of Medicine*, it is divided into 81 chapters in 24 volumes, dealing with nine classical needles, meridians and collaterals, acupoints, needling methods and therapies, etc. It is a classic of acupuncture, also an important medical literature for the study of acupuncture and medical theories of the Warring States Period.

灵台 Lingtai (GV10)

经穴名。属督脉。定位:在第六胸椎棘突下。主治:咳嗽,气喘,疔疮,背痛,项强等。操作:稍向上斜刺 0.5～1 寸;可灸。

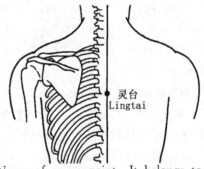

Name of an acupoint. It belongs to the Governor Vessel. Location: Below the spinous process of the 6th thoracic vertebra. Indications: Cough, asthma, furuncles, back pain, neck rigidity, etc. Method: Puncture obliquely upward 0.5-1 cun. Moxibustion is applicable.

灵墟 Lingxu (KI24)

经穴名。属足少阴肾经。定位:在第三肋间隙中,任脉旁开 2 寸处。主治:咳嗽,气喘,胸胁胀满,乳痈等。操作:斜刺或平刺 0.5～0.8 寸;可灸。

Name of an acupoint. It belongs to the Kidney Meridian of Foot-Shaoyin. Location: In the 3rd intercostal space, 2 cun

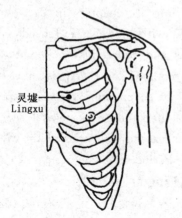

灵墟
Lingxu

lateral to the Conception Vessel. Indications: Cough, asthma, fullness in the chest and hypochondriac region, acute mastitis, etc. Method: Puncture horizontally or obliquely 0.5-0.8 cun. Moxibustion is applicable.

留针 retention of needle

指针刺入穴位后,将针留置在穴位内不动,经过一定时间后再拔针的方法。

To retain the inserted needle for a certain time.

流产 miscarriage

指妊娠妇女在胎儿成形前妊娠中断,由于气血虚弱或肝肾亏损所致。治宜补益肝肾、益气养血。取穴:关元、三阴交、肝俞、肾俞、足三里。

Interruption of pregnancy before the fetus has been formed, due to asthenia of qi and blood, or deficiency of the liver and kidney. Treatment principle: Tonify the liver and kindey, reinforce qi and nourish blood. Point selection: Guanyuan (CV4), Sanyinjiao (SP6), Ganshu (BL18), Shenshu (BL23), Zusanli (ST36).

流涎 salivation

又称流涎不收。指唾液分泌过多,常流出口外的症候。由脾热或脾胃虚寒所致。治宜健脾和中。取穴:地仓、颊车、合谷、中脘。

A sign of excessive secretion of saliva due to spleen-heat or asthenia cold of the spleen and stomach. Treatment principle: Strengthen the spleen and the stomach. Point selection: Dicang (ST4), Jiache (ST6), Hegu (LI4), Zhongwan (CV12).

流注八穴 eight influential points

即八脉八穴。

The eight crossing points of the eight extra vessels.

六腑 six fu-organs

指胆、胃、大肠、小肠、膀胱和三焦。

Referring to the gallbladder, stomach, large intestine, small intestine, urinary bladder and sanjiao.

六合 six pairs of combination

①指天地之间,上下四方为六合。②指十二经脉表里相合。③指十二经别,相互结为六对。

① The upside, the downside and the four directions between the heaven and the earth. ② The correlations between the exterior and the interior of the twelve regular meridians. ③The six correlations pairs between the twelve important branches of the twelve regular meridians.

六经 the six meridians

六类正经,即太阳经、阳明经、少阳经、太阴经、厥阴经、少阴经。

The six pairs of regular meri-dians, i. e., the Taiyang Meridians, the Yang-ming Meridians, the Shaoyang Meridi-ans, the Taiyin Meridians, the Jueyin Meridians, and the Shaoyin Meridians.

六经辨证 differentiation in accor-dance with the six meridians

外感病辨证方法之一。指据外感病传变情况将其划分为太阳病、阳明病、少阳病、太阴病、少阴病、厥阴病六种病证,作为辨证施治的提纲。

One of the methods of differentiating symptoms in exopathic diseases. Accor-ding to the transmission of the exogenous diseases, six syndromes were summed up and have been the guideline of identifying patterns and administering treatment. The six syndromes were the Taiyang dis-ease, the Yangming disease, the Shaoy-ang disease, the Taiyin disease, the Shaoyin disease, and the Jueyin disease.

六十六穴 the sixty-six points

十二经中井、荥、输、原、经、合各穴的总称,共有 66 个穴位。子午流注针法就是以此 66 穴为基础的。

The collective name of the Jing-Well points, the Xing-Spring points, the Shu-Stream points, the Yuan-Primary points, the Jing-River points and the He-Sea points of the twelve regular meridians, the midnight-noon ebb-flow doctrine in acupuncture is based on these points.

六淫 six evils

即风、寒、暑、湿、燥、火六种致病因子的合称。

A general term for the pathogenic a-gents, i. e., wind, cold, summer-heat, dampness, dryness and fire.

龙虎交战 dragon-tiger fighting

针刺手法名。龙即左转,虎即右转,左、右转反复进行称交战,左九右六,分浅、中、深三部重复进行。

Name of acupuncture manipulations. Dragon means rotating the needle left-ward while tiger means rotating the nee-dle rightward. It is called fighting be-cause the two-opposite-direction rotation is performed repeatedly and alternative-ly. The leftward rotation should be per-formed nine times while the rightward rotation six times, this can also be done in the shallow, middle and deep layers of the points repeatedly.

龙虎升降 dragon and tiger flying and diving

针刺手法名。龙虎指左右捻针;升降指气行上下。先用右手拇指向前捻针,入穴后以左手拇指向前捻针,得气后左右转针,并下按上提使气行。

Name of acupuncture manipulations. Dragon and tiger mean twisting the nee-dle leftward and rightward; flying and diving mean the movement of qi upward and downward. The needle is first twis-ted forward with the right hand thumb, then twisted forward by the left hand thumb after insertion. After the arrival of qi, the needle will be rotated leftward and rightward and will be lifted upward and thrusted downward to make qi move.

龙虎升腾 dragon and tiger rising and flying

①同龙虎升降。②在龙虎升降法上增加九六数的手法,用于气血凝滞诸证。

①The same manipulations as "dragon and tiger flying and diving". ② Nine times and six times of the manipulations are introduced into the above mentioned method to cure the various diseases of qi and blood stagnation.

龙泉 Longquan

然谷别名。又称龙渊。

The other name of Rangu (KI2), also called Longyuan.

聋哑 deaf-mutism

耳聋并口哑,多由热病后遗或先天缺陷所致。治宜通络开窍。取穴:聋取耳门、听会、听宫;哑取哑门、廉泉、通里。

A disorder resulting from the sequela of febrile diseases or congenital defect. Treatment principle:Remove obstruction in the meridians and open orifices. Point selection: Ermen (TE21), Ting-hui (GB2), Tinggong (SI19) for deafness, and Yamen(GV15), Lianquan(CV23), Tongli(HT5) for mutism.

癃闭 dysuria

指排尿困难,甚则尿闭的证候。实证多因肺气壅滞,湿热下注或瘀血、结石阻塞尿道所致;虚证多因脾肾阳虚,津液不得输化所致。实证治宜清利湿热、益气活血;虚证治宜温补脾肾、益气启闭。取穴:三阴交、阴陵泉、膀胱俞、中极、三焦俞、气海、肾俞。

Difficult urination or retention of urine caused by the stagnation of lung-qi, by the downward diffusing of damp-heat, or by the blockage of urinary tract resulting from blood stasis or stone in case of sthenia syndrome, and by the deficiency of spleen-yang and kidney-yang leading to the retention of fluid in case of asthenia syndrome. Treatment principle of excess syndrome: Clear heat and eliminate dampness, promote the qi and blood circulation. Treatment principle of deficiency syndrome: Warm and invigorate the spleen and kindey, replenish qi to promote uresis. Point selection: Sanyinjiao (SP6), Yinlingquan(SP9), Pangguangshu (BL28), Zhongji(CV3), Sanjiaoshu (BL22), Qihai(CV3), Shenshu(BL23).

漏谷 Lougu(SP7)

经穴名。属足太阴脾经。定位:在内踝尖与阴陵泉穴连线上,内踝尖上 6 寸,胫骨内侧缘后方。主治:腹胀肠鸣,膝腿厥冷、麻木不仁等。操作:直刺 0.5～0.8 寸;可灸。

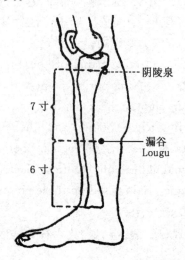

阴陵泉

7 寸

漏谷
Lougu

6 寸

Name of an acupoint. It belongs to the Spleen Meridian of Foot-Taiyin. Location:On the line connecting the tip of the medial malleolus and Yinlingquan(SP9), 6 cun above the tip of the medial malleolus, and on the posterior border of the medial aspect of the tibia. Indications: Abdominal distension, borborygmus, coldness, numbness and paralysis of the knee and leg, etc. Method:Puncture perpendicularly 0.5-0.8 cun. Moxibustion is applicable.

颅息 Luxi(TE19)

经穴名。属手少阳三焦经。定位:在翳风与角孙穴沿耳翼连线的上、中 1/3 交界处。主治:头痛,耳鸣,耳聋,耳痛,小儿惊风等。操作:平刺 0.3~0.5 寸;可灸。

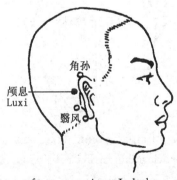

Name of an acupoint. It belongs to the Sanjiao Meridian of Hand-Shaoyang. Location:At the junction of the upper and middle third of the curve formed by Yifeng(TE17) and Jiaosun(TE20) behind the helix. Indications: Headache, tinnitus, deafness, earache, infantile convulsion, etc. Method:Puncture horizontally 0.3-0.5 cun. Moxibustion is applicable.

吕细 Lüxi

①太溪穴别名。②经外奇穴名。位于足内踝尖上,灸治牙痛。

① The other name of Taixi(KI3). ②Name of an extra point, it is located on the tip of the medial malleolus and used to cure toothache with moxibustion.

膂 paravertebral muscle of the back

部位名。指脊柱两旁的肌肉。

Name of the bodly part, i. e., the muscles lateral to the spinal column.

膂骨 paravertebral bone of the back

①椎骨之统称。②第一胸椎棘突。

① A collective term for vertebrae; ②The spinous process of the first thoracic vertebra.

轮 1-6 Helix 1-6

耳穴名。在耳轮上,自耳轮结节下缘至耳垂下缘中点划分为五等份,共 6 个点。由上而下依次为轮$_1$、轮$_2$、轮$_3$、轮$_4$、轮$_5$、轮$_6$。主治:发热,扁桃体炎,高血压。

Name of ear points. The points are at the region from the lower border of auricular tubercle to the midpoint of the lower of border of earlobe, and is divided into five equal parts. The points marking the divisions are respectively named Helix$_1$, Helix$_2$, Helix$_3$, Helix$_4$, Helix$_5$, Helix$_6$. Indications:Fever, tonsillitis, hypertension.

瘰疬 scrofula

多因肺肾阴虚,肝气久郁,虚火内灼,炼液为痰;或受风火邪毒,结于颈项、腋胯之间。初起结块如豆,无痛无热,后渐增大串生,久则微觉疼痛,或结块相互粘连,推之不移。若溃破,则脓汁稀薄,其中或夹有豆渣样物质,此愈彼起,久不收口,可形成窦道或瘘管。相当于淋巴结核或慢性淋巴结炎。治宜疏风清热、滋阴降火。取穴：曲池、支沟、肘尖、天井、少海、颈百劳。

Inflammation of the lymph nodes, dues to phlegm formation by the action of asthenic fire resulting from the deficiency of lung-yin and kidney-yin and prolonged stagnation of liver-qi, or due to exposure to wind-fire evil accumulation on the neck, armpit and hip. At first, the lymph nodes were in cluster painless and without heat, and then they adhere with each other and will not move. After a long time, the patient will feel slight pain. If the lymph nodes were broken, they will discharge thin purulent fluid containing bean-dregs like substance, and the fistula will form. It is equal to tuberculosis of lymph nodes or chronic lymphadenistis, etc. Treatment principle: Expel wind and clear heat, nourish yin to reduce pathogenic fire. Point selection: Quchi(LI11), Zhigou(TE6), Zhoujian (EX-UE1), Tianjing (TE10), Shaohai (HT3), Jingbailao(EX-HN15).

络刺 collateral puncture

九刺法之一。指用三棱针刺破皮下小血管放血。

One of the nine needling techniques, i. e., to cause bleeding by pricking the subcutaneous small blood vessels with a three-edged needle.

络脉 collateral

指经络系统中，从经脉分出的网络全身的细小分支脉络，有沟通经脉、运行气血的作用。

It referes to the branches all over the body separated from meridians, having the function of linking up meridians and circulating qi and blood.

络气 collateral qi

指行于络脉的气，与经气相对而言。

The qi moving in the collaterals, as distinguished from that moving in the meridians.

络却 Luoque(BL8)

经穴名。属足太阳膀胱经。定位：在前发际正中直上5.5寸，督脉旁开1.5寸处。主治：头晕，视物不清，耳鸣，癫狂等。操作：斜刺0.3～0.5寸；可灸。

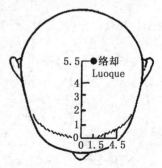

Name of an acupoint. It belongs to the Bladder Meridian of Foot-Taiyang. Location: 5.5 cun directly above the anterior hairline, 1.5 cun lateral to the Governor Vessel. Indications: Dizziness, blurred vision, tinnitus, mania, etc. Method: Puncture obliquely 0.3-0.5 cun. Moxibustion is applicable.

络穴 luo-connecting points

全身十五条大络中各有一个与经脉相联络的穴位。其中包括十四经脉发出的十四条络脉的穴位和脾脏分出的一条络脉的穴位，共十五个络穴。即：手太阴络——列缺穴；手少阴络——通里穴；手厥阴络——内关穴；手太阳络——支正穴；手阳明络——偏历穴；手少阳络——外关穴；足太阴络——公孙穴；足少阴络——大钟穴；足厥阴络——蠡沟穴；足太阳络——飞扬穴；足阳明络——丰隆穴；足少阳络——光明穴；任脉络——鸠尾穴；督脉络——长强穴；脾之大络——大包穴。

On each of the fifteen large collaterals there is one acupoint which is connected with the corresponding regular meridian. They are:For the Collateral of Hand-Taiyin—Lieque (LU7), for the Collateral of Hand-Shaoyin—Tongli (HT5), for the Collateral of Hand-Jueyin—Neiguan (PC6), for the Collateral of Hand-Taiyang—Zhizheng (SI7), for the Collateral of Hand-Yangming—Pianli (LI6), for the Collateral of Hand-Shaoyang—Waiguan (TE5), for the Collateral of Foot-Taiyin—Gongsun (SP4), for the Collateral of Foot-Shaoyin—Dazhong (KI4), for the Collateral of Foot-Jueyin—Ligou (LR5), for the Collateral of Foot-Taiyang—Feiyang (BL58), for the Collateral of Foot-Yangming—Fenglong (ST40), for the Collateral of Foot-Shaoyang—Guangming (GB37), for the Collateral of the Conception Vessel—Jiuwei (CV15), for the Collateral of the Governor Vessel—Changqiang (GV1), and for the Large Collateral of Spleen Meridian—Dabao (SP21).

M

马王堆汉墓帛书 brocade literatures unearthed from Mawangdui Tomb of the Han Dynasty

文献名。1973 年长沙马王堆汉墓出土大量帛书,其中有很多医学文献,抄写年代约在秦汉之际。

Name of literatures. In 1973, a large number of literatures including plenty of medical literatures were unearthed from Mawangdui Tomb of the Han Dynasty near Changsha. The literatures were copied roughly at the time of the transition from the Qin Dynasty to the Han Dynasty.

埋线法 suture-embedding therapy

指在无菌操作下,把羊肠线埋入一定的穴位中治疗疾病的方法。

With sterile manipulation, a length of catgut is embedded subcutaneously in a certain acupoint for therapeutic purposes.

埋针法 needle-embedding therapy

将特制的针刺入穴位内,用胶布封固后,留置较长时间的治疗方法。

Embedment and fixation of a needle in a point by adhesive plaster for a considerable period of time for therapeutic purposes.

麦粒灸 moxibustion with wheat grain-sized moxa cone

用麦粒大小的艾炷施行的灸法,即小炷灸。在某些部位,如头面部,需用此种灸法。

Certain parts of the human body, such as head and face, should be moxibusted with small moxa cones like wheat grains.

脉冲电刺激 electric-impulse stimulation

指运用电脉冲刺激穴位。

Stumulation of an acupoint with electric impulse.

脉度 measurement of meridians

经脉长短的度数,是古人测定人体经脉长度的一种数据记录。

Measuring and recording the lengths of meridians practised in ancient times.

脉会 influential point of vessels

即太渊穴。八会穴之一。

Taiyuan(LU9), one of the eight influential points.

芒针 elongated needle

针具名。取法于古代长针,近来用不锈钢制造,针身细长犹如麦芒,长可达 15 寸,用于深刺和皮下横刺。

A kind of needle derived from the ancient long needle. Recently this kind of needle is made of stainless steel, thin and long like the awn of wheat, the longest being 15 cun is used for deep acupuncture or subcutaneous horizontal acupuncture.

盲肠穴 Mangchangxue

经外奇穴名。位于髂前上棘与脐的连线中点。直刺或灸治肠痈、腹泻等。

Name of an extra point. Located at the midpoint of the line between the navel and the anterior superior iliac spine, perpendicular acupuncture or moxibustion is used to cure acute appendicitis, diarrhea, etc.

毛刺 shallow puncture

九刺法之一。指用短的毫针浅刺皮肤。

One of the nine needling techniques to puncture the skin superficially with a short filiform needle.

毛际 pubic margin

部位名，下腹部阴毛的边际。

A part of the body, referring to the margin of the pubic hair in the lower abdomen.

髦针 mao needle

即圆利针。古代九针之一。

The round-sharp needle, one of the nine classic needles in ancient times.

眉冲 Meichong(BL3)

经穴名。属足太阳膀胱经。定位：在攒竹穴直上，入发际 0.5 寸处。主治：头痛，眩晕，鼻塞等。操作：斜刺 0.3～0.5 寸；可灸。

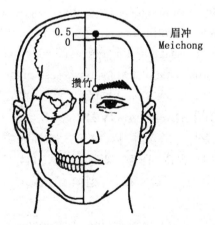

Name of an acupoint. It belongs to the Bladder Meridian of Foot-Taiyang. Location：Directly above Cuanzhu(BL2), 0.5 cun within the anterior hairline. Indica-tions：Headache, dizziness, nasal obstru-ction, etc. Method：Puncture obliquely 0.3-0.5 cun. Moxibustion is applicable.

眉枕线 eyebrow-occipital line

指眉中点上缘沿头侧部至枕外粗隆顶点下缘的连线。

It is the line connecting the upper margin of the midpoint of the eyebrow with the lower border of the external occipital tuberosity along the lateral aspect of the skull.

梅花针 plum-blossom needle

皮肤针的一种。又名七星针，针头由 5 或 7 枚水平排列的细针组成，用以叩击浅刺皮肤。

A kind of dermal needles. Also named seven-star needle. The tip is made of 5 or 7 needles arranged at the same level and is used to peck and prick the skin shal-lowly.

梦遗 nocturnal emission

指因梦交而遗精的证候。多因感情上的刺激，相火妄动或心火亢盛所致。治宜清心降火、滋阴涩精。取穴：心俞、肾俞、关元、神门、中封。

Involuntary discharge of semen during sleep, dues to hyperactivity of ministerial fire or heart-fire resulting from emotional irritation. Treatment principle：Clear heart-fire, nourish yin and astringe spermatorrhea. Point selection：Xinshu（BL15）, Shenshu（BL23）, Guanyuan（CV4）, Shenmen（HT7）, Zhongfeng(LR4).

面颊 Mianjia

耳穴名。在耳垂部眼穴的后上方。主治:面瘫,三叉神经痛,痤疮等。

Name of an ear point. It is on the ear lobe, at posterior and superior aspect of Yan. Indications: Facial paralysis, trigeminal neuralgia, acne, etc.

面王 Mianwang

素髎穴别名。

The other name of Suliao(GV25).

面针 facial acupuncture

将面部分为一定的区域进行针刺治疗疾病的方法。

The face is divided into several zones and acupuncture is performed in a certain zone to treat its related disease.

面针疗法 facial acupunture therapy

近代针刺疗法之一。针刺面部特定穴位,以治疗身体他处疾患。面部穴位与身体特定部位相关联。

Recently developed technique in which specific points on the face are needled to treat disorders elsewhere in the body. Relationship have been found between these points on the face and specific parts of the body.

胁 abdomen below hypochondrium

部位名。即腰侧,当胁肋与髂嵴之间的空软处。

Name of a body part. It is the soft space between lateral thorax and illiac crest. i. e. , the lateral side of the waist.

明灸 bright moxibustion

即直接灸。

The direct moxibustion.

明堂 bright hall

①古代帝王执政之堂。②指鼻部,因其位于面中央。③指有关针灸经穴的图书和模型。④指上星穴。

① The great hall of China ancient emperor's office. ②The nose, because it is situated at the center of the face. ③All the literatures and models about acupuncture, moxibustion, meridians and acupoints. ④Shangxing (GV23).

命关 Mingguan

①经外奇穴名。位于乳头直下,平脐上4寸处。灸治腹胀、水肿、小便不通、气喘、平卧呕吐反胃、痢疾、大便失禁等。②小儿按摩诊断用穴,指示指末节的掌侧横纹处。

①Name of an extra point. Located directly below the nipple, 4 cun above the level of navel. Moxibustion is used to cure abdominal distention, edema, difficult urination, asthma, vomiting and regurgitation when lying flat, dysentery, fecal incontinence, etc. ②Point for infantile massage and diagnosis, located at the palmar side of transverse crease of the index finger's final phalanx.

命门 Mingmen(GV4)

经穴名。属督脉,在第二腰椎棘突下。主治:腰痛,脊强,阳痿,遗精,月经不调,泄泻,带下等。操作:稍向上斜刺0.5～1寸;可灸。

Name of an acupoint. It belongs to the Governor Vessel. Located below the spinous process of the second lumbar vertebra. Indications: Lumbago, stiffness of the back, impotence, nocturnal emis-

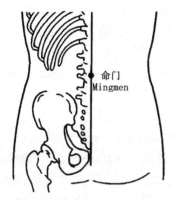

命门
Mingmen

sion，irregular menstration，lekorrhea，etc. Method：Puncture obliquely upward 0.3-0.5 cun. Moxibustion is applicable.

缪刺 contralateral puncture

古代刺法之一,左病刺右,右病刺左。现在以浅刺井穴和体表瘀血的络脉为主。

One of the ancient acupuncture techniques. The technique originally involved needling points contralateral to the disorder side of the body. Presently contralateral puncture is practiced by superficially puncturing Jing-Well points and small superficial veins with blood stasis.

摩法 palm-rubbing technique

按摩手法。用手掌紧贴皮肤做环形活动的治疗方法。

Rubbing the affected part in a circular motion with the palm pressing tightly against the skin as a therapeutic method.

抹法 wiping manipulation

按摩手法。用拇指指腹或手掌面紧贴皮肤,略用力做上下或左右缓慢的往返移动,有疏气活血作用。

A manipulation of massage, performed by rubbing the skin with the palmar side of the operator's thumbs or the palms up and down or right and left with moderate force to promote flow of qi and blood.

拇指寸 thumb cun

取穴比例寸之一。以拇指指间关节的宽度为 1 寸。

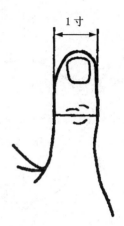

1 寸

One of the proportional measurement units for locating points, i. e., the width of the interphalangeal joint of the thumb is taken as 1 cun.

踇趾里横纹 Muzhilihengwen

经外奇穴名。位于踇趾掌侧横纹中点处。直刺或灸治疝气。

Name of an extra point. Located at the midpoint of the palmar transverse crease of the big toe. Vertical acupuncture or moxibustion is used to cure hernia.

目₁ Mu 1

耳穴名。在耳垂前面,屏间切迹前下方。主治:青光眼,假性近视等。

Name of an ear point. Located in the anterior earlobe, on posterior and inferior side of intertragic notch. Indications：Glaucoma, pseudomyopia, etc.

目₂ Mu 2

耳穴名。在耳垂前面,屏间切迹后下方。主治:散光、假性近视等。

Name of an ear point. Located in the anterior earlobe, on anterior and inferior side of intertragic notch. Indications：Astigmatism, pseudomyopia, etc.

目窗 Muchuang(GB16)

经穴名。属足少阳胆经。定位:在头部,前发际上 1.5 寸,头正中线旁开 2.25 寸。主治:头痛,眩晕,目赤痛,鼻塞等。操作:平刺 0.3~0.8 寸;可灸。

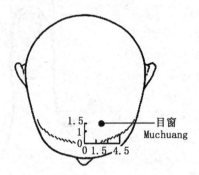

Name of an acupoint. It belongs to the Gallbladder Meridian of Foot-Shaoyang. Location:On the head, 1.5 cun above the anterior hairline, 2.25 cun lateral to the midline of the head. Indications:Headache, vertigo, red and painful eyes, nasal obstruction, etc. Method:Puncture horizontally 0.3-0.8 cun. Moxibustion is applicable.

目寸 eye cun

奇穴取穴的比量法之一。系以患者本人的内眼角至外眼角的距离作为 1 寸。

One of the proportional measurement for locating extra point, i. e. , taking the distance between the internal and external canthus of the patient as 1 cun.

目干涩 eye dryness

眼结膜干涩不适的一种症状,可由肺阴不足或肝肾阴虚所致。治宜补益肝肾。取穴:睛明、合谷、三阴交、照海。

A symptom characterized by dryness of the conjunctiva, dues to defficiency of lung-yin or asthenia of the liver-yin and kidney-yin. Treatment principle:Tonify the liver and kindey. Point selection:Jingming(BL1), Hegu(LI4), Sanyinjiao(SP6), Zhaohai(KI6).

目昏 Blurred vision

视物模糊不清的症状。多因脏腑精气虚损、不能上注于目所致。治宜补益肝肾。取穴:睛明、足三里、肝俞、肾俞。

A symptom caused by the consumption of visceral essential qi which fail to nourish the eyes. Treatment principle:Tonify the liver and kindey. Point selection:Jingming(BL1), Zusanli(ST36), Ganshu(BL18), Shenshu(BL23).

目窠 eye orbit

眼的凹陷处,容纳眼球的地方。

The depression for the eyeballs.

目上纲 upper eye outline

又名目上弦。指上眼睑的边缘部。

It refers to the margin of the upper eyelid.

目系 eye system

又名目本。指眼球连于脑的脉络,即今之视神经、血管。

Also named the root of the eyes. Referring to the ocular nerve and blood vessels by which the eyes and brain connect.

目下纲 lower eye outline

又名目下弦。指下眼睑的边缘部。

It refers to the margin of the lower eyelid.

目痒 eye itching

由风火、湿热或血虚引起。以眼结膜奇

痒为主证。治宜祛风清热。取穴：太冲、太阳、合谷、风池。

A symptom characterized by intense itching of the conjunctiva, caused by the attack of wind-fire or damp-heat evil, or by blood deficiency. Treatment principle: Dispel wind to clear heat. Point selection: Taichong (LR3), Taiyang (EX-HN5), Hegu(LI4), Fengchi(GB20).

目眦 canthus

即眼角。是上下眼睑连结的部位。

The angle at either end of the fissure between the eyelids.

募穴 Front-Mu points

指脏腑经气汇聚于胸腹部的一类特定穴，与脏腑的生理、病理反应密切相关。即肺募——中府穴；心募——巨阙穴；肝募——期门穴；脾募——章门穴；肾募——京门穴；心包募——膻中穴；胆募——日月穴；胃募——中脘穴；大肠募——天枢穴；小肠募——关元穴；三焦募——石门穴；膀胱募——中极穴。

A kind of specific points located on the chest and abdomen where the qi of the zang-fu organs infuses. They are reflect the physiologic and pathologic changes of the viscera. They are: Zhongfu(LU1), Front-Mu point of the lung; Juque(CV14), Front-Mu point of the heart; Qimen (LR14), Front-Mu point of the liver; Zhangmen (LR13), Front-Mu point of the spleen; Jingmen (GB25), Front-Mu point of the kidney; Danzhong(CV17), Front-Mu point of the pericardium; Riyue(GB24), Front-Mu point of the gallbladder; Zhongwan (CV12), Front-Mu point of the stomach; Tianshu (ST25), Front-Mu point of the large intestine; Guanyuan(CV4), Front-Mu point of the small intestine; Shimen(CV5), Front-Mu point of Sanjiao, and Zhongji (CV3), Front-Mu point of the urinary bladder.

募原 Muyuan

①指膏之原（鸠尾）和肓之原（气海）。②概指病邪蕴结之处。

①Jiuwei (CV15) and Qihai (CV6). ② The location where evils accumulate.

N

拿法 grasping manipulation

操作者用一手或两手提拿患处肌肉加以压挤,或提后迅速放手的一种按摩手法。

A massage maneuver by lifting and squeezing or lifting and rapidly releasing the affected muscles with one or both hands of the operator.

纳干法 method of combining the Heavenly Stems

子午流注针法内容之一。指十二经配合十天干以按时取穴。

One of the contents of the midnight-noon and ebb-flow correlated method, i. e., the combination of the 10 Heavenly Stems with the 12 meridians to select points according to the calculated time.

纳气法 qi-keeping method

针刺手法名。即先按九六数紧按慢提,得气后,将针尖斜对病痛处,使气上行,然后将针直起,向下按纳,不使气回流。

A term of acupuncture manipulation, i. e., first, quickly thrust and slowly lift the needle by six or nine times, after arrival of qi, make the needle tip oblique to the diseased part to make qi move upwards, finally, lift the needle upright and press it downward to avoid reflux of qi.

纳支法 method of combining the earthly branches

子午流注针法内容之一。指十二经配合十二地支按时取穴。

One of the contents of the midnight-noon and ebb-flow correlated method, i. e., the combination of the 12 Earthly Branches with the 12 meridians to select points according to the calculated time.

难产 difficult labour

在分娩过程中,胎儿难以产出,可因产道狭窄、胎位不正、胎儿过大或宫缩无力等引起。治宜理气行血、调气催产。取穴:合谷、三阴交、独阴、至阴。

Difficult childbirth, caused by deformaties of the birth canal, abnormities of position or size of the fetus, or uterine inertia, etc. Treatment principle: Regulate qi and circulate blood, tonify qi to promote labor. Point selection: Hegu (LI4), Sanyinjiao (SP6), Duyin (EX-LE11), Zhiyin(BL67).

难经 *Classic of Difficult Issues*

为中医重要古籍之一。作者名佚,托名秦越人,撰于秦汉之际。本书以问答形式阐述《内经》的医学难题。

An important medical classic which appeared around the Qin and Han Dynasty, with its authorship ascribed to Qin Yueren. Its real author is unkown. The book is arranged in catechism dealing mainly with medical problems in *Huangdi's Canon of Medicine*.

难经集注 *The Variorum of Classic of Difficult Issues*

宋代王惟一编撰,明代王九思等编辑,为《难经》现存最早的集注本。

The earliest variorum on *Classic of Difficult Issues*, compiled by Wang

Weiyi in the Song Dynasty and edited by Wang Jiusi in the Ming Dynasty.

脑 brain

奇恒之腑之一。中医认为脑的生长发育及正常功能与肾精有密切关系,是主管人的高级神经活动的极其重要的器官,其功能也与心、肝有关。

One of the extraordinary fu-organs. It is considered that its growth and normal function bear a close relation to the kidney essence. The brain is a vital organ of human body and serves as the center controlling the mental activities. Its function is also related to the heart and liver.

脑户 Naohu(GV17)

经穴名。属督脉。定位:后发际正中直上 2.5 寸,风府穴直上 1.5 寸,枕骨粗隆上缘凹陷处。主治:癫病,头晕,项强等。操作:平刺 0.5~1 寸;可灸。

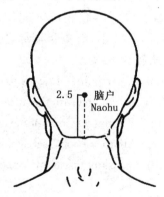

Name of an acupoint. It belongs to the Governor Vessel. Location: 2.5 cun directly above the midpoint of the posterior hairline, 1.5 cun directly above Fengfu (GV16), in the depression of the u-pper border of the occipital protuberance. Indications: epilepsy, dizziness, stiff neck,

etc. Method: Puncture horizontally 0.5-1 cun. Moxibustion is applicable.

脑空 Naokong(GB19)

经穴名。属足少阳胆经。定位:在头部,枕外隆突的上缘外侧,头正中线旁开 2.25 寸,与脑户穴相平处。主治:头痛项强,眩晕,眼痛,耳鸣,癫痫等。操作:平刺 0.3~0.5 寸;可灸。

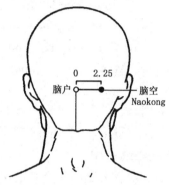

Name of an acupoint. It belongs to the Gallbladder Meridian of Foot-Shaoyang. Location: On the head, lateral to the upper border of external occipital protuberance, 2.25 cun lateral to the midline of the head, at the level with Naohu(GV17). Indications: Headache, stiff neck, vertigo, painful eyes, tinnitus, epilepsy, etc. Method: Puncture horizontally 0.3-0.5 cun. Moxibustion is applicable.

臑 nao

部位名。指上臂。

Name of the body part, i. e., the upper arm.

臑会 Naohui(TE13)

经穴名。属手少阳三焦经。定位:在臂外侧,当肩髎穴与天井穴连线上,肩髎穴下 3 寸,当三角肌的后下缘。主治:瘿气,肩臂痛等。操作:直刺 0.8～1.2 寸;可灸。

Name of an acupoint. It belongs to the Sanjiao Meridian of Hand-Shaoyang. Location:On the lateral side of the arm, 3 cun below Jianliao(TE14), on the line connecting Jianliao(TE14) and Tianjing (TE10), at the posterior and inferior border of the deltoid muscle. Indications: Goiter, pain in the shoulder and arm, etc. Method: Puncture perpendicularly 0.8-1.2 cun. Moxibustion is applicable.

臑交 Naojiao

臑会穴别名。

The other name of Naohui (TE13).

臑俞 Naoshu(SI10)

经穴名。属手太阳小肠经。定位:当上臂内收,从肩贞穴直上,在肩胛冈下缘凹陷中。主治:肩肿,肩臂痛无力等。操作:直刺 1～1.5 寸;可灸。

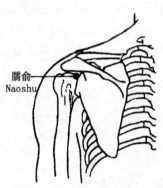

臑俞
Naoshu

Name of an acupoint. It belongs to the Small Intestine Meridian of Hand-Taiyang. Location:When the arm is adducted, the point is directly above Jianzhen (SI9), in the depression inferior to the scapular spine. Indications: Swelling of the shoulder, aching and weekness of the shoulder and arm, etc. Method:Puncture perpendicularly 1-1.5 cun. Moxibustion is applicable.

内鼻 Neibi

耳穴名。在耳屏内侧面下 1/2 处。主治:过敏性鼻炎、上颌窦炎、鼻衄等。

Name of an ear point. Location:At the lower half of medial aspect of tragus. Indications: Allergic thinitis, maxillary sinusitis, epistaxis, etc.

内耳 Neier

耳穴名。在耳垂 6 区。主治:内耳性眩晕、耳鸣、听力减退等。

Name of an ear point. Location:In the area 6 of the ear lobe. Indications:Auditory vertigo, tinnitus, impaired hearing, etc.

内分泌 Neifenmi

耳穴名。在耳甲腔底部屏间切迹内。主治:痛经,月经不调,更年期综合征,间日疟,皮肤病,阳痿等。

Name of an ear point. Location:At the base of cavum conchae in the intertragic notch. Indications:Dysmenorrhea, irregular menstruation, menopausal syndromes, tertian malaria, skin diseases, impotence, etc.

内关 Neiguan(PC6)

经穴名。属手厥阴心包经。本经络穴,八脉交会穴之一,通于阴维脉。定位:在腕横纹上 2 寸,掌长肌腱与桡侧腕屈肌腱之间。主治:心痛,心悸,胸闷,胁痛,胃痛,恶心,呕吐,呃逆,癫狂痫,失眠,热病,烦躁,疟疾,臂肘挛痛等。操作:直刺

0.5~1寸;可灸。

The acupoint and the Luo-Connecting point of the Pericardium Meridian of Hand-Jueyin. One of the eight confluence points, communicate with the Yin Link Vessel. Location: 2

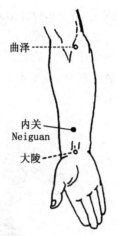

曲泽

内关
Neiguan

大陵

cun above the transverse crease of the wrist, between the tendons of the long palmar muscle and radial flexor muscle of the wrist. Indications: Cardiac pain, palpitation, stuffy chest, pain in the hypochondriac region, stomachache, nausea, vomiting, hiccup, manic and depressive psychosis, epilepsy, insomnia, malaria, spasm and pain of the elbow and arm, etc. Method: Puncture perpendicularly 0.5-1 cun. Moxibustion is applicable.

内筋 Neijin

交信穴别名。

The other name of Jiaoxin (KI8).

内经 *Canon of Medicine*

①《黄帝内经》的简称。②指内行于脏腑的经脉,与外行于肢节的经脉相对而言。

① Abbreviated name of *Huangdi's Canon of Medicine*. ② The meridians moving into the internal organs, as contrasted with the meridians moving into the extremities and joints.

内睛明 Neijingming

经外奇穴名。位于目内眦之泪埠上。沿眶内侧壁直刺0.5~1寸深,勿捻转提插。主治:目赤肿痛、视力模糊、视神经萎缩、视网膜出血等。

Name of an extra point. Located on the lacrimal caruncle of medial canthus. It can be punctured perpendicularly to the depth of 0.5-1 cun close to the medial orbital side, but twisting, twirling, lifting and thrusting manipulations are prohibited. Indications: Redness, swelling and pain of the eyes, blurred vision, optical nerve atrophy, retinal bleeding, etc.

内灸 internal moxibustion

指吞服生大蒜的疗法。

A kind of therapy by swallowing fresh gralic.

内昆仑 Neikunlun

①太溪穴别名。②经外奇穴名,位于内踝后五分。

① The other name of Taixi (KI3). ②Name of the extra point located 0.5 cun behind the medial ankle.

内龙眼 Neilongyan

经外奇穴名。即内膝眼。位于膝关节髌骨内侧下缘凹陷处。主治膝关节炎及周围软组织炎。治疗常用针斜刺。

Name of the extra point, i. e., Neixiyan, located at the depression near the medial inferior margin of the patella. Main indications are knee arthritis and the soft tissue inflammation around the knees, using oblique needling.

内庭 Neiting(ST44)

经穴名。属足阳明胃经,本经荥穴。定位:在足背第二、三趾间,趾蹼缘后方,赤白

肉际处。主
治：牙痛，面
痛，口㖞，咽喉
肿痛，鼻衄，胃
痛，吐酸，腹胀
泄泻，痢疾，便
秘，足背肿痛，
热病 等。操
作：直刺 0.3～
0.5寸；可灸。

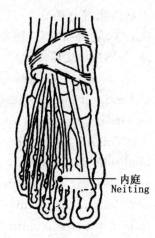

内庭
Neiting

The acu-
point and the Xing-Spring point of the
Stomach Meridian of Foot-Yangming.
Location：Posterior to the web margin between the second and third toes, at the
junction of the dorso-ventral boundary of
the foot. Indications：Toothache, pain in
the face, deviation of the mouth, sore
throat, epistaxis, gastric pain, acid regurgitation, abdominal distension, diarrhea, dysentery, constipation, swelling
and pain of the dorsum of the foot, febrile
diseases, etc. Method：Puncture perpendicularly 0.3-0.5 cun. Moxibustion is applicable.

内阳池 Neiyangchi

经外奇穴名。位于掌后横纹大陵穴上 1
寸。主治：口腔炎，咽喉痛，小儿惊风等。
治疗常用直刺或灸治。

Name of an extra point. Location：A-
bove the transverse crease of the wrist, 1
cun above Daling（PC7）. Indications：
Stomatitis, sore throat, infantile convulsion, etc. , by perpendicular acupuncture
or moxibustion.

内迎香 Neiyingxiang（EX-HN9）

经外奇穴名。位于鼻孔内，当鼻翼软骨
与鼻甲交界的黏膜处。主治：目赤肿痛，
鼻痒鼻塞，咽喉肿痛，中暑，头痛等。点刺
出血。

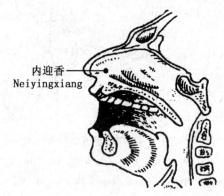

内迎香
Neiyingxiang

Name of an extra point. Location：On
the mucosa in the nostril, at the junction
between the alar cartilage of the nose and
the nasal bone. Indications：Redness,
swelling and pain of the eyes, nasal itching and stuffiness, sore throat, sunstroke, headache, etc. , by pricking to let
out blood.

内至阴 Neizhiyin

经外奇穴名。位于足小趾内侧，甲根脚
旁约 0.1 寸，与至阴穴内外相对。主治：
小儿惊风，晕厥等。治疗常用直刺或三棱
针点刺出血。

Name of an extra point. Located at the
medial side of the small toe, 0.1 cun a-
way from the corner of the nail just opposite Zhiyin（BL67）on the lateral side.
Main indications are infantile convulsion,
syncope, etc, using perpendicular acupuncture or letting out blood with a
three-edged needle.

泥丸宫 palace

①指脑部。②指百会穴。

①The cerebral part. ②Baihui (GV20).

逆灸 preventing moxbustion

指无病而灸,以预防疾病和增强抗病能力。

A kind of moxibustion not to cure but to prevent diseases and increase body's resistance to disease.

腻苔 greasy fur

苔质颗粒细腻而致密,边薄中厚,紧贴舌面,刮之不易脱落。多见于湿浊困阻于内或消化不良及痰饮内阻的疾病。

It refers to that the papillae of the tongue fur are greasy and dense, which are thick in the center while thin at the edge and can't be scraped off easily, usually seen in case of dampness-evil or phlegm, or dyspepsia.

捻法 holding and twisting

推拿手法。用拇指和示指捏住一定部位[主要是指(趾)小关节和浅表皮肤]做捻线状揉搓,以疏通关节,使气血畅通。

A manipulation of massage by holding a digital or toe joint or the skin with the thumb and the index finger and twisting it as if twisting a thread, used to relieve rigidity of joints and ensure natural flow of qi and blood.

捻针 twirling of the needle

将针刺入体内后进行捻转的方法。

One of the acupuncture techniques, i. e. , to twirl the needle after it has been inserted into the body.

捻转补泻 twirling supplementation and draining

针刺补泻方法,右手持针,左转行补法,即捻转时拇指向前,示指向后;右转行泻法,即捻转时示指向前,拇指向后。

A reinforcing-reducing method of acupuncture. Hold the needle with the right hand, twirling it left with the thumb moving forward and index finger backward is "supplementation", while twirling the needle right with the thumb moving backward and index finger forward is "draining".

捻转法 twirling method

针刺入穴位后,将针转动的手法,又称捻针。

A manipulaiton of acupuncture by twirling the needle after insertion, also named twirling of the needle.

捻转进针 twirling insertion

进针法之一。保持针身挺直,以手指小幅度捻转可快速进针,减少透皮时的疼痛。

One of the inserting methods, i. e. , holding the needle upright and twirling the needle in a small range to insert it quickly to diminish the pain when the needle passes through the skin.

尿道 Niaodao

耳穴名。在与对耳轮下脚下缘相对的耳轮处。主治:尿频、尿急、尿痛、尿潴留。

Name of an ear point. It is on helix, at the level with the lower border of inferior antihelix. Indications: Frequent, urgent and painful urination, retention of urine.

尿血 hematuria

指小便中混有血液。因阴虚火旺者,症见尿血鲜红,腰腿酸软、耳鸣眼花、心烦口干、舌质红、脉细数;脾肾两亏者,症见尿血淡红、面色萎黄、饮食减少、腰酸肢冷、舌质淡、脉虚软。治宜养阴清热、降火止血。取穴:关元、阴谷、太溪、大敦。

Blood in the urine. If it is due to deficiency of yin with hyperactivity of fire, it is manifested as bright red blood in the urine, soreness of the loins and legs, tinnitus, dizziness, restlessness, thirst, reddish tongue, and thin, rapid pulse. If it is due to asthenia of both the spleen and the kidney, it is manifested as pink blood in the urine, sallow complexion, loss of appetite, lumbago, cold limbs, pale tongue, and weak, soft pulse. Treatment principle: Nourish yin, remove heat and reduce pathogenic fire to stop bleeding. Point selection: Guanyuan (CV4), Yingu(KI10), Taixi(KI3), Dadun(LR1).

尿血穴 Niaoxue point

经外奇穴名。位于第七胸椎棘突旁开5寸。斜刺或灸治尿血。

Name of an extra point. Location: 5 cun lateral to the 7th spinous process of thoracic vertebra. Oblique acupuncture or moxibustion is used to treat hematuria.

捏骨疗法 spine pinching method

用手指捏小儿脊肌以治疗疳积的方法。

A method of treating infantile malnutrition by pinching or massaging the muscles along the spine.

颞 Nie

耳穴名。又名太阳。在对耳屏外侧面的中部,额与枕穴之间。主治偏头痛。

Name of an ear point. The other name of this point is Taiyang. It is in the centre of the lateral aspect of antitragus, between E and Zhen, and used for treating migraine.

颞颥 temple

眼眶的外后方颧骨弓上方的部位。

The region on either side of the head above the zygomatic arch.

牛皮癣 psoriasis

因风、湿、热毒蕴于肌肤所致的苔藓样皮肤病。皮损初起为大小不等的扁平丘疹,呈淡褐色,逐渐融合成片,呈苔藓样改变,干燥肥厚,有阵发性奇痒。病程呈慢性经过,其发作与精神因素有关,类似于神经性皮炎。治宜疏风、清热、利湿。取穴:阴陵泉、太白、太渊、风池、阿是穴。

A lichenoid dermatosis caused by stagnation of wind, dampness and heat-evils in the muscle and skin. At onset, the lesions appear as brownish papules of various sizes, which coalesce together gradually to form dry, thick and itchy lichenoid patches. The course of the disease is prolonged and its outbreak is related to emotional upsets. Treatment principle: Dispel wind, clear heat and promote diuresis. Point selection: Yinlingquan (SP9), Taibai(SP3), Taiyuan(LU9), Fengchi (GB20), Ashi points.

女膝 Nüxi

经外奇穴名。别名女须。定位:位于足

后跟，当根骨之中点处。主治：吐泻、足痛、齿龈炎、精神病等。治疗常用直刺或灸治。

Name of an extra point. The other name of it is Nüxu. Location：On the heel，at the center of the heel bone. Perpendicular acupuncture or moxibustion is usually used for treating vomiting，diarrhea，gingivitis，mental diseases，etc.

女子胞 uterus

奇恒之腑之一。包括女性整个生殖系统，主管月经、受孕及胎儿发育，与心、肝、脾、肾等有密切关系。

One of the extraordinary fu-organs. It controlls the menstruation，pregnancy and the growth of the fetus and bears a close relation to the heart，liver，spleen and kidney.

衄血 hemorrhage

①非外伤所致的某些外部出血的证候，如眼衄、耳衄、鼻衄、齿衄、舌衄、肌衄等。②指鼻出血。

①Bleeding not due to injury，such as bleeding from the eye，ear，nose，tooth，tongue，muscle，etc. ②Referring especially to epistaxis.

疟疾 malaria

阵发性寒战、高热、出汗为特征的一种疾病。治宜祛邪截疟、和解表里。取穴：丘墟、陶道、液门、曲池、间使。

A disease characterized by paroxysms of chills，high fever，and sweating. Treatment principle：Eliminate malarial pathogen to prevent reoccurrence of malaria，regulate the interior and exterior. Point selection：Qiuxu（GB40），Taodao（GV13），Yemen（TE2），Quchi（LI11），Jianshi（PC5）.

D

呕吐 vomiting

饮食、痰涎从胃中上涌自口而出，因胃失和降、胃气上逆所致。治宜疏肝和胃。取穴：上脘、阳陵泉、太冲、梁丘、神门。

Throwing up of food and sputum from the stomach through the mouth; due to adverse rising of the stomach-qi resulting from the dysfunction of the stomach. Treantment principle: Dispersing stagnated liver-qi for regulating stomach. Point selection: Shangwan (CV13), Yanglingquan(GB34), Taichong (LR3), Liangqiu(ST34), Shenmen(HT7).

偶刺 coupled needling

十二刺法之一。用于治疗心痹（心胸痛）。方法是在疼痛的前胸和后背部相对应的部位用手按住，前后各斜刺一针。但要防止直刺和深刺，以免伤及内脏。

One of the twelve needling techniques used for treating precordial pain (angina pectoris). It consists of palpating the painful areas on the chest and the corresponding area on the back, puncturing these areas obliquely with one needle each, but care must be taken to avoid perpendicular and deep puncture causing damages to the viscera.

P

排罐法 multiple cupping in alignment

拔罐疗法之一。在一个较大治疗面积上同时吸拔数个火罐以增加疗效。常用于较大范围的软组织病变,如腰肌劳损、肩背疼痛等。

A form of cupping therapy for treating soft tissue diseases of large area such as injury of the back muscles, back and shoulder pain, by applying a number of cups on the affected area.

盘法 circular turning method

针刺手法名。浅刺皮下后,针身倾斜,将针柄做圆周形盘转,主要用于腹部,左盘按针为补,右盘提针为泻。

Name of an acupuncture manipulation. After inserting the needle shallowly into the skin, slightly bend the needle and turn the needle handle in circles, turning the needle left and thrusting after is reinforcing method; turning the needle right and lifting after is educing method. The technique is mostly used on the abdomen.

旁廷 Pangting

经外奇穴名。定位:在腋下四肋间,与乳平。斜刺或灸治胸胁胀满、呕吐、喘逆、咽干、胁痛等。

Name of an extra point. Location: At the 4th intercostal space below the armpit, at the same level as the nipple. Oblique acupuncture or moxibustion is used to cure fullness in chest and hypochondri-um, vomiting, asthma, dry throat, hypochondriac pain, etc.

膀胱 bladder; Pangguang

①六腑之一。位于盆腔的前方,它的功能是贮藏和排泄尿液。②耳穴名。在对耳轮下脚的下缘,大肠穴直上方。主治:遗尿,尿潴留,坐骨神经痛,腰痛,膀胱炎等。

①One of the six fu-organs, located at the anterior part of the pelvic cavity with the function of storing and discharging urine. ②Name of an ear point. It is on the lower border of the inferior antihelix crus, directly above Dachang. Indicaitons: Enuresis, retention of urine, sciatica, lumbargo, cystitis, etc.

膀胱经 Bladder Meridian

足太阳膀胱经的简称。

Abbreviation of the Bladder Meridian of Foot-Taiyang.

膀胱俞 Pangguangshu (BL28)

经穴名。属足太阳膀胱经,膀胱背俞穴。定位:平第二骶后孔,后正中线旁开1.5寸处。主治:小便不利,遗尿,尿频,泄泻,便秘,腰脊强痛等。操作:直刺0.8～1.5寸;可灸。

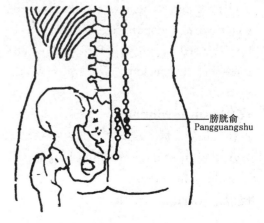

膀胱俞
Pangguangshu

Name of an acupoint. It belongs to the Bladder Meridian of Foot-Taiyang. It is the Back-Shu point of the bladder. Location: 1. 5 cun lateral to the posterior midline, at the same level as the second posterior sacral foramen. Indications: Retention of urine, enuresis, frequent urination, diarrhea, constipation, stiffness and pain of the lower back and spine, etc. Method: Puncture perpendicularly 0. 8-1. 5 cun. Moxibustion is applicable.

配穴 adjunct acupuncture points

指针刺配方中起辅助治疗作用的穴位。

The auxiliary points in a prescription of acupuncture.

配穴法 point prescription

针灸治疗时,穴位相互配合的方法。

Method of selecting related points to be used in combination during acupuncture treatment.

铍针 sword-like needle

古代九针之一。针的下端如宝剑形,两面有刃。多用于外科,以刺破痈疽,排出脓血。

One of the nine classic needles of the ancient times. The lower end is sword-shape with a double-edged blade. It is mainly used in surgery for piercing abscess and carbuncle to discharge pus and blood.

皮刺 skin needling

在穴位处皮肤上浅刺。

A kind of shallow needling by puncturing the skin surface.

皮肤针 dermal needle

又称梅花针或七星针,由 5 或 7 根不锈钢针镶嵌在手柄的一端制成。用于叩刺皮肤表面,以激发经络之气,调整脏腑功能。

Also named plum-blossom needle or seven-star needle, which is made of 5 or 7 stainless steel needles inlaid into the end of a handle. It is used to prick the skin superficially by tapping to stimulate qi of the meridians and regulate the functions of the zang-fu organs.

皮内针 intradermal needle

指埋置在皮肤下的一种针具。可用于治疗慢性或疼痛性疾病。

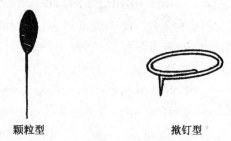

颗粒型　　　　　　　撳钉型

Small needles could be embedded underneath the skin. They can be used in treating chronic or painful diseases.

皮质下 Pizhixia

耳穴名。在对耳屏内侧面。主治痛症,神经衰弱,失眠,炎症,肾虚耳鸣,多梦等。

Name of an ear point. Located at the medial aspect of antitragus. Indications: Pain, neurasthenia, insomnia, inflammation, tinnitus due to kidney deficiency, dreaminess, etc.

琵琶 Pipa

经外奇穴名。位于肩井下,巨骨旁凹陷中。直刺或灸治肩痛,上肢不举等。

Name of extra points. Located at the depression below Jianjing （GB21） and next to Jugu （LI16）. Perpendicular acupuncture or moxibustion is used to cure shoulder pain，inability to raise hands，etc.

脾 spleen；Pi

①五脏之一。中医学的脾不能与现代医学的脾的构造、解剖位置和功能等同起来。它有吸收、输送营养物质到机体各组织器官和参与水液代谢及统摄血液使其循行于血管内等生理功能。如某些消化系统疾病、水肿、慢性出血性疾病都可能与脾功能的紊乱有关。②耳穴名。定位：在耳甲腔的后上方。主治：腹泻，腹胀，消化不良，胃炎，功能性子宫出血等。

①One of the five zang organs in TCM which does not completely match the organ in western medicine regarding its structure，location and function. It has the functions of digesting food，transforming and transporting nutrients to the body tissues. The spleen also takes part in regulation of fluid metabolism and serves to control the blood and to keep the blood circulating within the vessels. Some diseases of the digestive system，edema and chronic hemorrhagic diseases are usually attributable to malfunction of the spleen. ②Name of an ear point. Location：At the posterior and superior aspect of cavum conchae. Indications：Diarrhea，abdominal distension，indigestion，gastritis，functional uterus bleeding，etc.

脾气虚 spleen qi deficiency

脾的功能低下，消化及吸收功能障碍的病理。症见食欲减退或食后腹胀，伴有眩晕、倦怠、面色萎黄等。

A disorder of digestion and absorption due to disfunction of the spleen；manifested as poor appetite，or abdominal distension after meal，dizziness，fatigue，sallow complexion，etc.

脾肾两虚 deficiency of both spleen and kidney

由肾阳虚衰，不能温养脾阳或脾阳久虚而导致脾肾阳气俱虚的一种病理变化。症见形寒肢冷，面色㿠白，腰膝或少腹冷痛，泄泻，完谷不化，或五更泻，浮肿，小便不利或多尿，舌质淡嫩，苔白润，脉沉弱等。

A morbid condition due to deficiency of kidney-yang which fails to support spleen-yang，or vice versa；manifested as chilly sensation of the whole body，especially the limbs，pale complexion，cold sensation and pain of the loins and knees or lower abdomen，lienteric diarrhea or predawn diarrhea，edema，dysuria or polyuria，pale and tender tongue with whitish and moist fur，deep and weak pulse，etc.

脾俞 Pishu （BL20）

经穴名。属足太阳膀胱经，脾的背俞穴。定位：在第十一胸椎棘突下，后正中线旁开1.5寸处。主治：上腹疼痛，腹胀，黄疸，呕吐，泄泻，痢疾，便血，月经量多，水肿，厌食，背痛。操作：向内斜刺0.5～1寸；可灸。

Name of an acupoint. It belongs to the

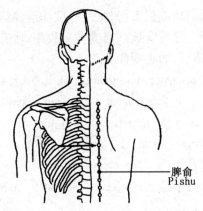

脾俞
Pishu

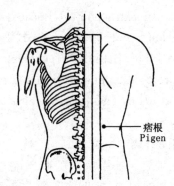

痞根
Pigen

Bladder Meridian of Foot-Taiyang. It is the Back-Shu point of spleen. Location: At the same level as the lower border of the spinous process of the 11th thoracic vertebra, 1.5 cun lateral to the posterior midline. Indications: Epigastric pain, abdominal distension, jaundice, vomiting, diarrhea, dysentery, bloody stools, profuse menstruation, edema, anorexia, backache, etc. Method: Puncture obliquely 0.5-0.8 cun toward the interspace of the spine. Moxibustion is applicable.

脾之大络 the Large Collateral of Spleen Meridian

十五条大络脉之一,穴名大包。从渊液下3寸分出,散络于胸肋部。

One of the fifteen large collaterals, the corresponding acupoint is named Dabao (SP21), separated from the main meridian 3 cun below Yuanye(GB22), dispersed in the chest and hypoihondrium region.

痞根 Pigen (EX-B4)

经外奇穴名。在第一腰椎棘突下旁开3.5寸处。主治:肝脾大,腰痛等。

Name of an extra point. Located 3.5 cun lateral to the inferior spinous process of the 1st lumbar vertebra. Indications: Hepatosplenomegaly, lumbago, etc.

偏历 Pianli (LI6)

经穴名。属手阳明大肠经,本经络穴。定位:在阳溪穴与曲池穴连线上,阳溪穴上3寸。主治:目赤,耳聋,鼻衄,喉痛,手臂酸痛等。操作:直刺或斜刺0.5～0.8寸;可灸。

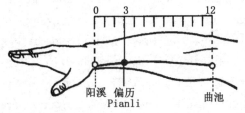

阳溪　偏历　曲池
Pianli

The acupoint, Luo-Connecting point, belongs to the Large Intestine Meridian of Hand-Yangming. Location: On the line connecting Yangxi(LI5) and Quchi (LI11), 3 cun above Yangxi(LI5). Indications: Redness of the eyes, deafness, epistaxis, sore throat, aching of the hand and arm, etc. Method: Puncture perpendicularly or obliquely 0.5-0.8 cun. Moxibustion is applicable.

偏瘫 hemiplegia

又称偏风、偏枯。指一侧肢体偏废不

用,久则见患肢肌肉枯瘦。多由营卫俱虚、真气不能充于全身,或兼邪气侵袭所致。治宜通经活络、补益肝肾。取穴:肩髃、曲池、合谷、阳溪、髀关、梁丘、足三里、解溪、肝俞、肾俞。

Paralysis of one side of the body, accompanied with muscular atrophy of the affected side in chronic cases; caused by deficiency of nutrient-qi and defensive-qi leading to the disorder of genuine qi circulation, or by the attack of evils simultaneously. Treatment principle:Clear and activate the meridians and co-llaterals, tonify the liver and kindey. Point selection:Jianyu(LI15), Quchi(LI11), Hegu(LI4), Yangxi(LI5), Biguan(ST31), Liangqiu(ST34), Zusanli(ST36), Jiexi(ST41), Ganshu(BL18), Shenshu(BL23).

偏头风 migraine

即偏头痛。其痛多在一侧颞部,有时痛连目或视力受损,或兼恶心呕吐。多因风邪侵于少阳或肝虚痰火郁结所致。治宜平肝潜阳。取穴:悬颅、太冲、太溪、率谷。

A recurrent, intense headache usually confined to one side of the temporal region, occasionally affecting the eye or leading to impaired vision or accompanied with nausea and vomiting; mostly due to attack of wind-evil to Shaoyang or stagnation of phlegm-fire resulting from asthenia of the liver. Treatment principle: Calm the liver and suppress hyperactivity of the liver-yang. Point selection:Xuanlu(GB5), Taichong(LR3), Taixi(KI3), Shuaigu(GB8).

平补平泻 neutral reinforcement and reduction

①指手法较轻、刺激量较小的针刺手法,与大补大泻相对。②指先泻后补的针刺手法。即先泻邪气,后补正气,以协调阴阳。③指不分补泻的针刺手法,类似于平针法。

① A kind of acupuncture technique with gentle manipulations and moderate stimulation as contrasted with vigorous reinforcing and reducing. ②A kind of acupuncture technique by reducing first and reinforcing after, i. e., expelling the pathogenic qi first and reinforcing the vital qi after to harmonize yin and yang. ③ A kind of acupuncture technique without performing the reinforcing or reducing manipulations, similar to the even needling.

平肝熄风 calming the liver to inhibit the wind-evil

又称镇肝熄风。用于肝肾阴虚,肝阳上亢,引动内风的治法。症见头痛、头晕目眩、口眼歪斜、肢体发麻或震颤、舌体活动不灵或偏斜、语言不清,甚至突然昏倒、手足抽搐、舌质红、苔薄、脉弦等。

A treatment for endogenous wind-syndrome due to deficiency of liver-yin and kidney-yin, and abnormal rising of liver-yang, applicable to cases manifested as headache, dizziness, deviation of eyes and mouth, numbness or tremor of the extremities, stiffness or deviation of the tongue, dysphasia, or even syncope and convulsion, red tongue with thin fur, wiry pulse, etc.

平衡区 equilibrium zone

自枕外粗隆旁平齐旁开 3.5 cm 处，向下与正中线平行做 4 cm 长的直线，所围成的区域即为本区。主治小脑疾病引起的平衡失调。

A line 4 cm long drawn downwards and parallel to the posterior midline from a point at the same level with the external occipital protuberance 3.5 cm lateral to the midline. It is used for treating disturbance of equilibrium of carabellum origin.

平针法 even needling

针刺手法名。指进针后以达到得气为主而不分补泻的方法。

Name of acupuncture technique, i. e., to obtain the sensation of needling without performing the reinforcing or reducing manipulations.

屏尖 Pingjian

耳穴名。定位：在耳屏上部隆起的尖端。主治：发热，牙痛。

Name of an ear point. Location: At the tip of the protuberance on the upper border of tragus. Indications: Fever, toothache.

屏间切迹 intertragic notch

解剖名称。指耳屏与对耳屏之间的凹陷。

Terminologia anatomica. The depression between the tragus and antitragus.

屏轮切迹 helix notch

解剖名称。指对耳屏与对耳轮之间的凹陷。

Terminologia anatomica. The depression between the tragus and antihelix.

屏上切迹 supratragic notch

解剖名称。指耳屏上缘与耳轮脚之间的凹陷。

Terminologia anatomica. The depression between the helix crus and the upper border of the tragus.

魄户 Pohu(BL42)

经穴名。属足太阳膀胱经。定位：在第三胸椎棘突下，后正中线旁开 3 寸处。主治：肺痨，咯血，咳嗽，气喘，项强，肩背痛等。操作：斜刺 0.5～0.8 寸；可灸。

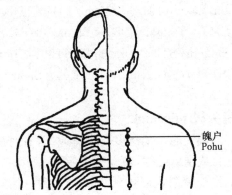

魄户
Pohu

Name of an acupoint. It belongs to the Bladder Meridian of Foot-Taiyang. Location: At the same level as the lower border of the spinous process of the 3rd thoracic vertebra, 3 cun lateral to the posterior midline. Indications: Pulmonary tuberculosis, hemoptysis, cough, asthma, stiff neck, pain in the shoulder and back, etc. Method: Puncture obliquely 0.5-0.8 cun. Moxibustion is applicable.

魄门 pomen

即肛门。为七冲门之一。

The anus. One of the seven important openings of the digestive system.

仆参 Pucan (BL61)

经穴名。属足太阳膀胱经。定位：在昆仑穴直下，跟骨外侧赤白肉际处。主治：下肢痿痹，足跟痛等。操作：直刺 0.3～0.5 寸；可灸。

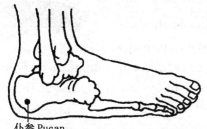

仆参 Pucan

Name of an acupoint. It belongs to the Bladder Meridian of Foot-Taiyang. Location: Directly below Kunlun(BL60), on the dorso-ventral boundary of the foot lateral to the calcaneum. Indications: Muscular atrophy and weakness of the lower extremities, heel pain, etc. Method: Puncture perpendicularly 0. 3-0. 5 cun. Moxibustion is applicable.

普济方 *General Benevolent Prescriptions*

医书名。明代朱橚主编。为我国现存的最大方书。

Name of the medical book compiled chiefly by Zhu Su in the Ming Dynasty. It is the most comprehensive prescription book conserved till now.

Q

七星针 seven-star needle

皮肤针的一种,形如小锤,由数枚细针组成,用以叩击浅刺皮肤。

One of the dermal needles which looks like a small hammer made up of several fine needles and can be used to tap and prick shallowly on the skin.

期门 Qimen (LR14)

经穴名。属足厥阴肝经,肝的募穴。定位:在乳头直下,第六肋间隙中。主治:胁痛,腹胀,呃逆,吞酸,乳痈,热病等。操作:斜刺或平刺 0.5～1 寸;可灸。

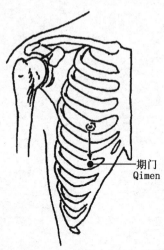

期门
Qimen

The acupoint, Front-Mu point, belongs to the Liver Meridian of Foot-Jueyin. Location: Directly below the nipple, in the 6th intercostal space. Indications: Hypochondriac pain, abdominal distension, hiccup, acid regurgitation, acute mastitis, febrile diseases, etc. Method: Puncture perpendicularly or obliquely 0.

5-1 cun. Moxibustion is a-pplicable.

齐刺 triple puncture

十二刺法之一。用于治疗部位较小和较深的寒痹。方法是在患处中央刺一针,两旁各刺一针。

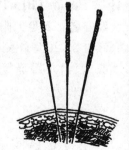

One of the twelve needling techniques for treating cold bi (obstruction of pathogenic cold factor to the body) with a relatively small and deep area. The method is to puncture the centre of the area with one needle and both sides with two needles.

岐伯 Qibo

传说中的古代医学家,为黄帝之师。

An ancient physician in Chinese legend. It is said that he was the teacher of Huangdi.

岐黄 Qihuang

名医岐伯与黄帝的合称。中国古代传说黄帝令岐伯研究医药而立经方,故歧黄也作中医学的同义语。

A combined term of Qibo (a well-known physician) and Huangdi (an Emperor in ancient China). A legend says that Qibo was entrusted by Huangdi to study medicine and establish classic prescriptions. Hence, the term Qihuang has been used as synonym for traditional Chinese medicine.

奇经 extra meridians

奇经八脉的简称。

The simplified name of the eight extra meridians.

奇经八脉 eight extra meridians

奇经是督脉、任脉、冲脉、带脉、阳维脉、阴维脉、阳跷脉、阴跷脉八脉的总称。它们的特点是：与脏腑没有直接联系，它们之间也无表里配合，是调节气血运行的一些特殊通路，可补充十二经脉的不足。

The collective term for the Governor Vessel, the Conception Vessel, the Thoroughfare Vessel, the Belt Vessel, Yang Heel Vessel, Yin Heel Vessel, Yang Link Vessel, Yin Link Vessel. They are characterized by not related with the viscera, and without the interior-exterior relationship among themselves. They are special paths for regulating the flow of qi and blood, which can supplement the deficiency of the twelve meridians.

奇经八脉考 Study on The Eight Extra Meridians

明代李时珍撰，1578 年成书。作者对历代有关奇经八脉的文献做了全面考证，对每条奇经的循行和功用分别进行了说明。

A book of an overall textual research on the past literature about the eight extra meridians with comments on the course and function of each meridian in detail, composed by Li Shizhen in the Ming Dynasty (1578).

奇恒之腑 extraordinary fu organs

即脑、髓、骨、脉、胆、女子胞，形态中空似腑，而功能藏精气如脏，故名。

Referring to the brain, marrow, bones, vessels, gallbladder and uterus. They are hollow like the fu organs and they store essence like the zang organs.

奇输 qi acupoints

①指治热病的五十九俞。②指经外奇穴。

①The collective name of the 59 acupoints specially used to cure febrile diseases. ②The other name of extra points.

奇穴 extra points

即经外奇穴。指既有一定的穴名，又有明确的位置，但尚未归入十四经系统的腧穴。

It refers to the points with certain names and clear locations, but not included in the fourteen-meridian system.

脐 umbilicus

腹壁中央的陷窝，为出生后脐带断落结疤所形成。

The depression at the center of abdominal formed by the detachment of the umbilical cord after birth.

脐上下 Qishangxia

经外奇穴名。位于脐上下各半寸。直刺或灸治小儿囟陷、囟门不合、肠炎、水肿、疝气、下痢等。

Name of extra points. Location：0. 5 cun above and below the navel. Perpendicular acupuncture or moxibustion is used to cure infantile sunken fontanel, unclosed fontanel, enteritis, edema, hernia, dysentery, etc.

脐四边 Qisibian

经外奇穴名。位于脐中及其上、下、左、右各 1 寸处，共 5 穴。直刺（脐中除外）或灸治急慢性胃肠炎、胃痉挛、水肿、消化不良等。

Name of the extra points, including Shenque (CV8) and the other 4 points located 1 cun above, below, and lateral to the center of the navel. Five acupoints in total. Perpendicular acupuncture (except Shenque) or moxibustion is used to cure acute or chronic gastroenteritis, gastric spasm, edema, indigestion, etc.

脐中 Qizhong

即神阙穴。

The other name of Shenque (CV8).

骑竹马灸 Qizhuma jiu

经外奇穴名。定位:位于筋缩穴两侧各1寸处。灸治无名肿毒、发背、脑疽、肠痈、牙痛、痰核、瘰疬、四肢下部各种痈疮等。

Name of extra points. Location:1 cun lateral to Jinsuo (GV8). Moxibustion is used to cure innominate inflammations, back carbuncles and nape carbuncles, acute appendicitis, toothache, phlegm nodule, scrofula, different kinds of sores and suppurative inflammations in the lower extremities, etc.

气 air; qi

①指呼吸过程中进出人体的空气。②体内流动着的富有营养的精微物质。③人体及脏器组织的功能。

①The air breathing in and out of the body during respiration. ②Refined and nutritious substances flowing in the body. ③The functions of various organs and tissues of the body.

气冲 Qichong(ST30)

经穴名。属足阳明胃经。定位:在脐下5寸,前正中线旁开2寸处。主治:腹痛,肠鸣,疝气,外阴肿痛,痛经,月经不调等。操作:直刺0.5~1寸;可灸。

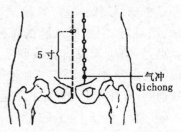

Name of an acupoint. It belongs to the Stomach Meridian of Foot-Yangming. Location:5 cun below the umbilicus, 2 cun lateral to the anterior midline. Indications:Abdominal pain, borborygmus, hernia, swelling and pain of the external genitalia, dysmeno-rrhea, irregular menstruation, etc. Me-thod:Puncture perpendicularly 0. 5-1 cun. Moxibustion is applicable.

气端 Qiduan

经外奇穴名。定位:在足十趾尖端,距趾甲游离缘0.1寸,左右共10穴。主治:脚气,足趾麻痹,足背红肿,急救等。治疗常常用直刺深0.1~0.2寸,

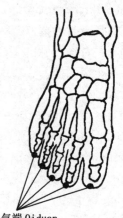

三棱针点刺出血或者灸治。

Name of extra points. Location:At the tip of the ten toes, 0. 1 cun from the edge of each toenail, ten points in all. Main indications are beriberi, toe numbness, sore foot, emergncies, etc. , by perpendicular acupuncture to the depth of 0. 1-0. 2 cun, letting out blood with a three-edged needle or moxibustion.

气短 shortness of breath

呼吸无力、浅表、急促的症状。常由于气虚所致。治宜补脾益气。取穴：脾俞、足三里、气海、太渊。

A State of weak, shallow and rapid respiration, usually due to deficiency of qi. Treatment principle: Invigorate the spleen and replenish qi. Point selection: Pishu(BL20), Zusanli(ST36), Qihai(CV6), Taiyuan(LU9).

气反 opposite qi

《内经》取穴法之一。指取穴与病所位置相反，如上病下取，下病上取，中病旁取。

One of the point-selecting principles in *Huangdi's Canon of Medicine*, which is to choose the points opposite to the sites of the diseases, such as taking the lower points to cure the upper diseases, the upper points to cure the lower diseases, the peripheral points to cure the central diseases.

气功 Qigong

是运用意识的引导作用，通过调节呼吸、意守等，对生命过程实行自我调节、控制，以达到防治疾病、强身延年的一种自我身心锻炼方法。

A mental and physical self-training for the prevention and treatment of diseases, and also for health care and prolongation of life. It includes intention, breathing exercise and mediation, etc.

气功疗法 Qigong therapy

利用气功治疗某些疾病的方法。

The treatment of disease by breathing exercise.

气管 Qiguan

耳穴名。在外耳道口与心穴之间。主治：咳嗽，气喘等。

Name of an ear point. The point is between the opening of external auditory meatus and the ear point Xin. Indications:Cough, asthma, etc.

气海 Qihai(CV6)

①穴名。属任脉。定位：在腹中线上，脐下1.5寸处。主治：腹痛，泄泻，遗尿，遗精，阳痿，疝气，水肿，痢疾，便秘，气喘，痛经，崩漏，月经不调，闭经，白带，产后出血等。操作：直刺0.5～1.5寸；可灸。②即膻中。

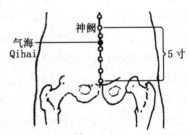

①Name of an acupoint. It belongs to the Conception Vessel. Location:On the midline of the abdomen, 1. 5 cun below the umbilicus. Indications: Abdominal pain, diarrhea, enuresis, nocturnal emission, impotence, hernia, edema, dysentery, constipation, asthma, dysmenorrhea, uterine bleeding, irregular menstruation, amenorrhea, leukorrhea disease, postpartum hemorrhage, etc. Method: Puncture perpendicularly 0.5-1.5 cun. Moxibustion is applicable. ② Danzhong(CV17).

气海俞 Qihaishu (BL24)

经穴名。属足太阳膀胱经。定位:在第三腰椎棘突下,后正中线旁开 1.5 寸处。主治:腰痛,月经不调,痛经,气喘等。操作:直刺0.8～1.5寸;可灸。

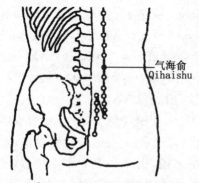

气海俞 Qihaishu

Name of an acupoint. It belongs to the Bladder Meridian of Foot-Taiyang. Location:At the level of the lower border of the spinous process of the 3rd lumbar vertebra, 1.5 cun lateral to the posterior midline. Indications: Lumbago, irregular menstruation, dysmenorrhea, asthma, etc. Method:Puncture perpendicularly 0.8-1.5 cun. Moxibustion is applicable.

气候 climatic condition

天气变化的气象,如风、寒、暑、湿、燥、火,或泛指天气变化。

Meteorological phenomena of the climatic changes such as wind, cold, heat, dampness, dryness and fire, or the climatic variation in general.

气户 Qihu (ST13)

经穴名。属足阳明胃经。定位:在锁骨下缘,前正中线旁开 4 寸处。主治:胸满、气喘,咳嗽,呃逆,胸胁疼痛等。操作:斜刺0.5～0.8寸;可灸。

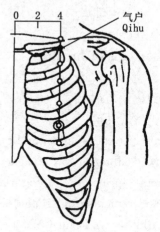

气户 Qihu

Name of an acupoint. It belongs to the Stomach Meridian of Foot-Yangming. Location:At the lower border of the clavicle, 4 cun lateral to the anterior midline. Indications: Fullness in the chest, asthma, cough, hiccup, pain in the chest and hypochondrium, etc. Method: Puncture obliquely 0.5-0.8 cun. Moxibustion is applicable.

气会 influential point of qi

八会穴之一,即膻中穴。

It refers to Danzhong(CV17), one of the eight influential points.

气街 qi thoroughfare

①经络之气通行的经络,分四气街。②指气冲部。③指气冲穴。

①The passageways of qi in the meridians and collaterals classsified into 4 kinds. ② The part where exists Qichong (ST30). ③Qichong(ST30).

气门 Qimen

经外奇穴名。定位：在关元穴旁 3 寸。主治不孕、崩漏、阴挺、尿闭、小肠疝气。治疗常用直刺深 1～1.5 寸或灸治。孕妇禁刺。

Name of an extra point. Location: 3 cun lateral to Guanyuan(CV4). Indications: Infertility, metrorrhagia, uterine prolapse, anuria, inguinal hernia, etc. , by perpendicular acupuncture to the depth of 1-1.5 cun or moxibustion. Acupuncture here is prohibited in pregnant women.

气舍 Qishe(ST11)

经穴名。属足阳明胃经。定位：在锁骨内侧端的上缘，胸锁乳突肌的胸骨头与锁骨头之间。主治：颈项强痛，咽喉肿痛，气喘，呃逆，瘿气等。操作：直刺 0.3～0.5 寸；可灸。

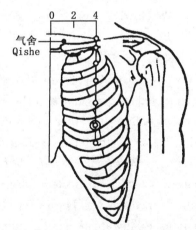

Name of an acupoint. It belongs to the Stomach Meridian of Foot-Yangming. Location: At the superior border of the medial end of the clavicle, between the sternal head and clavicular head of musculi sternocleidomastoideus. Indications: Pain and rigidity of the neck, sore throat, asthma, hiccup, goiter, etc. Method: Puncture perpendicularly 0.3-0.5 cun. Moxibustion is applicable.

气俞 Qishu

京骨穴别名。

The other name of Jinggu(BL64).

气为血帅 qi as the commander of blood

说明气和血液的运行有密切的关系，即气为血液运行的动力。中医学认为血能够在经脉中不停地循环，是依靠气作为它的动力。

A term referring to the close relationship between qi and blood, i. e. , qi is the motive force of the blood flow and is responsible for the persistent circulation of the blood in the vessels.

气虚 deficiency of qi

①脏腑虚损、元气损耗所致的一种病状。症见面色㿠白、头眩耳鸣、心悸气短、倦怠乏力、自汗、脉虚无力等。②指肺气虚。症见面色淡白、气短、声音低弱、畏风、自汗等。治宜补脾益气。取穴：脾俞、足三里、气海、太渊。

①A morbid state due to impairment of the viscera and consumption of primordial qi, manifested as pale complexion, dizziness, tinnitus, palpitation, shortness of breath, lassitude, spontaneous sweating, weak and feeble pulse, ect. ② Referring specially to deficiency of lung-qi, manifested as pale complexion, shortness of breath, lower voice, intolerance of wind, spontaneous sweating, ect. Treatment principle: Invigorate the spleen and replenish qi.

Point selection：Pishu（BL20），Zusanli（ST36），Qihai(CV6)，Taiyuan(LU9)．

气穴 Qixue(LI13)

经穴名。属足少阴肾经。定位：在脐下3寸，前正中线旁开0.5寸处。主治：月经不调，痛经，小便不利，腹痛，泄泻等。操作：直刺1～1.5寸；可灸。

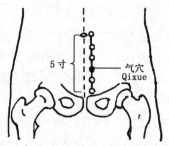

Name of an acupoint. It belongs to the Kidney Meridian of Foot-Shaoyin. Location：3 cun below the umbilicus，0.5 cun lateral to the anterior midline. Indication：Irregular menstruation，dysmenorrhea，dysuria，abdominal pain，diarrhea，etc. Method：Puncture perpendicularly 1-1.5 cun. Moxibustion is applicable.

气原 Qiyuan

中极穴别名。

The other name of Zhongji(CV3)

气至病所 arrival of qi at the affected area

指针刺感应趋向病痛所在部位。

Qi(here refers to the sensation by acupuncture)should reach the site of the disease.

气滞 qi stagnation

即气运行不畅，通常指某一组织器官功能障碍。常见局部胀满或疼痛。治宜疏肝理气。取穴：肝俞、太冲、内关、膻中。

A disorder of the activitiy of qi，usually referring to the dysfunction of a tissue or organ，manifested as local distention or pain. Treatment principle：Relieve the depressed liver and regulate the flow of qi. Point selection：Ganshu（BL18），Taichong(LR3），Neiguan(PC6），Danzhong(CV17).

掐法 nipping manipulation

推拿手法。用指甲按压穴位，产生强刺激。通常用于晕厥、惊风等证。

A manipulation of massage by pressing at a point with a finger-nail to produce a strong stimulation，usually used in the treatment of syncope，convulsion，etc.

千金要方 Essential Prescriptions Worth Thousand Gold

书名。原名《备急千金要方》。唐代孙思邈著，共30卷。广辑唐以前的医药资料，其中针灸疗法尤多。

Name of a Chinese classical medical book compiled by Sun Simiao in the Tang Dynasty including altogether 30 volumes. The full name of the book is *Essential Prescriptions Worth Thousand Gold for Emergency*，which collected large amounts of medical data before the Tang Dynasty especially about acupuncture and moxibustion.

千金翼方 Supplement to Essential Prescriptions Worth Thousand Gold for Emergency

孙思邈撰。《千金要方》的补篇，包括医学各科。此书与《千金要方》同被视为唐代医学代表著作。

A book dealing with various branches of medicine appended to *Essential Prescriptions Worth Thousand Gold for Emergency* by Sun Simiao. Both books are recognized as the representative medicial works of the Tang Dynasty.

牵正 Qianzheng

经外奇穴名。定位:在耳垂前 0.5～1 寸处。主治:口眼歪斜,口舌生疮等。

Name of an extra point. Location: 0.5-1 cun anterior to the earlobe. Indications: Deviation of eyes and mouth, ulceration on tongue and in the mouth, etc.

前顶 Qianding(GV21)

经穴名。属督脉。定位:在头正中线上,百会穴前 1.5 寸处。主治:癫痫,头晕,视物昏花,头顶痛,鼻渊等。操作:平刺 0.5～0.8 寸;可灸。

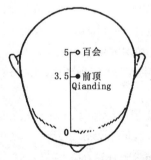

Name of an acupoint. It belongs to the Governor Vessel. Location: On the midline of the head, 1.5 cun anterior to Baihui (GV20). Indications: Epilepsy, dizziness, blurred vision, vertex headache, nasosinusitis, etc. Method: Puncture horizontally 0.5-0.8 cun. Moxibustion is applicable.

前发际 Qianfaji

经外奇穴名。位于太阳穴直上 3 寸。沿皮刺或灸治颜面疔疮。

Name of an extra point. Located 3 cun directly aboue Taiyang(EX-HN5). Subcutaneous acupuncture or moxibusion is used to cure facial boils and sores.

前谷 Qiangu(SI2)

经穴名。属手太阳小肠经,本经荥穴。定位:微握拳,在第五掌指关节前尺侧,掌指横纹头赤白肉际处。主治:热病,耳鸣,头痛,咽喉肿痛,乳痛,乳汁少等。操作:直刺 0.3～0.5 寸;可灸。

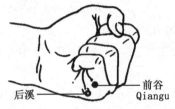

The acupoint, Xing-Spring point of the Small Intestine Meridian of Hand-Taiyang. Location: On the ulnar side, distal to the 5th metacarpophalagal joint, on the dorso-ventra boundary of the end of the metacarpophalangeal transverse crease when a loose fist is made. Indications: Febrile diseases, tinnitus, headache, sore throat, acute mastitis, insufficient lactation, etc. Method: Puncture perpendicularly 0.3-0.5 cun. Moxibustion is applicable.

前后配穴法 anterior and posterior point-combining method

配穴法之一。指头面、胸腹部的穴位与枕项、腰背部的穴位配合应用。多用于五官及内科疾病。

One of the point-combining methods, i. e., the combination of the points located on the head, face, thorax and abdomen with the points located on the occipital, neck, waist and back are often used to treat the five sense organs diseases and the internal diseases.

前后正中线 anterior and posterior midline

指从眉间至枕外粗隆顶点下缘的连线，即头颅中线。

It is the line extending from the midpoint between the eyebrows to the lower border of the external occipital protuberance, i. e. , the midline of the skull.

前阴 anterior Yin

指外生殖器，与后阴（肛门）相对，合称二阴。

The external genitalia, as contrasted with the posterior Yin(anus), both given a collective name"two Yin".

强间 Qiangjian(GV18)

经穴名，属督脉。定位：后发际正中直上4寸，脑户穴直上1.5寸处。主治：头痛项强，视物昏花，癫狂等。操作：平刺0.5～1寸；可灸。

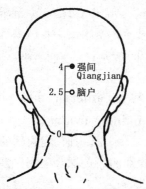

Name of an acupoint. It belongs to the Governor Vessel. Location：4 cun directly above the midpoint of the posterior hairline, 1. 5 cun directly above Naohu(GV17). Indications：Headache, neck rigidity, blurred vision, mania, ect. Method：Puncture horizontally 0. 5-1 cun. Moxibustion is applicable.

强阳 Qiangyang

络却穴别名。

The other name of Luoque(BL8).

切法 nail pressing method

针刺辅助手法。指进针前用指甲于穴位部做切按动作，以宣散气血。

Supplementary manipulation in acupuncture which is to apply pressure with finger nails on the point before insertion of the needle in order to dissipate qi and blood.

秦越人 Qin Yueren

即扁鹊，战国时著名医学家。

The other name of Bianque, the well-known physician during the Warring States.

揿针 thumbtack needle

指形如图钉的一种针具，可供皮下埋置用。

A kind of needle like a thumbtack for subcutancous embedding.

青灵 Qingling(HT2)

经穴名。属手少阴心经。定位：在少海穴与极泉穴的连线上，肘横纹上3寸，肱二头肌内侧沟中。主治：胸胁肩臂痛。操作：直刺0.5～0.8寸；可灸。

Name of an acupoint. It belongs to the Heart Meridian of Hand-Shaoyin. Location：On the line connecting Shaohai (HT3) and Jiquan(HT1), 3 cun above the cubital transverse crease, in the

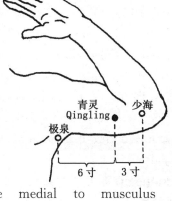

青灵 Qingling 少海

极泉

6寸 3寸

groove medial to musculus biceps brachii. It is used for treating pain in the cardiac and hypochondriac region, shouder and arm, etc. Method: Puncture perpendicularly 0. 5-0. 8 cun. Moxibustion is applicable.

青灵泉 Qinglingquan

青灵穴别名。

The other name of Qingling(HT2).

清泠渊 Qinglingyuan(TE11)

经穴名,属手少阳三焦经。定位:在臂外侧,屈肘,当肘尖直上2寸,天井穴上1寸。主治:肩肘痛不能举,偏头痛等。操作:直刺 0.8～1.2 寸;可灸。

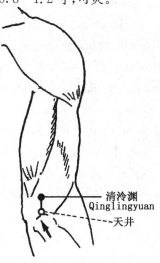

清泠渊 Qinglingyuan

天井

Name of an acupoint. It belongs to the Sanjiao Meridian of Hand-Shaoyang. Location:On the lateral side of the arm, 2 cun directly above the tip of the elbow, 1 cun above Tianjing(TE10) when the elbow is flexed. Indications:Motor impairment and pain of the shouder and arm, migraine, etc. Method:Puncture perpendicularly 0. 8-1. 2 cun. Moxibustion is applicable.

青龙摆尾 green dragon wagging its tail

针刺手法名。飞经走气法之一,与"白虎摇头"相对。即斜向浅刺,针尖向病痛处,将针尾做左右摆动;或结合下按动作,反复九数或二十七数,以行卫气。

Name of an acupuncture technique, one of the techniques of moving qi throughout the meridians, as contrasted with the "white tiger shaking its head", i. e., oblique, shallow puncture with the needle pointing end in the direction of the di-sease while swaying the needle side to side, sometimes combined with the thrusting manipulations repeatedly for nine or twenty-seven times to move the defense qi.

清热解毒 clearing heat and removing toxin

用清热邪、解热毒的药物,治疗热性病里热亢盛及皮肤、软组织化脓性感染或斑疹的一种方法。

A treatment for febrile diseases with excessive interior heat, pathogenic infection of skin and soft tissue, or skin eruptions by using the herbs for elimination the heat-evil.

清热开窍 clear heat to open the orifices

又称清心开窍。治疗温热病神智昏迷的方法。适用于温病高热，神志昏迷，烦躁不安，胡言乱语，四肢抽搐等。

A treatment for coma in febrile disease, applicable to the case manifested as high fever, loss of consciousness, restlessness, delirium, twitching of the four limbs, etc.

清热利湿 clear heat and drain dampness

使用清热利湿、通利小便的药物，治疗湿热之邪蕴结下焦的一种方法。适用于下焦湿热者，症见小腹急胀，尿少，尿痛或小便混浊，舌苔黄腻等。

A treatment for the accumulation of damp-heat evil in the lower jiao by the application of herbs for clearing away the heat and dampness-evils and promoting diuresis, applicable to the case with damp-heat syndrome of the lower jiao, manifested as sudden onset of fullness of the lower abdomen, oliguria, dysuria, discharge of turbid urine, yellowish and greasy fur on the tongue, etc.

清泻肝火 clearing the liver-fire

又称泻肝、清肝火。用苦寒药物清泻肝火的方法。常用于肝的实火上升者。症见头痛眩晕，耳聋耳鸣，面红目赤，口干口苦，胁部疼痛，甚则吐血，急躁易怒，便秘，苔黄，脉弦数等。

A treament for the elimination of liver-fire by the application of herbs with bitter taste and cold nature, applicable to cases with abnormal rising of the liver-fire manifested as headache, dizziness, deafness, tinnitus, flushed face, red eyes, dry mouth with bitter taste, hypochondriac pain, hematemesis, irritability, constipation, yellowish fur on the tongue, wiry and rapid pulse, etc.

穷骨 qionggu

指骶骨和尾骨。

The sacral and coccgeal bones.

丘墟 Qiuxu(GB40)

经穴名。属足少阳胆经，本经原穴。定位：在外踝前下方，趾长伸肌腱外侧凹陷中。主治：项痛，腋肿，胁痛，目赤肿痛，目翳，下肢痿痹，外踝肿痛，疟疾等。操作：直刺0.5～1寸；可灸。

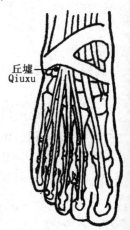

丘墟 Qiuxu

The acupoint, Yuan-Primary point of the Gallbladder Meridian of Foot-Shaoyang. Location: Anterior and inferior to the external malleolus, in the depression on the lateral side of the tendon of extensor digitiform longus. Indications: Neck pain, swelling in the axillary region, pain in the hypochondriac region, redness, swelling and pain of the eyes, cloudiness of cornea, muscular atrophy of the lower limbs, pain and swelling of the external malleolus, malaria, etc. Method: Puncture perpendicularly 0. 5-1 cun. Moxibustion is applicable.

球后 Qiuhou (EX-HN7)

经外奇穴名。在目眶下缘外 1/4 与内 3/4 交界处。主治目疾。

Name of an extra point. Location: At the junction of the lateral 1/4 and the medial 3/4 of the infraorbital margin. It

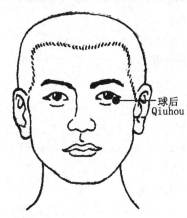

is used for treating eye diseases.

曲鬓 Qubin(GB7)

经穴名。属足少阳胆经。定位:在头部,当耳前鬓角发际后缘的垂线与耳尖水平线交点处。主治:偏头痛,颊肿,小儿惊风等。操作:向后平刺 0.5~0.8 寸;可灸。

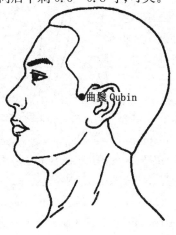

Name of an acupoint. It belongs to the Gallbladder Meridian of Foot-Shaoyang. Location: On the head, at the crossing point of the posterior border of the temple hairline and horizontal line level with the ear apex. Indications: Migraine, swelling of the cheek, infantile convulsion, ect. Method: Puncture horizontally backward 0. 5-0. 8 cun. Moxibustion is applicable.

曲差 Qucha(BL4)

经穴名。属足太阳膀胱经。定位:前发际正中直上 0.5 寸,旁开 1.5 寸,神庭与头维穴连线的内 1/3 与外 2/3 交界处。主治:头痛,鼻塞,鼻衄,视物不清等。操作:斜刺 0.3~0.5 寸;可灸。

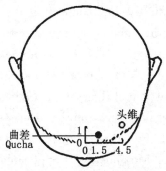

Name of an acupoint. It belong to the Bladder Meridian of Foot-Taiyang. Location: 1. 5 cun lateral to the point 0. 5 cun directly above the center of the anterior hairline, at the junction of the medial 1/3 and the lateral 2/3 of the line connecting Shenting(GV24) and Touwei(ST8). Indications: Headache, nasal obstruction, epistaxis, blurred vision, ect. Method: Puncture obliquely 0. 3-0. 5 cun. Moxibustion is applicable.

曲池 Quchi(LI11)

经穴名。属手阳明大肠经，本经合穴。定位：屈肘成直角，在肘横纹外侧端与肱骨外上髁连线的中点。主治：咽喉肿痛，齿痛，目赤痛，腹痛，呕吐，泄泻，热病等。操作：直刺0.5～1.5寸；可灸。

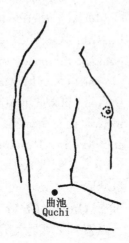

The acupoint and the He-Sea point of the Large Intestine Meridian of Hand-Yangming. Location：When the elbow is flexed to a right angle, the point is at the middle of the the line connecting the lateral end of the cubital transverse crease and the lateral epicondyle of the humerus. Indications：Sore throat, toothache, redness and pain of the eye, abdominal pain, vomiting, diarrhea, febrile diseases, etc. Method：Puncture perpendicularly 0.5-1.5 cun. Moxibustion is applicable.

曲骨 Qugu(CV2)

经穴名。属任脉。定位：在耻骨联合上缘中点。主治：小便不利，遗精，阳痿，带下，月经不调。操作：直刺0.5～1寸；可灸。

Name of an acupoint. It belongs to the Conception Vessel. Location：At the midpoint of the upper border of the pubic symphysis. Indications：Dysuria, nocturnal emission, impotence, leukorrhea, irregular menstuation. Method：Puncture perpen-

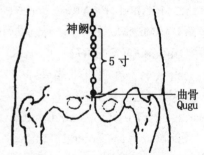

dicularly 0.5-1 cun. Moxibustion is applicable.

曲颊 angulus mandibulae

指下颌骨角。

The mandible angle.

曲节 Qujie

少海穴别名。

The other name of Shaohai(HT3).

曲眉 Qumei

印堂穴别名。

The other name of Yintang(GV29).

曲泉 Ququan (LR8)

经穴名。属足厥阴肝经，本经合穴。定位：屈膝，在膝内侧横纹头上方，半膜肌、半腱肌止端的前缘凹陷处。主治：阴挺，少腹痛，小便不利，遗精，腿膝内侧痛等。操作：直刺1～1.5寸；可灸。

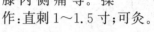

The acupoint, He-Sea point of the Liver Meridian of Foot-Jueyin. Location：When the knee is flexed, it is on the medial side of the knee, superior to the end of the transverse crease, in the depression of the anterior border of the ends of the semimembranosus and semitendinous. Indications：Prolapse of uterus, lower abdominal pain, retention of urine, nocturnal emission, pain in the medial aspect of the knee and thigh, etc. Method：Puncture perpendicularly 1-1. 5 cun. Moxibustion is applicable.

曲牙 Quya

颊车穴别名。

The other name of Jiache(ST6).

曲垣 Quyuan (SI13)

经穴名。属手太阳小肠经。定位：在肩胛部，冈上窝内侧端，当臑俞穴与第二胸椎棘突连线的中点处。主治：肩胛疼痛。操作：直刺 0.5 寸或斜刺 0.5～1 寸；可灸。

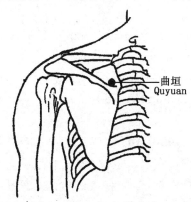

Name of an acupoint. It belongs to the Small Intestine Meridian of Hand-Taiyang. Location：On the scapula, at the midpoint of the line connecting Naoshu (SI10) and the spinous process of the 2nd thoracic vertebra. Indications：Pain of the scapular region. Method：Puncture perpendicularly 0. 5 cun or puncture obliquely 0. 5-1 cun. Moxibustion is applicable.

曲泽 Quze(PC3)

经穴名。属手厥阴心包经，本经合穴。

定位：在肘横纹中，当肱二头肌肌腱的尺侧缘。主治：心痛，心悸，热病，烦躁，胃痛，呕吐，肘臂痛等。操作：直刺 0.8～1 寸；可灸。

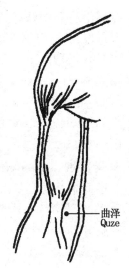

The acupoint, He-Sea point of the Pericardium Meridian of Hand-Jueyin. Location：At the midpoint of the cubital transverse crease, on the ulnar side of the tendon of the biceps brachii. Indications：Cardiac pain, palpitation, febrile diseases, irritability, stomachache, vomiting, pain in the elbow and arm, etc. Method：Puncture perpendicularly 0. 8-1 cun. Moxibustion is applicable.

屈骨端 Quguduan

经外奇穴名。别名横骨。定位：位于耻骨联合中点。主治：虚弱，遗精，尿频，遗尿，尿闭，腹中胀满，泄泻等。治疗常用斜刺或灸。

Name of an extra point, also known as Henggu(KI11). Location：At the midpoint of the pubic symphysis. Oblique acupuncture or moxibustion is used to cure weakness, nocturnal emission, frequent urination, enuresis, urodialysis, abdominal fullness, diarrhea, etc.

祛邪扶正 eliminating evils to support vital qi

治则名。扶正指扶助正气，正气强盛则

有利于病邪的祛除;驱邪指祛除邪气,病邪得以祛除,有利于正气的恢复。

Term of treatment principle. Strengthening vital qi may help to eliminate pathogenic factors, while eliminating pathogenic factors may benefit the restore of the vital qi.

全身浮肿 anasarca

指遍体浮肿。多由脾肾虚弱,水液代谢障碍,水湿潴留,外溢肌肤所致。治宜健脾温肾、助阳利水。取穴:脾俞、肾俞、气海、水分、足三里。

Generalized whole body edema caused by asthenia of the spleen and kidney leading to the disturbance of fluid metabolism and the abnormal accumulation of fluid in the subcutaneous tissues. Treatment principle:Strengthen the spleen and warm the kidney, support yang and remove dampness by diuresis. Point selection: Pishu (BL20), Shenshu(BL23), Qihai(CV6), Shuifen(CV9), Zusanli(ST36).

全身无力 general weakness

即全身疲困乏力。本症多由气血俱虚或湿邪内阻引起。临床上伴有相应的症状。治宜健脾补肾、益气养血。取穴:足三里、关元、气海、脾俞。

A symptom usually caused by the deficiency of qi and blood or the stagnation of dampness-evil, usually accompanied with the corresponding clinical manifestations. Treatment principle:Strengthen the spleen and tonify the kindey, reinforce qi and nourish blood. Point selection:Zusanli (ST36), Guanyuan(CV4), Qihai(CV6),

Pishu(BL20).

泉门 Quanmen

经外奇穴名。定位:位于女性阴唇前联合上缘。直刺或灸治不孕、漏下赤白、月经不调、闭经等。

Name of an extra point. Location:At the top margin of the anterior commissure of labia in female. Perpendicular acupuncture or moxibustion is used to cure infertility, red and white vaginal discharge, irregular menstruation, amenorrhea, etc.

泉阴 Quanyin

经外奇穴名。定位:位于耻骨联合中点旁开 3 寸处。直刺或灸治疝气、睾丸炎等。

Name of an extra point. Location: 3 cun lateral to the midpoint of the pubic symphysis. Perpendicular acupuncture or moxibustion is used to cure hernia, testitis, etc.

拳尖 Quanjian

经外奇穴名。定位:位于手背第三掌骨小头高点处,握拳取之。灸治目赤、目痛、白癜风等。

Name of extra points. Location:At the dorsal side of the hands, on the prominence of the 3rd metacarpal bone. Locate the point when making a fist. Moxibustion is used to cure red and sore eyes, vitiligo, etc.

颧髎 Quanliao(SI18)

经穴名。属手太阳小肠经。定位:在面部,当目外眦直下,颧骨下缘凹陷处。主治:面瘫,眼球瞤动,面痛,齿痛,颊肿,目黄等。操作:直刺 0.3～0.5寸;可灸。

Name of an acupoint. It belongs to the Small Intestine Meridian of Hand-Tai-yang. Location:On the face, directly be-

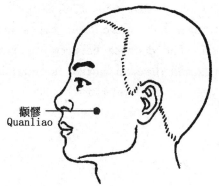

low the outer canthus, in the depression below the zygomatic bone. Indications: Facial paralysis, twitching of eyelid, pain in the face, toothache, swelling of the cheek, yellowish sclera, etc. Method: Puncture perpendicularly 0.3-0.5 cun. Moxibustion is applicable.

缺盆 Quepen(ST12)

经穴名。属足阳明胃经。定位:在锁骨上窝中央,距前正中线4寸。主治:咳嗽,气喘,咽喉肿痛,缺盆中痛等。操作:直刺0.3～0.5寸;可灸。

Name of an acupoint. It belongs to the Stomach Meridian of Foot-Yangming. Location:At the center of the supracla-vicular fossa, 4 cun lateral to the anterior midline. Indications: Cough, asthma, sore throat, pain in the supraclavicular fossa, etc. Method:Puncture perpendicu-larly 0.3-0.5 cun. Moxibustion is appli-cable.

阙中 glabella

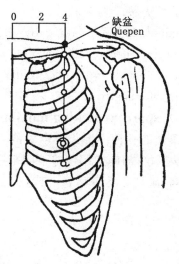

部位名。指两眉之间,印堂穴位于此。

Name of the body part between the two eyebrows, where is situated Yintang (GV29).

雀斑 freckle

发于颜面、颈和手背等处,呈黑褐色或淡黑色散在斑点,小如针尖或大至绿豆。多由火郁孙络血分,复感风邪凝滞;或肺经血热所致。治宜清热和营。取穴:风府、曲池、血海、足三里。

Dark brown or light black spots occur-ring over the face, neck and the dorsum of the hand, varying from a pinpoint to a mung bean in size; due to the stagnation of fire-evil in the small collaterals and the blood and also the attack of wind-evil, or due to blood-heat in the Lung Meridian. Treatment principle:Clear heat and regu-late the nutrient qi. Point selection: Fengfu (GV16), Quchi (LI11), Xuehai (SP10),Zusanli(ST36).

雀啄法 sparrow-pecking needling

针刺入穴位后,做有规律的小幅度上下

提插的手法,如雀啄米状。

Manipulation of needling by rhythmical-repeated lifting and thrusting of the needle in a small amplitude similar to the pecking of a sparrow.

雀啄灸 sparrow-pecking moxibustion

艾条灸的一种。将艾条燃着的一端对着施灸部位,与施灸部位并不固定在一定的距离,而是像鸟雀啄食一样,一上一下地移动,给予较强的断续的热刺激。

A form of moxa-stick moxibustion. Burn one end of a moxa-stick and move it up and down in a way similar to the pecking of a sparrow in order to provide a stronger and intermittent hot stimulation. The distance between the moxa-stick and the skin surface is determined by the patient's tolerance for heat.

R

然谷 Rangu (KI2)

经穴名。属足少阴肾经,本经荥穴。定位:在足内缘,足舟骨粗隆下方,赤白肉际处。主治:月经不调,阴挺,遗精,咯血,口渴,泄泻,足背肿痛,小儿脐风等。操作:直刺 0.5~1 寸;可灸。

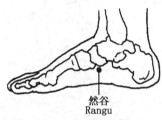

然谷
Rangu

The acupoint, Xing-Spring point of the Kidney Meridian of Foot-Shaoyin. Location: On the medial border of the foot, below the tuberosity of the navicular bone, on the dorso-ventral boundary of the foot. Indications: Irregular menstruation, prolapse of uterus, nocturnal mission, hemoptysis, thirst, diarrhea, swelling and pain of the dorsum of the foot, tetanus neonatorum, etc. Method: Puncture perpendicularly 0. 5-1 cun. Moxibustion is applicable.

热 heat

①即热邪。②即八纲之一。指各种原因引起的阳气亢盛,表现为热象如发热、面红、目赤、口渴等。③治法之一。即温法或祛寒法。④药物的四气之一。

①Referring to the heat-evil. ②One of the eight principle syndromes, a syndrome of hyperfunction of yang-qi, mani-fested as heat syndrome such as fever, flushed face, red eyes and thirst, etc. ③A therapeutic method, i. e., the therapy by warming or by expelling cold. ④One of the four characters of Chinese medicines.

热病五十九俞 fifty-nine points for febrile diseases

治疗热病应取的 59 个效穴,详见《黄帝内经》。

The fifty-nine effective acupoints in curing the febrile disease, see *Huangdi's Canon of Medicine* for details.

热敷 hot compress

用热药使患部产生温热的外敷方法。

Application of warm herb to the affected area in order to raise its temperature.

热极生寒 extreme heat engendering cold

当热证病情发展到热极阶段,因热邪内盛,阳气闭郁于内,不能外达四肢而出现四肢逆冷、脉沉等假寒的现象。

The occurrence of a false cold syndrome when the heat syndrome develops to a serious stage, in which the heat-evil is hyperactive in the interior, and the yang-qi is trapped in the body and fails to distribute to the extremities; manifested as cold extremities, deep pulse, etc.

热灸 hot moxibustion

指利用各种形式的热能灸治的方法,与"冷灸(发泡灸)"相对。

Moxibustion using various kinds of heat sources, as contrasted with "cold moxibustion (blistering moxibustion)".

热则疾之 quick needling for heat

sydrome

针刺治疗原则之一。指对热病应浅刺快出针,与"寒则留之"相对。

One of the principles in acupuncture, i. e. , needle shallowly and withdraw the needle quickly to cure heat syndrome as contrasted with "slow needling for cold syndrome".

人部 human level

又称人才。穴位深浅分部名,指中层,当肌肉之中。

Also called rencai, a name showing the depth of the points in acupuncture, namely, referring to the medium depth of the points inside the muscles.

人横 Renheng

大横穴的别名。

The other name of Daheng(SP15).

人神 Renshen

古代针灸宜忌说之一。意指人神按时巡行各部,其所在部位忌用针灸。

Theory of indications and contra-indications of acupuncture in ancient China. Renshen (human spirit) moves regularly through all parts of the human body, and where it stays, acupuncture and moxibustion are prohibited.

人事不省 unconsciousness

意识丧失的状态。治宜醒脑开窍。取穴:水沟、十二井穴、太冲、丰隆、劳宫。

A condition of unconsciousness. Treatment principle:Activate the brain and regain consciousness. Point selection:Shuigou (GV26), the twelve Jing-Well points, Taichong (LR3), Fenglong (ST40), Laogong(PC8).

人迎 Renying (ST9)

经穴名。属足阳明胃经。定位:在颈部,结喉旁,当胸锁乳突肌的前缘,颈总动脉搏动处。主治:咽喉肿痛,气喘,瘿气等。操作:直刺 0.3～0.8 寸,避开颈总动脉;可灸。

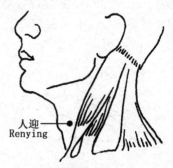

人迎
Renying

Name of an acupoint. It belongs to the Stomach Meridian of Foot-Yangming. Location:On the neck, near the Adam's apple, on the anterior border of the sternocleidomastoid, just on the pulsation point of the common carotid artery. Indications:Sore throat, asthma, goiter, etc. Method:Puncture perpendicularly 0. 3-0. 8 cun avoiding the common carotid artery. Moxibustion is applicable.

人中 philtrum; Renzhong

①上唇正中凹陷处。②水沟穴。

① Depression in the middle of the upper lip. ②Shuigou(GV26).

任脉 Conception Vessel

奇经八脉之一。起于小腹内,沿着脊椎骨内部上行。同时又出会阴部,上到阴毛部,沿腹部正中线,通过脐部,上至胸部、颈部,至下唇中央,由此分为左右两支,止于眼部。在循行过程中和诸阴经相联系,是阴经经脉的总纲。本经病症主要有疝气、赤白带、腹内肿块、胸腹部内脏功能失调、元气虚弱等。

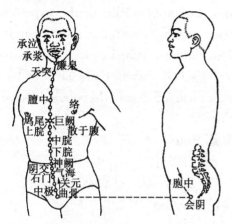

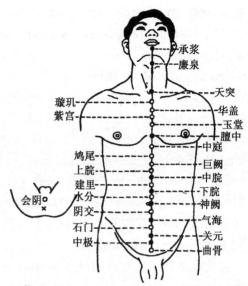

One of the eight extra meridians. It originates in the pelvis, and runs upward inside the vertebrae. At the same time, it runs out of the perineum, and to the pubic hair area, upward along the midline of the abdomen, via the umbilicus, to the chest, neck and the middle of the lower lip, where it divides into two branches, ends at the eyes. In the course of its circulation, it connects with all the yin meridians. It is the commander of all the yin meridians. When it is diseased, it can manifest symptoms such as hernia, red and white vaginal discharge, mass in the abdomen, dysfunction of the viscera in the chest and abdomen, deficiency of primordial qi.

任脉穴 points of the Conception Vessel

①任脉所属共 24 穴。②指列缺穴，为八脉交会穴之一。

① The 24 points of the Conception Vessel. ②Lieque(LU7), one of the eight confluence points.

妊娠恶阻 hyperemesis gravidarum

指妊娠早期出现的不同程度的反应。轻者仅觉轻微恶心、呕吐、不能进食。本病多由受孕后冲脉之气冲逆，胃失和降所致。治宜健脾和中、调气降逆。取穴：足三里、上脘、中脘、公孙。

Nausea or vomiting during early pregnancy, considered as a physiological response in mild cases. Severe cases with anorexia is caused by the dysfunction of stomach as a result of abnormal circulation of the Thoroughfare Vessel qi. Treatment principle:Strengthen the spleen and the stomach, regulate qi and lower the adverse flow of stomach-qi. Point selection:Zusanli(ST36), Shangwan(CV13), Zhongwan(CV12), Gongsun(SP4).

妊娠水肿 pregnancy edema

即妊娠肿胀。指妊娠 6 个月以后肌肤肢体肿胀。多因脾肾阳虚，水湿停聚，泛溢肌肤所致。治宜健脾益肾、调气行水。

取穴:脾俞、肾俞、水分、复溜、公孙。

Edema during pregnancy. A condition usually occurring after six months of pregnancy, caused by deficiency of spleen-yang and kidney-yang leading to retention of fluid in the body. Treatment principle: Strengthen the spleen and tonify the kindey, promote qi circulation and enhance water discharge. Point selection: Pishu(BL20), Shenshu(BL23), Shuifen (CV9), Fuliu(KI7), Gongsun(SP4).

日光灸 solar moxibustion

将艾绒平铺于腹部在日光下暴晒的一种疗法。

A kind of therapy by applying the mugwort floss on the abdomen and then being exposed to the sunlight.

日月 Riyue(GB24)

经穴名。属足少阳胆经,胆的募穴。定位:在上腹部,当乳头直下,第七肋间隙,前正中线旁开4寸。主治:胁痛,呕吐,吞酸,呃逆,黄疸,乳痈等。操作:平刺或斜刺0.5～0.8寸;可灸。

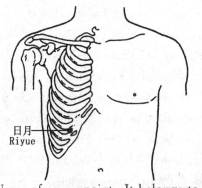

日月
Riyue

Name of an acupoint. It belongs to the Gallbladder Meridian of Foot-Shaoyang. It is the Front-Mu point of gallbladder.

Location: On the upper abdomen, directly below the nipple, in the 7th intercostal space, 4 cun lateral to the anterior midline. Indications: Pain in the hypochondriac region, vomiting, acid regurgitation, hiccup, jaundice, acute mastitis, etc. Method: Puncture obliquely or horizontally 0.5-0.8 cun. Moxibustion is applicable.

肉郄 Rouxi

承扶穴别名。

The other name of Chengfu(BL36).

肉柱 Rouzhu

承山穴别名。

The other name of Chengshan(BL57).

濡脉 soft pulse

浅表、细而柔软的脉象。轻按可触知,重按反不明显。多见于失血伤阴或湿邪滞留的患者。

A pulse condition characterized by superficial, thin and soft beats which are palpable when pressing lightly, but become indistinct when pressing heavily; commonly seen in case of consumption of yin after hemorrhage or stagnation of dampness-evil.

乳癖 lump in breast

多由思虑伤脾,郁怒伤肝,以致气滞痰凝而成。症见乳房中生肿块,形如梅李、鸡卵,或呈结节状,质硬压痛,推之可移,皮色不变,可随喜怒消长。类似于乳腺增生及乳腺良性肿瘤。治宜清热散结、疏肝理气。取穴:行间、肩井、膻中、丰隆、少泽。

A condition due to the stagnation of qi

and phlegm resulting from the damage of spleen by anxiety and from the damage of liver by anger; characterized by multiple lumps in the breast which are round or oval, indurated, tender, movable, covered with normal skin and vary in size with emotional changes; similar to hyperplasia of the mammary gland and benign tumor of the breast. Treatment principle: Clear heat and resolve masses, smooth the liver and regulate the circulation of qi. Point selection: Xingjian (LR2), Jianjing (GB21), Danzhong (CV17), Fenglong (ST40), Shaoze(SI1).

乳根 Rugen(ST18)

经穴名。属足阳明胃经。定位：在胸部，乳头直下，当第五肋间隙，距前正中线4寸。主治：胸痛，咳喘，气喘，乳痈，乳汁少等。操作：斜刺 0.5～0.8 寸；可灸。

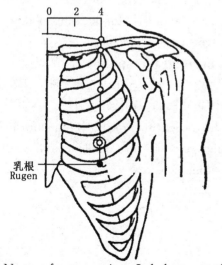

Name of an acupoint. It belongs to the Stomach Meridian of Foot-Yangming. Location: On the chest, directly below the nipple, on the lower border of the breast, in the 5th intercostals space, 4 cun lateral to the anterior midline. Indications: Pain in the chest, cough, asthma, acute mastitis, insufficient lactation. Method: Puncture obliquely 0.5-0.8 cun. Moxibustion is applicable.

乳上 Rushang

经外奇穴名。定位：位于乳头直上1寸处。灸治乳病及胸痛等。

Name of extra points. Location: 1 cun directly above the nipple. Moxibustion is used to cure breast diseases, chest pain, etc.

乳下 Ruxia

经外奇穴名。定位：位于乳头直下1寸处。常用灸治腹痛、腹满、胁痛、乳肿、乳汁少、久咳、反胃、干呕、胃痛、闭经等。

Name of extra points. Location: 1 cun below the nipple. Moxibustion is adopted to cure abdominal pain and fullness, hypochondriac pain, swelling breast, insufficient lactation, prolonged cough, regurgitation, retching, stomachache, amenorrhea, etc.

乳痈 acute mastitis

多由肝气郁结，胃热壅滞而成。初起乳房出现硬块，肿痛，乳汁不畅，全身可有恶寒发热，继则肿块增大，焮红剧痛，寒热不退，蕴酿成脓。治宜清热散结、疏肝理气。取穴：行间、肩井、膻中、丰隆、少泽。

A condition caused by the stagnation of liver-qi and accumulation of heat-evil in the stomach; characterized by indurated nodules, distending pain and inhibited flow of milk, accompanied with chills and fever, followed by enlargement of the nodules with erythema, intense pain and pustulation. Treatment principle: Clear heat and resolve masses, smooth the liver and regulate the circulation of qi. Point selection: Xingjian (LR2), Jianjing (GB21), Danzhong(CV17), Fenglong (ST40), Shaoze(SI1).

乳汁不足 insufficient lactation

乳汁分泌过少,多因产后气血亏虚、乳汁化源不足或肝郁气滞,乳汁壅滞不行所致。治宜益气补血,或疏肝解郁,佐以通乳。取穴:乳根、膻中、脾俞、足三里、少泽、太冲。

A condition mostly due to the deficiency of qi and blood after childbirth, or obstruction of the mammary ducts resulting from the stagnation of liver-qi. Treatment principle: Supplement qi and enrich the blood, or smooth the liver and regulate the circulation of qi, combine with promoting lactation. Point selection: Rugen(ST18), Danzhong (CV17), Pishu (BL20), Zusanli(ST36), Shaoze(SI1), Taichong(LR3).

乳中 Ruzhong(ST17)

经穴名。属足阳明胃经。定位:在胸部,当第四肋间隙,乳头中央,距前正中线4寸。此穴不针灸,只作胸腹部取穴的定位标志。

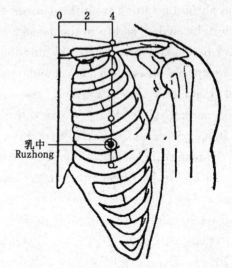

Name of an acupoint. It belongs to the Stomach Meridian of Foot-Yangming. Location: On the chest, in the 4th intercostal space, at the center of the nipple, 4 cun lateral to the anterior midline. Acupuncture and moxibustion on this point are contraindicated. This point serves only as a landmark for locating points on the chest and abdomen.

煏 burning therapy

古代用火针、温针或石针加热,用于刺激体表局部的一种治疗方法。

An ancient therapeutic method for local stimulation with fire needle, warm needle, or stone needle.

三变刺 three special kinds of acupuncture

刺法分类名。指针刺出血、出气和针后纳热三法。

Name of three special acupuncture skills which consist in bleeding, letting out qi and applying heat after needling.

三部九候 three positions and nine pulse-takings

诊脉分部名。①诊脉所用动脉分人迎、寸口、趺阳三部，每部又分天、地、人三候，合而为九。从此九部动脉诊候内脏及有关部位气血的盛衰。②诊寸口脉，以寸、关、尺为三部，每部又分轻按、中按、重按三候，共九候。

Different parts for checking pulse. ① The arteries for checking pulse can be divided into renying, cunkou and fuyang parts, and each part can be further divided into heaven, earth and man levels. Hence, three multiplied by three is nine. Diagnosis of sthenia and asthenia of qi and blood in the viscera and related parts can be made by feeling the arteries in these parts and levels. ②It refers to the cunkou diagnostic method, which includes cun, guan and chi parts. The pulse at each part can also be felt with slight pressure, moderate pressure and heavy pressure, total nine methods.

三部穴 three part points

指大包、天枢、地机三穴。此三穴位于人体上、中、下三部的重要位置，在治疗中具有重要意义。

Referring to Dabao (SP21), Tianshu (ST25) and Diji (SP8). These three points are situated on the very important sites of the upper, middle and lower parts of the human body and have remarkable significance in the treatment.

三才 three factors

原意指天、人、地。针灸中用作上、中、下或浅、中、深的分部名。

Three factors originally refer to the heaven, the man and the earth. In acupuncture and moxibustion, it means the top, the middle and the bottom level or the shallow, middle and deep.

三才穴 sancai points

指百会、璇玑、涌泉三穴，因其各分布在头、胸、足，故而得名。

It is the collective name of Baihui(GV20), Xuanji(CV21) and Yongquan(KI1), because these three points are situated on the head, the chest and the feet.

三池 Sanchi

经外奇穴名，即曲池及其上、下各一寸处，共三穴。主治：热病，鼻渊，肘臂酸痛，上肢不遂等。治疗常用针刺或温灸。

Name of extra points which consists of three points, including Quchi(LI11) and the points 1 cun above and below it. Indications: Febrile diseases, nasosinusitis, pain in elbow and arm, paresis of the upper arm. Method: Perpendicular acupuncture or warm moxibustion.

三刺 three-level needling

①指古代按皮下浅、中、深三层进行针刺的方法。②"齐刺"的别称。

① It is the technique used by ancient physicians to needling according to the superficial, medium and deep level beneath the skin. ② Another name of "triple needling".

三伏 sanfu

时令名。为阴历 1 年中最热的时期,约当阳历 7 月中旬至 8 月中旬。针灸临床常于三伏天治疗慢性疾病。

Season name. Sanfu is the hottest days of the year in the Chinese lunar calendar, roughly corresponding to the period from the middle of July to the middle of August. During these days acupuncture and moxibustion are often performed clinically to cure chronic diseases.

三间 Sanjian(LI3)

经穴名。属手阳明大肠经,本经输穴。定位:微握拳,在示指桡侧,第二掌指关节后凹陷处。主治:齿痛,咽喉肿痛,手指、手背红肿

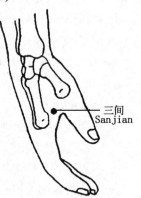

等。操作:直刺 0.3～0.5 寸;可灸。

The acupoint, Shu-Stream point of the Large Intestine Meridian of Hand-Yangming. Location: On the radial side of the index finger, in the depression of the 2nd metacarpophalangeal joint when a loose fist is made. Indications: Toothache, sore throat, redness and swelling of finger and the dorsum of the hand, etc. Method: Puncture perpendicularly 0.3-0.5 cun. Moxibustion is applicable.

三焦 sanjiao

①六腑之一,分上、中、下三个部位。具有调节各脏腑机能活动和参与调节体液代谢的功能。②耳穴名。在耳甲腔底部内分泌穴上方。主治:便秘、腹胀、上肢外侧痛等。

① One of the six fu organs, separated into upper, middle and lower portions. It has the function of regulating the activities of other viscera and participating in the control of fluid metabolism. ② Name of an ear point. On the base of the cavum conchae, superior to Neifenmi. Indications: Constipation, abdominal distension, pain in lateral aspect of upper limb, etc.

三焦辨证 sanjiao pattern differentiation

按温热病的病理过程及其传变情况,以上焦、中焦、下焦三个阶段作为辨证纲领,判断病变的部位、病情轻重及预后的一种辨证方法。

A principle of diagnosis for determining the involved part, severity and prognosis of a warm-heat disease by classifying the course of the disease into three stages, i. e., upper jiao, middle jiao and lower jiao.

三焦经 Sanjiao Meridian

手少阳三焦经的简称。

Abbreviation for the Sanjiao Meridian

of Hand-Shaoyang.

三焦俞 Sanjiaoshu(BL22)

经穴名。属足太阳膀胱经，三焦背俞穴。定位：在腰部，第一腰椎棘突下，旁开1.5寸。主治：肠鸣腹胀，呕吐，泄泻，痢疾，水肿，腰背强痛等。操作：直刺0.8～1.5寸；可灸。

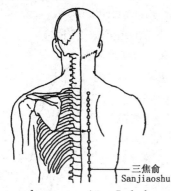

三焦俞
Sanjiaoshu

Name of an acupoint. It belongs to the Bladder Meridian of Foot-Taiyang. It is also the Back-Shu point of sanjiao. Location: On the waist, below the spinous process of the 1st lumbar vertebra, 1.5 cun lateral to the posterior midline. Indications: Borborygmus, abdominal distension, vomiting, diarrhea, dysentery, edema, pain and stiffness of the back and waist. Method: Puncture perpendicularly 0.8-1.5 cun. Moxibustion is applicable.

三角窝 triangular fossa

解剖名称。指对耳轮上下脚之间构成的三角形凹窝。

Terminologia anatomica. The triangular depression between the two crura of the antihelix.

三结交 Sanjiejiao

指关元穴。因任脉、足阳明、足太阴之脉皆结于此。

The other name of Guanyuan(CV4). It is the crossing point of the Conception Vessel, Foot-Yangming Meridian and Foot-Taiyin Meridian.

三进一退 three thrusting and one lifting

刺法用语。补法的进退针方法，"烧山火"中常用此法。此法与"一进三退"的泻法相对，分三层进针，一次退针直接到浅层。可反复施行。

A term of acupuncture which is one of the needle-manipulating methods for reinforcing. It is often used in the acupuncture skill "mountain-burning method", contrary to "one thrusting and three lifting" for reduction consists of thrusting in three levels and lifting the needle once directly to the shallow level of the point. This operation can be done repeatedly.

三棱针 three-edged needle

针具名。一般用不锈钢制成，针柄呈圆柱状，针身呈三角形而有刃，临床上用以刺破浅表静脉，放出少量血液来治病。多用于热病、炎症、中暑、昏迷等。

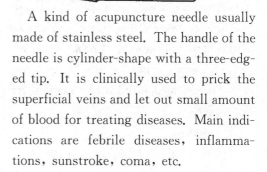

A kind of acupuncture needle usually made of stainless steel. The handle of the needle is cylinder-shape with a three-edged tip. It is clinically used to prick the superficial veins and let out small amount of blood for treating diseases. Main indications are febrile diseases, inflammations, sunstroke, coma, etc.

三里 Sanli

经穴名。有二：一属足阳明胃经，一属手阳明大肠经。前者为足三里，后者为手三里。一般多指前者而言。

Name of acupoints. There are two points both called Sanli, one belongs to the Stomach Meridian, the other to the Large Intestine Meridian. The former is called Zusanli (ST36), the latter is called Shousanli (LI10). It usually refers to the former.

三毛 clump hair

聚生于踇趾第一节背面皮肤的汗毛。

Hair growing in thick cluster on the dorsal aspect of the proximal phalange of the big toe.

三商 Sanshang

经外奇穴名。即老商、中商、少商。在拇指甲根后 0.1 寸处，三穴并列，中商居中，老商居尺侧甲根角外，少商居桡侧甲根角外。主治：昏迷，高热，流行性感冒，急性扁桃体炎，腮腺炎等。三棱针点刺出血。

Collective name of three extra points, i. e., Laoshang, Zhongshang and Shaoshang, located 0. 1 cun behind the nail root of the thumb at the same level with Zhongshang in the middle, Laoshang on the ulnar side of the corner of the nail and Shaoshang on the radial side of the corner of the nail. Indications: Coma, high fever, influenza, acute tonsillitis, mumps, etc. Three-edged needles are used to let out blood.

三水 sanshui

三水者，三阴，即太阴。又指肝、脾、肾。

It refers to the third yin, namely the Taiyin Meridians, or to the liver, spleen and kidney.

三阳经 three yang meridians

太阳、阳明和少阳三经的总称。

A collective term for the Taiyang Meridians, the Yangming Meridians, and the Shaoyang Meridians.

三阳络 Sanyangluo (TE8)

经穴名。属手少阳三焦经。定位：在前臂背侧，桡、尺骨之间，腕背横纹上 4 寸。主治：耳聋，暴喑，胸胁痛，手臂痛，齿痛等。操作：直刺 0.5～1寸，可灸。

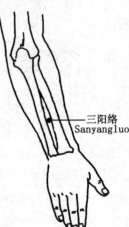

三阳络
Sanyangluo

Name of an acupoint. It belongs to the Sanjiao Meridian of Hand-Shaoyang. Location: On the dorsal side of the forearm, 4 cun above the transverse crease of the dorsum of the wrist, between the radius and ulna. Indications: Deafness, sudden loss of voice, pain in the chest and hypochondriac region, pain in the arm, toothache, etc. Method: Puncture perpendicularly 0. 5-1 cun. Moxibustion is applicable.

三阳五会 Sanyangwuhui

百会穴别名。

The other name of Baihui(GV20).

三阳在头 three yang on the head

指三阳经脉的动力集中反映于足阳明

胃经在头颈部的人迎动脉,相当于颈总动脉搏动处。

The motive force of three yang meridians are collectively reflected at renying artery of the Stomach Meridian of Foot-Yangming in the neck, corresponding to the point where the pulsation of the common carotid artery can be felt.

三阴交 Sanyinjiao(SP6)

经穴名。属足太阴脾经。定位:在小腿内侧,当足内踝尖上 3 寸,胫骨内侧缘后方。主治:腹痛肠鸣,腹胀泄泻,痛经,月经不调,尿血,带下,阴挺,滞产,不

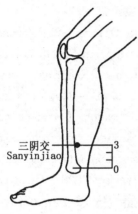

三阴交 Sanyinjiao

孕,遗精,阳痿,遗尿,水肿,疝气,心悸,失眠,高血压,下肢痿痹等。操作:直刺 0.5〜1 寸;可灸。

Name of an acupoint. It belongs to the Spleen Meridian of Foot-Taiyin. Location: On the medial side of the leg, 3 cun above the tip of the medial malleolus, posterior to the medial border of the tibia. Indications: Abdominal pain, borborygmus, abdominal distension, diarrhea, dysmenorrhea, irregular menstruation, hematuria, leukorrhea, prolapse of the uterus, prolonged labour, sterility, nocturnal emission, impotence, enuresis, edema, hernia, palpitation, insomnia, hepertension, paralysis and weakness of the lower limbs, etc. Method: Puncture perpendicularly 0.5-1 cun. Moxibustion is applicable.

三阴经 three yin meridians

太阴、少阴和厥阴三经的总称。

A collective term for the Taiyin Meridian, the Shaoyin Meridian, and the Jueyin Meridian.

三阴在手 three yin in the hand

指三阴经脉的动力集中反映于手太阴肺经在手腕部的寸口动脉,相当于桡动脉搏动处。

The motive force of the three yin meridians are collectively reflected at cunkou artery of the Lung Meridian of the Hand-Taiyin at the wrist, corresponding to the point where the pulsation of the radial artery can be felt.

散刺 scattered needling

刺法之一。指在穴位及其周围进行散在的多点浅刺。

One of the needling techniques, i. e., perform multiple scattered shallow acupuncture at the point and surrounding area.

散脉 scattered pulse

脉象名。散脉浮散无根,脉率不齐,至数不清,浮取应指,稍按则无,脉势软弱。多见于元气耗散,脏腑精气将绝,虚阳外越的重病。

A kind of pulse. It refers to a rootlessly scattered pulse with irregular and uncountable beats. It is feeble in nature, likely to be felt by touching and becomes indistinctive on pressure, usually seen in critical syndromes of scattering of primordial qi, exhaustion of essential qi from zang-fu organs and outward going of yang-qi in a deficiency condition.

散俞 scattered acupoints

即各经散在的腧穴,多用于春季点刺出血。

The scattered acupoints of the meridians, mostly used in spring for bleeding.

散笑 Sanxiao

经外奇穴名。位于鼻唇沟中点处。沿皮刺,主治鼻塞、颜面疔疮、口眼歪斜等。

Name of an extra point. Located at the midpoint of the nasolabial groove. Subcutaneous acupuncture is used to cure stuffy nose, facial sores, deviation of eyes and mouth, etc.

散针法 scattered needling method

指在病痛部位针刺,而不拘泥于流注。

One kind of needling method which needles directly at the points of the diseased part not necessarily considering the midnight-noon and ebb-flow acupoint selection.

涩脉 choppy pulse

脉搏不流畅,细而往来艰涩的一种脉象。多因津血亏损,气滞血瘀所致。

A pulse condition which is not fluent, thin, and comes and goes in difficulty, caused by consumption of blood and body fluid, stagnation of qi and blood stasis.

山根 shangen

部位名。指鼻根部,约与两眼内眦相平。

Name of the body part, i. e., the nasal root, roughly at the same level with the two inner canthi of the eyes.

闪罐 quick cupping

即快速拔罐,快速撤下,反复多次,直至局部皮肤潮红为止的一种治疗方法。

The technique of repeatedly applying and swiftly removing the cup until the skin of that area becomes hyperemic.

疝 hernia

①指体腔内容物向外突出的病。②指外生殖器如睾丸、阴囊部位的病变。③指腹部剧烈疼痛,兼有二便不通的病。治宜补气升陷、止痛。取穴:归来、带脉、维道、关元。

①Hernia. ②Referring to the diseases of the external genitalia such as testis and scrotum. ③Referring to severe abdominal pain accompanied with difficulty in urination and defecation. Treatment principle: Tonify and elevate the spleen-qi and alleviate pain. Point selection: Guilai (ST29), Daimai (GB26), Weidao(GB28), Guanyuan(CV4).

疝气穴 Shanqi point

经外奇穴名。取穴法:以口寸组成等边三角形,其顶端置于脐,底边两角为穴。灸治疝气、冷气心痛等。

Name of extra points. Location: Make an equilateral triangle with the length of one mouth cun and put the tip of the triangle at the navel, the apex of the two base angles are the points. Moxibustion is used to cure hernia, cardiac pain caused by cold-evil, etc.

伤寒杂病论 Treatise on Cold Damage and Miscellaneous Diseases

东汉末张仲景撰(公元 3 世纪初)。分为《伤寒论》和《金匮要略》两部分,是中医学的一部经典著作。

A classic medical work, written by the

outstanding physician Zhang Zhongjing in the late Eastern Han Dynasty（in the early 3rd century AD）. It contains two parts，one entitled *Treatise on Cold Damage Diseases*，the other，*Synopsis of Prescriptions of the Golden Chamber*.

商丘 Shangqiu（SP5）

经穴名。属足太阴脾经,本经经穴。定位:在足内踝前下方凹陷中,当舟骨结节与内踝尖连线的中点处。主治:腹胀,便秘,泄泻,肠鸣,舌本强痛,足踝痛等。操作:直刺 0.3～0.5 寸;可灸。

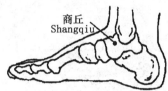

The acupoint，Jing-River point of the Spleen Meridian of Foot-Taiyin. Location：In the depression，anterior and inferior to the medial malleolus，at the midpoint of the line connecting the tuberosity of the navicular bone and the tip of the medical malleous. Indications：Abdominal distension，constipation，diarrhea，borborygmus，pain and rigidity of the tongue，pain in the ankles，etc. Method：Puncture perpendicularly 0.3-0.5 cun. Moxibustion is applicable.

商曲 Shangqu（KI17）

经穴名。属足少阴肾经。定位:在上腹部,当脐中上 2 寸,前正中线旁开 0.5 寸。主治:腹痛,腹泻,便秘等。操作:直刺 1～1.5 寸;可灸。

Name of an acupoint. It belongs to the Kidney Meridian of Foot-Shaoyin. Location：

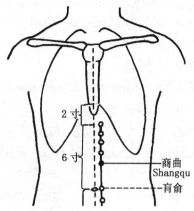

On the upper abdomen，2 cun above the center of the umbilicus，and 0.5 cun lateral to the anterior midline. Indications：Abdominal pain，diarrhea，constipation，etc. Method：Puncture perpendicularly 1-1.5 cun. Moxibustion is applicable.

商阳 Shangyang（LI1）

经穴名。属手阳明大肠经,本经井穴。定位:在手示指末节桡侧,距指甲角 0.1 寸。主治:齿痛,咽喉肿痛,颌肿,手指麻木,热病昏迷等。操作:浅刺 0.1 寸,或三棱针点刺出血。

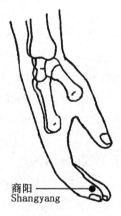

The acupoint，Jing-Well point of the Large Intestine Meridian of Hand-Yangming. Location：On the radial side of the distal segment of the index finger，0.1 cun from the corner of the nail. Indications：Toothache，sore throat，swelling of the submandibular region，numbness of finger, coma caused by febrile diseases, etc. Method: Puncture shallowly 0.1 cun or prick with the three-edged needle to cause bleeding.

上病下取 taking the lower points to cure the upper diseases

取穴法之一,指上部的病症取用下部穴。

One of the point-selecting methods which consists in choosing the lower part points to cure the upper part diseases.

上都 Shangdu

经外奇穴名。八邪之一。

Name of an extra point. It is one of the Baxie (EX-UE9).

上腭 Shang'e

经外奇穴名。定位:位于上腭齿龈上缘中点。斜刺或三棱针点刺出血治黄疸、热病等。

Name of an extra point. Location: At the midpoint of the upper margin of the gingiva of the palate. Obligue acupuncture or letting out blood with a three-edged needle is used to cure jaundice, febrile diseases, etc.

上耳背 Shangerbei

耳穴名。主治:皮肤病,坐骨神经痛,背痛等。

Name of an ear point. Indications: Skin diseases, sciatica, back pain, etc.

上耳根 Shangergen

①解剖名称。指耳廓上缘与头皮附着处。②耳穴名。又称郁中、脊髓。在耳根最上缘,主治头痛、腹痛、气喘、衄血等。

①Terminologia anatomica. It refers to the area where the superior border of au-

ricle attaches to the scalp. ②Name of an ear point. It also named Yuzhong, Jisui. It is on the top edge of the auricular. Indications: Headache, abdominal pain, asthma, bleeding from five sense organs or subcutaneous tissue, etc.

上关 Shangguan(GB3)

经穴名。属足少阳胆经。定位:在耳前,下关穴直上,当颧弓的上缘凹陷处。主治:头痛,耳鸣,耳聋,齿痛,口眼歪斜等。操作:直刺0.5～0.8寸;可灸。

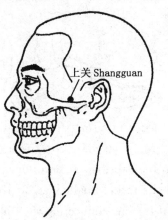

上关 Shangguan

Name of an acupoint. It belongs to the Gallbladder Meridian of Foot-Taiyang. Location: Anterior to the ear, directly above Xiaguan(ST7), in the depression above the upper border of the zygomatic arch. Indications: Headache, tinnitus, deafness, toothache, deviation of eyes and mouth, etc. Method: Puncture perpendicularly 0.5-0.8 cun. Moxibustion is applicable.

上焦 upper jiao

三焦的上部,从咽喉至胸膈,心肺位于其中,具有将脾胃传输而来的营养物均匀地分布到全身的作用。

The upper part of sanjiao, corresponding to the body cavity above the diaphragm, where the heart and lung are located. It possesses the function of evenly distributing the nutrients absorbed by the stomach and spleen to the whole body.

上巨虚 Shangjuxu(ST37)

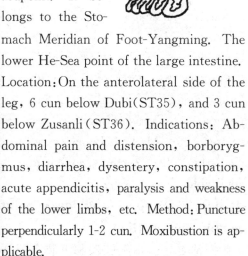

经穴名。属足阳明胃经,大肠下合穴。定位:在小腿前外侧,当犊鼻穴下 6 寸,足三里穴下 3 寸。主治:腹痛腹胀,肠鸣泄泻,痢疾,便秘,肠痈,下肢痿痹等。操作:直刺 1～2 寸;可灸。

上巨虚
Shangjuxu

Name of an acupoint. It belongs to the Stomach Meridian of Foot-Yangming. The lower He-Sea point of the large intestine. Location: On the anterolateral side of the leg, 6 cun below Dubi(ST35), and 3 cun below Zusanli(ST36). Indications: Abdominal pain and distension, borborygmus, diarrhea, dysentery, constipation, acute appendicitis, paralysis and weakness of the lower limbs, etc. Method: Puncture perpendicularly 1-2 cun. Moxibustion is applicable.

上廉 Shanglian(LI9)

经穴名。属手阳明大肠经。定位:在前臂背面桡侧,当阳溪与曲池连线上,肘横纹下 3 寸。主治:肩臂酸痛,手臂麻木,腹痛肠鸣等。操作:直刺 0.5～1 寸;可灸。

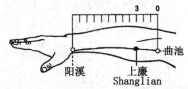

阳溪　　上廉
Shanglian

Name of an acupoint. It belongs to the Large Intestine Meridian of Hand-Yangming. Location: On the radial side of the dorsal side of the forearm and on the line connecting Yangxi (LI5) and Quchi (LI11), 3 cun below the cubital transverse crease. Indications: Aching of the shoulder and arm, numbness of the arm, abdominal pain, borborygmus, etc. Method: Puncture perpendicularly 0. 5-1 cun. Moxibustion is applicable.

上廉泉 Shanglianquan

经外奇穴名。定位:在下颌中点下缘 1 寸,当下颌下缘与舌骨体之间凹陷处。主治:喑哑,流涎,舌强,咽痛,吞咽困难,失音等。

Name of an extra point. Location: 1 cun below the midpoint of the lower jaw, in the depression between the hyoid bone and the lower border of the jaw. Indications: Alalia, salivation, stiff tongue, sore throat, difficulty in swallowing, loss of voice, etc.

上髎 Shangliao(BL31)

经穴名。属足太阳膀胱经。定位:在骶部,当髂后上棘与后正中线之间,适对第一骶后孔处。主治:腰痛,小便不利,便秘,月经不调,带下,阴挺等。操作:直刺 0.8～1.2 寸;可灸。

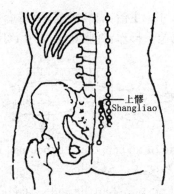

Name of an acupoint. It belongs to the Bladder Meridian of Foot-Taiyang. Location：On the sacrum, at the midpoint between the posterior superior iliac spine and the posterior midline, just at the 1st posterior sacral foramen. Indications： Lumbago, dysuria, constipation, irregular menstruation, leukorrhea, prolapse of the uterus, etc. Method：Puncture perpendicularly 0. 8-1. 2 cun. Moxibustion is applicable.

上林 Shanglin

上巨虚穴别名。

The other name of Shangjuxu(ST37).

上门 Shangmen

幽门穴别称。

The other name of Youmen(KI21).

上气海 Shangqihai

膻中穴别名。

The other name of Danzhong(CV17).

上实下虚 upper excess and lower deficiency

①指邪气实于上、正气虚于下的一种病理现象。②指肝肾阴虚、肝阳上亢的病理。

①A morbid condition with hyperactivity of the evil in the upper part and deficiency of vital qi in the lower part. ②A morbid condition with deficiency of liver-yin, kidney-yin, and hyperfunction of liver-yang.

上脘 Shangwan (CV13)

经穴名。属任脉。定位：在上腹部，前正中线上，当脐中上 5 寸。主治：胃痛，腹胀，恶心，呕吐，癫痫，失眠等。操作：直刺 0.8～1.2寸；可灸。

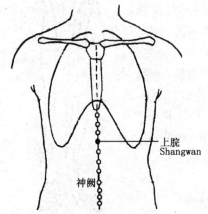

Name of an acupoint. It belongs to the Conception Vessel. Location：On the upper abdomen, on the anterior midline, 5 cun above the center of the umbilicus. Indications：Stomachache, abdominal distension, nausea, vomiting, epilepsy, insomnia, etc. Method：Puncture perpendicularly 0. 8-1. 2 cun. Moxibustion is applicable.

上下配穴法 upper and lower point combination method

配穴法之一。指上肢穴和下肢穴配合应用。

One of the point combination methods, namely, the combination of points in the arms and the legs.

上星 Shangxing(GV23)

经穴名。属督脉。定位：在头部，当前发际正中之上 1 寸。主治：头痛，目痛，鼽衄，癫狂等。操作：平刺 0.3～0.5 寸；可灸。

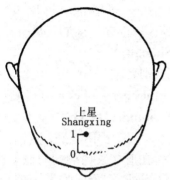

Name of an acupoint. It belongs to the Governor Vessel. Location：On the head，1 cun directly above the midpoint of the anterior hairline. Indications：Headache，eye pain，nasal obstruction，epistaxis，mental disorder，etc. Method：Puncture horizontally 0.3-0.5 cun. Moxibustion is applicable.

上龈里 Shangyinli

经外奇穴名。位于上唇黏膜正中，外与水沟穴相对处。直刺或三棱针点刺出血治黄疸、热病等。

Name of an extra point. Location：At the center of the upper lip mucosa, corresponding to Shuigou(GV26) on the exterior. Perpendicular acupuncture or letting out blood with a three-edged needle is used to cure jaundice, febrile diseases, etc.

上迎香 Shangyingxiang(EX-HN8)

经外奇穴名。也称鼻穿或鼻通穴。位于鼻骨下凹陷中，鼻唇沟上端尽处。主治：久流冷泪，火眼，鼻炎，鼻窦炎等。沿皮刺。

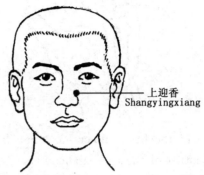

Name of an extra point, also called Bichuan or Bitong, situated at the depression of the nasal bone or at the upper end of the nasolabial groove. Subcutaneous acupuncture is used to cure chronic cold lacrimation, acute conjunctivitis, rhinitis, nasosinusitis, etc.

烧山火 mountain-burning method

指针刺入皮下后，按照浅、中、深的顺序三进一退，反复操作，使患者出现热感的方法。

After the needle is inserted, repeatedly thrust it three times through the superficial, medium and deep levels, and lift it once so as to make the patient feel warm.

少冲 Shaochong(HT9)

经穴名。属手少阴心经，本经井穴。定位：在手小指末节桡侧，距指甲角 0.1 寸。主治：心悸，心痛，胸胁痛，癫狂，热病，昏迷等。操作：浅刺 0.1 寸，或三棱针点刺出血；可灸。

The acupoint, Jing-Well point of the Heart Meridian of Hand-Shaoyin. Location：On the radial side of the distal seg-

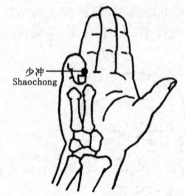

ment of the litter finger, 0.1 cun from the corner of the nail. Indications: Palpitation, cardiac pain, pain in the chest and hypochondriac regions, mania, febrile diseases, coma, etc. Method: Puncture shallowly 0.1 cun or prick with a three-edged needle to cause bleeding. Moxibustion is applicable.

少府 Shaofu(HT8)

经穴名。属手少阴心经,本经荥穴。定位:在手掌面,第四、五掌骨之间,握拳时,当小指尖处。主治:心悸,胸痛,小指挛痛,掌中热,小便不利,遗尿,阴痒等。操作:直刺0.3～0.5寸;可灸。

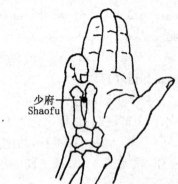

The acupoint, Xing-Spring point of the Heart Meridian of Hand-Shaoyin. Location: In the palm, between the 4th and 5th metacarpal bones, at the tip of the litter finger when a fist is made. Indications: Palpitation, pain in the chest, spasmodic pain of the little finger, feverish sensation in the palm, dysuria, enuresis, pruritus of the vulvae, etc. Method: Puncture perpendicularly 0.3-0.5 cun. Moxibustion is applicable.

少谷 Shaogu

三间穴别名。

The other name of Sanjian(LI3).

少海 Shaohai (HT3)

经穴名。属手少阴心经,本经合穴。定位:屈肘,在肘横纹内侧端与肱骨内上髁连线的中点处。主治:心痛,肘臂挛痛,手颤,瘰疬,腋肿胁痛等。操作:直刺0.5～1寸;可灸。

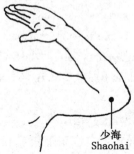

The acupoint, He-Sea point of the Heart Meridian of Hand-Shaoyin. Location: When the elbow is flexed, it is at the midpoint of the line connecting the medial end of the cubital transverse crease and the medial epicondyle of the humerus. Indications: Cardiac pain, spasmodic pain and numbness of the arm, tremor of the hand, scrofula, swelling of the axilla, pain in hypochondriac regions, etc. Method: Puncture perpendicularly 0.5-1 cun. Moxibustion is applicable.

少吉 Shaoji

少泽穴别名。

The other name of Shaoze(SI1).

少商 Shaoshang(LU11)

经穴名。属手太
阴肺经,本经井穴。
定位:在手拇指末
节桡侧,距指甲角
0.1 寸。主治:咽
喉肿痛,咳嗽,气
喘,鼻衄,发热,昏
迷等。操作:浅刺
0.1寸,或三棱针点刺出血;可灸。

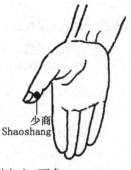
少商
Shaoshang

The acupoint, Jing-Well point of the Lung Meridian of Hand-Taiyin. Location:On the radial side of the distal segment of the thumb, 0.1 cun from the corner of the finger nail. Indications:Sore throat, cough, asthma, epistaxis, fever, coma, etc. Method:Puncture shallowly 0.1 cun or prick with a three-edged needle to cause bleeding. Moxibustion is applicable.

少阳 Shaoyang

有阳气减弱之意。

It means that the yang-qi is diminishing.

少阳经 Shaoyang Meridian

三阳经之一,手少阳三焦经与足少阳胆经的总称。

One of the three yang meridians, i.e., a joint name of the Sanjiao Meridian of Hand-Shaoyang and the Gallbladder Meridian of Foot-Shaoyang.

少阳为枢 the Shaoyang Meridians are pivots

指少阳经位于身体三阳经的表里之间,起枢纽作用。

The Shaoyang Meridians are located between the outside and the inside of the three yang meridians, acting as pivots or switches.

少阴 Shaoyin

有阴气减弱之意。

It means that the yin-qi is diminishing.

少阴经 Shaoyin Meridian

手少阴心经与足少阴肾经的总称。

A joint name of the Heart Meridian of Hand-Shaoyin and the Kidney Meridian of Foot-Shaoyin.

少阴俞 Shaoyinshu

肾俞穴别名。

The other name of Shenshu(BL23).

少阴为枢 Shaoyin Meridians are pivots

指少阴经位于三阴经的中间部位,起枢纽作用。

The Shaoyin Meridians are located in the middle of the three yin meridians, acting as pivots or switches.

少泽 Shaoze (SI1)

经穴名。属手太
阳小肠经,本经井
穴。定位:在手小
指末节尺侧,距指
甲角 0.1 寸。主
治:头痛,热病,昏
迷,乳汁少,咽喉
痛,目赤膜翳等。

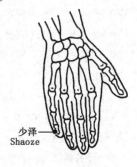
少泽
Shaoze

操作:浅刺 0.1 寸,或三棱针点刺出血;可灸。

The acupoint, Jing-Well point of the Small Intestine Meridian of Hand-Taiyang. Location: On the ulnar side of the distal segment of the little finger, 0.1 cun from the corner of the nail. Indications: Headache, febrile diseases, coma, insufficient lactation, sore throat, redness of the eyes, cloudiness of the cornea, etc. Method: Puncture shallowly 0.1 cun or prick with a three-edged needled to cause bleeding. Moxibustion is applicable.

舌 tongue; She

①在口腔内活动的肌性器官,对味有特别的感觉,有助于咀嚼、吞咽、发音。与心的功能有密切关系。观察舌的色、质、形态及舌苔变化是中医望诊的重要内容之一。②耳穴名,在耳垂2区正中,主治舌炎。

①The movable, muscular organ on the floor of the mouth, subserving a special sense for taste and aiding in mastication, deglutition, and the articulation of sound. It is considered that the condition of the tongue is closely related to the function of the heart. The inspection of the colour, nature, appearance and fur of the tongue serves as a principle aspect in the diagnosis of diseases. ②Name of an ear point. It is in the center of zone 2 of lobe. It is used for treating glossitis.

舌本 root of tongue; Sheben

①即舌根。舌体靠近咽喉的部位,数条经脉行经该部,与各经脉及内脏有密切关系。②风府穴和廉泉穴的别称。

①It's the part of the tongue attached to the the throat, through which several meridians pass. It is closely related to the conditions of various meridians and viscera. ② Another name for Fengfu(GV16) or Lianquan(CV23).

舌绛 crimson tongue

舌质呈深红色,是温病热邪侵入营分的舌象。深红而舌中心干,是胃火伤津;深红色光亮而无苔,则属胃阴已亡;深红而舌质干枯不鲜者,是肾阴涸竭的征象。

A deep red colour of the tongue, indicating the attack of heat-evil to the nutrient aspect during warm diseases. Dryness at the center signifies the consumption of body fluid by stomach-fire; bright and uncoated appearance signifies the exhaustion of stomach-yin; dryness all over the tongue signifies the exhaustion of kidney-yin.

舌强 stiff tongue

舌体强硬,转动不灵,多兼见语言謇涩不清。若伴肢体瘫痪、口眼歪斜等症,多属中风;若舌质红绛、神昏谵语,多属温热病热入心包或高热伤津所致。治宜通经活络。取穴:哑门、廉泉、通里。

Immovability of the tongue usually associated with dysphasia. If accompanied with paralysis of the limbs and deviation of eyes and mouth, it is often seen in apoplexy; if accompanied with crimson tongue and delirium, it is often seen in warm-heat diseases when the pericardium is attacked by the heat-evil, or the body fluid is consumed during high fever.

Treatment principle：Activate the meridians and the collaterals. Point selection：Yamen（GV15）, Lianquan（CV23）, Tongli(HT5).

舌苔 tongue fur

舌质表面的一层苔状物。通过观察舌苔的变化,可以判断病情,了解病邪的深浅及津液的存亡,是望诊的重要内容之一。

A coating over the surface of the tongue, serving as an important criteria for the diagnosis, the estimation of the severity of a disease and of the fluid amount of the body.

舌歪 deviation of the tongue

舌伸出时偏于一侧,歪斜不正,常与四肢瘫痪、口眼歪斜同时出现,多因肝风内动或风邪中络所致。治宜通经活络。取穴:哑门、廉泉、通里、金津、玉液。

A sign characterized by deviation of tongue to one side when it is stuck out, usually accompanied with paralysis of the limbs and deviation of the eyes and mouth；caused by the liver-wind stirring in the interior or the wind-evil invading the collaterals. Treatment principle：Activate the meridians and the collaterals. Point selection：Yamen（GV15）, Lianquan(CV23）, Tongli(HT5), Jinjin(EX-HN12）, Yuye(EX-HN13).

舌诊 tongue diagnosis

望诊的主要内容。即通过观察舌质及舌的形态、色泽、润燥等的变化,来辨别病情,帮助诊断。

A main inspection by observing the texture, colour and moisture of the tongue for making a diagnosis.

舌柱 Shezhu

①指舌系带。②经外奇穴名。位于舌系带上方。用三棱针点刺出血。

①The lingual frenulum. ②Name of an extra point. It is located at the upper part of the lingual frenulum. Letting out blood with a three-edged needle is usually adopted.

摄法 pinching technique

针刺补助手法。即用手指甲掐、切、抓、捏经络部位,以催气行血。

One of the acupuncture supplementary technique, i. e., pinching, incising, grasping and kneading the part where the meridians pass with fingernails to induce the needling sensations and promote the blood circulation.

申脉 Shenmai(BL62)

经穴名。属足太阳膀胱经,八脉交会穴之一,通于阳跷脉。定位:在足外侧部,外踝直下方凹陷中。主治:癫狂,痫证,头痛,眩晕,失眠,背痛,腰腿酸痛等。操作:直刺0.3~0.5寸;可灸。

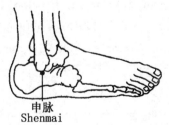

申脉
Shenmai

Name of an acupoint. It belongs to the Bladder Meridian of Foot-Taiyang. One of the eight confluence points, communicates with the Yang Heel Vessel. Location：On the lateral side of the foot, in the depression directly below the external malleolus. Indications：Mania, epilepsy, headache, dizziness, insomnia, backache, aching of the waist and legs, etc. Method：Puncture perpendicularly 0. 3-0. 5 cun. Moxibustion is applicable.

身柱 Shenzhu (GV12)

经穴名。属督脉。定位：在背部，当后正中线上，第三胸椎棘突下凹陷中。主治：咳嗽，气喘，癫痫，脊强背痛，疔疮等。操作：稍向上斜刺0.5～1寸；可灸。

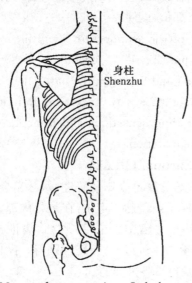

身柱
Shenzhu

Name of an acupoint. It belongs to the Governor Vessel. Location：On the back, on the posterior midline, in the depression below the spinous process of the 3rd thoracic vertebra. Indications：Cough, asthma, epilepsy, pain and stiffness of the back, hard furuncles, etc. Method：Puncture obliquely upward 0. 5-1 cun. Moxibustion is applicable.

神 vitality

①人体生命活动的总称，包括显露于外的生理性或病理性征象，是望诊的重要内容之一。②指思维意识活动。

①Spirit：A general term for the life activities, including the external appearances of the physiological or pathological condition of the body, which are major criteria for diagnosis. ②Mind：Referring to thought and state of consciousness.

神藏 Shencang(KI25)

经穴名。属足少阴肾经。定位：在胸部，当第二肋间隙，前正中线旁开2寸。主治：咳嗽，气喘，胸痛等。操作：斜刺或平刺0.5～0.8寸；可灸。

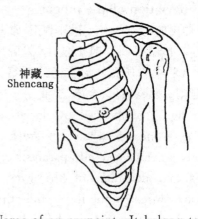

神藏
Shencang

Name of an acupoint. It belong to the Kidney Meridian of Foot-Shaoyin. Location：On the chest, in the 2nd intercostal space, 2 cun lateral to the anterior midline. Indications：Cough, asthma, chest pain, etc. Method：Puncture obliquely or horizontally 0. 5-0. 8 cun. Moxibustion is applicable.

神聪 Shencong

经外奇穴名。位于百会穴四面，各相去1寸。共四穴，又名四神聪。沿皮肤刺或灸治中风、头痛、晕眩、癫痫、狂乱及神经衰弱等。操作:平刺 0.5～0.8 寸;可灸。

Name of extra points. They are located 1 cun lateral to Baihui(GV20) on the four sides, four points in all, so also known as Sishencong(EX-HN1). Subcutaneous acupuncture or moxibustion is used to cure apoplexy, headache, vertigo, epilepsy, mania, neurasthenia, etc. Method:Puncture horizontally 0.5-0.8 cun. Moxibustion is applicable.

神道 Shendao(GV11)

经穴名。属督脉。定位:在背部,当后正中线上,第五胸椎棘突下凹陷中。主治:健忘,心悸,脊背强痛,咳嗽,心痛等。操作:稍向上斜刺 0.5～1 寸;可灸。

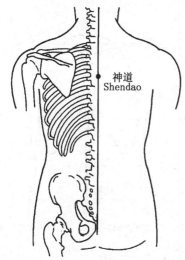

Name of an acupoint. It belongs to the Governor Vessel. Location:On the back, on the posterior midline, in the depression below the spinous process of the 5th thoracic vertebra. Indications:Amnesia, palpitation, pain and stiffness of the back, cough, cardiac pain, etc. Method:Puncture obliquely upward 0.5-1 cun.

Moxibustion is applicable.

神封 Shenfeng(KI23)

经穴名。属足少阴肾经。定位:在胸部,当第四肋间隙,前正中线旁开 2 寸。主治:咳嗽,气喘,胸胁胀满,乳痛等。操作:斜刺或平刺 0.5～0.8 寸;可灸。

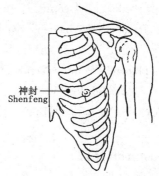

Name of an acupoint. It belongs to the Kidney Meridian of Foot-Shaoyin. Location:On the chest, in the 4th intercostals space, 2 cun lateral to the anterior midline. Indications:Cough, asthma, fullness in the chest and hypochondriac region, acute mastitis, etc. Method:Puncture obliquely or horizontally 0.5-0.8 cun. Moxibustion is applicable.

神府 Shenfu

经外奇穴名。定位:位于中庭穴下 0.3 寸。沿皮刺或艾灸主治心痛。

Name of an extra point. Location: 0.3 cun below Zhongting(CV16). Subcutaneous acupuncture or moxibustion is used to cure cardiac pain.

神光 Shenguang

日月穴别名。

The other name of Riyue(GB24).

神昏 coma

指神志昏迷,意识不清,往往由邪热内

陷心包,或湿热、痰浊蒙蔽清窍所引起。治宜熄风开窍、清心豁痰。取穴:水沟、十二井穴、太冲、丰隆、劳宫。

A state of unconsciousness, usually caused by heat-evil attacking the pericardium or by damp-heat evil and phlegm blocking the upper orifices. Treatment principle: Calm the endopathic wind and regain consciousness, remove heat from the heart and eliminate phlegm. Point selection: Shuigou (GV26), the twelve Jing-Well points, Taichong (LR3), Fenglong (ST40), Laogong (PC8).

神门 Shenmen(HT7)

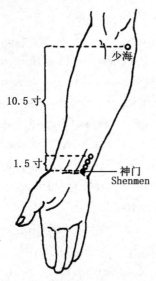

经穴名。属手少阴心经,本经输穴、原穴。定位:在腕部,腕横纹尺侧端,尺侧腕屈肌腱的桡侧凹陷处。主治:心痛,心烦,心悸,癔病,失眠健忘,癫狂,痫证,胸胁痛,高血压等。操作:直刺或斜刺0.3~0.5寸;可灸。

The acupoint, Shu-Stream and Yuan-Primary point of the Heart Meridian of Hand-Shaoyin. Location: On the wrist, at the ulnar end of the wrist transverse crease, in the depression of the radial side of the tendon of the ulnar flexor muscle of the wrist. Indications: Cardiac pain, irritability, palpitation, hysteria, insomnia, amnesia, mania, epilepsy, pain in the chest and hypochondriac region, hypertension, etc. Method: Puncture perpendicularly or obliquely 0.3-0.5 cun. Moxibustion is applicable.

神阙 Shenque(CV8)

经穴名。属任脉。定位:在脐中。主治:腹痛肠鸣,泄泻脱肛等。操作:禁针;可灸。

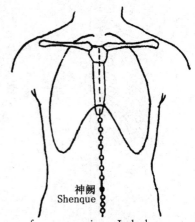

Name of an acupoint. It belongs to the Conception Vessel. Location: At the center of the umbilicus. Indications: Abdominal pain, borborygmus, diarrhea, prolapse of the rectum, etc. Method: Puncture is prohibited. Moxibustion is applicable.

神堂 Shentang(BL44)

经穴名。属足太阳膀胱经。定位:在背部,当第五胸椎棘突下,后正中线旁开3

寸。主治：气喘，心痛，心悸，胸闷，咳嗽，脊背强痛等。操作：斜刺 0.5～0.8 寸；可灸。

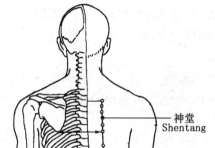

神堂
Shentang

Name of an acupoint. It belongs to the Bladder Meridian of Foot-Taiyang. Location：On the back，below the spinous process of the 5th thoracic vertebra，3 cun lateral to the posterior midline. Indications：Asthma，cardiac pain，palpitation，stuffy chest，cough，stiffness and pain in the back，etc. Method：Puncture obliquely 0.5-0.8 cun. Moxibustion is applicable.

神庭 Shenting(GV24)

经穴名。属督脉。定位：在头部，当前发际正中直上 0.5 寸。主治：癫痫，心悸，健忘，头痛，眩晕，鼻渊等。操作：平刺 0.3～0.5 寸；可灸。

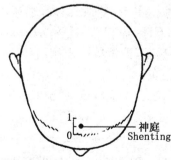

神庭
Shenting

Name of an acupoint. It belongs to the Governor Vessel. Location：On the head，

0.5 cun directly above the midpoint of the anterior hairline. Indications：Epilepsy，palpitation，amnesia，headache，vertigo，nasosinusitis，etc. Method：Puncture horizontally 0.3-0.5 cun. Moxibustion is applicable.

神应王 Shenyingwang

指中国古代名医扁鹊，后指医生。

An official rank given to the famous ancient Chinese doctor Bianque and later it refers to doctors.

肾 kidney；Shen

①五脏之一。中医学的肾不能与现代医学的肾的解剖位置和生理功能等同。它的主要功能是：主藏精，滋养脏器、骨和脑。肾精的盛衰对个体的生长发育（包括胚胎时期）有着极重要的意义。肾和肺、脾两脏共同参与人体水液的代谢，是调节人体水液代谢的重要器官。中医学的肾大体上包括了泌尿生殖系统及内分泌系统、造血系统、中枢神经系统的部分功能。②耳穴名。在对耳轮下脚下缘，小肠穴直上方。主治：腰痛，耳鸣，神经衰弱，哮喘，夜尿症，月经不调，遗精，阳痿，早泄等。

①One of the five viscera. In TCM, the kidney does not completely match that of western medicine from the standpoint of anatomy and physiology. Its main function is storing the essence of life to nourish the viscera，bones and brain. The kidney essence is important for the growth and development of an individual，including the embryonic stage. The kidney is an important organ in participating in the metabolism of body fluids together with the lung and the spleen. In general, the kidney in TCM mainly performs partial functions of urogenital system, endocrine system, hematopoietic system and central nervous system. ② Name of an ear point which is on the lower of inferior antihelix crus, directly above Xiaochang. Indications: Lumbago, tinnitus, neurasthenia, asthma, nocturia, irregular menstruation, nocturnal emission, impotence, premature ejaculation, etc.

肾肝之部 hepatonephric part

针刺的分部,指肌肉深层,与"心肺之部"相对。

Acupuncture section, i. e. , the deep part in the muscles in contrast with "cardiopulmonary part".

肾合膀胱 kidney being connected with bladder

指肾与膀胱之间的相互关联和影响。它们通过经络的联系,互为表里,在生理上互相协调,在病理上互相影响。如肾与膀胱互相配合共同完成尿的生成、贮藏和排出。若肾的功能失常,往往影响膀胱的功能而出现尿液排泄障碍。

The paired relationship between kidney and bladder which are connected by the network of meridians. They cooperate in function and involve each other when diseased. For instance, the formation, storage and discharge of urine are completed by the kidney and the bladder coordinately, and dysfunction of the kidney may cause disorders of the bladder leading to the impediment of urination.

肾间动气 motive qi between the kidneys

生理学术语。两肾所藏之真气,即命门相火。人体脏腑经络的正常功能、三焦气化及抵御外邪均赖此动气,故又称生气之原。

A terminology of physiology. Referring to the genuine qi stored between the kidneys, i. e. , the ministerial fire of the life gate. It is necessary for the activities of zang-fu organs, meridians and collaterals, qi-transformation of sanjiao and eliminating the exogenous evils, so is said to be the source of qi.

肾上腺 Shenshangxian

耳穴名。定位:在耳屏下部隆起的尖端。主治:低血压,风湿性关节炎,腮腺炎,休克等。

Name of an ear point. Location: At the tip of the tubercle on the lower broder of the tragus. Indications: Hypotension, rheumatoid arthritis, mumps, shock, etc.

肾俞 Shenshu(BL23)

经穴名。属足太阳膀胱经,肾的背俞穴。定位:在腰部,当第二腰椎棘突下,旁开 1.5 寸。主治:梦遗,阳痿,遗尿,月经不调,带下,腰痛膝软,目昏头晕,耳聋耳鸣,水肿喘咳,泄泻等。操作:直刺 0.8～1.5 寸;可灸。

Name of an acupoint. It belongs to the Kidney Meridian of Foot-Taiyang. Back-Shu point of the kidney. Location: On the lower back, below the spinous process of the 2nd lumbar vertebra, 1.5 cun lateral to the posterior midline. Indications:

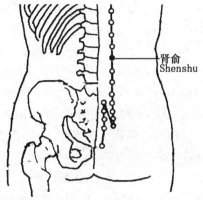

肾俞
Shenshu

Nocturnal emission, impotence, enuresis, irregular menstruation, leukorrhea, lumbago, weakness of the knees, blurred vision, dizziness, deafness, tinnitus, edema, asthma, diarrhea, etc. Method: Puncture perpendicularly 0.8-1.5 cun. Moxibustion is applicable.

肾俞五十七穴 fifty-seven points related to the kidney

指治疗水病的五十七穴,皆与肾有关。

The 57 acupoints used to cure the water-diseases related to the kidney.

肾系 Shenxi

经外奇穴名。位于伏兔穴下 1 寸。针灸治消渴、便数。

Name of an extra point. Located 1 cun below Futu (ST32). Acupuncture or moxibustion can be adopted to cure consumptive thirst, polyuria, etc.

肾虚 asthenia of kidney

又称肾亏。通常指肾脏精气不足。症见精神疲乏、头晕耳鸣、健忘、腰酸、遗精等。治宜补肾益精。取穴:肾俞、太溪、命门、关元。

A morbid state of insufficiency of e-ssence and qi of the kidney; manifested as fatigue, dizziness, tinnitus, amnesia, soreness of loins, nocturnal emission, etc. Treatment principle: Tonify the kindey and nourish the essence. Point selection: Shenshu (BL23), Taixi (KI3), Mingmen(GV4), Guanyuan(CV4).

肾阳虚 deficiency of kidney-yang

肾脏生理功能低下,也是人体生命活动功能低下的病理。症见身寒、怕冷、腰酸、阳痿、夜尿多,甚则浮肿、气喘等。治宜补益肾阳。取穴:肾俞、命门、关元、大椎。

A morbid state of renal hypofunction and decreased vital activities; manifested as low body temperature, intolerance of cold, soreness of loins, impotence, frequent urination at night or even edema, asthma, etc. Treatment principle: Strengthen the kidney-yang. Point selection:Shenshu(BL23), Mingmen(GV4), Guanyuan(CV4), Dazhui(GV14).

肾阴虚 deficiency of kidney-yin

又称肾阴不足,即肾脏阴精不足,可引起肾脏病理性亢进。症见腰酸疲乏、头晕耳鸣、遗精早泄、口干咽痛,五心烦热或午后潮热、舌红少苔、脉细数等。治宜补益肾阴。取穴:肾俞、太溪、照海、三阴交。

A morbid state of insufficiencyof kidney-yin, usually leading to pathological hyperfunction of the kidney; manifested as soreness of loins, fatigue, dizziness, tinnitus, nocturnal emission, premature ejaculation, dry mouth, sore throat, dysphoria with feverish sensation in chest, palms and soles, or afternoon tidal fever, red uncoated tongue, thin and rapid pulse, etc. Treatment principle: Nourish the kindey-yin. Point selection: Shenshu (BL23), Taixi(KI3), Zhaohai(KI6), Sanyinjiao(SP6).

肾之府 residence of kidney

指腰部。因肾在其中。

The loins where the kidney exists.

肾主水 kidney controls water

肾的主要生理功能之一。肾主体内水液的分布与排泄,在调节体液平衡中起着极为重要的作用。

One of the main functions of the kidney. Kidney controls the distribution and excretion of body fluid and also plays an important role in the regulation of body fluid equilibrium.

升提中气 lifting up the middle qi

治疗中气下陷的方法。适用于脾虚中气下陷引起的久泻、脱肛、子宫脱垂等病症。

A treatment for the collapse of middle qi, applicable to cases caused by spleen deficiency and collapse of middle qi, such as chronic diarrhea, prolapse of rectum, uterine prolapse, etc.

生成数 sheng-cheng numbers

古代一、二、三、四、五称作"生数",六、七、八、九、十称为"成数"。其中奇数属天,偶数属地,相互配合应用于针刺的补泻手法中。

In ancient China, the numbers from one to five were named "sheng-numbers" while the numbers from six to ten were named "cheng-numbers". The odd numbers among them belong to the heaven and the even numbers among them belong to the earth. These numbers were combined in different ways and used in the reinforcing or reducing acupuncture.

生熟 weak or strong moxibustion

灸法用语。生指少灸和小火灸,熟指多灸和旺火灸。

A term used in moxibustion. Weak moxibustion refers to short time and weak fire moxibustion while strong moxibustion refers to long time and intense fire moxibustion.

圣济总录 Complete Records of Holy Benevolence

医书名。宋朝官修,共 200 卷。其中 191～194 卷为针灸内容。

Name of a medical book. Compiled by the government of the Song Dynasty, 200 volumes in all. The 4 volumes from No. 191 to No. 194 deals with acupuncture and moxibustion.

盛者泻之 treating excess with purgation

针灸治疗原则之一。意指对实证应行泻法,与"虚者补之"相对。

One of the principles in acupuncture and moxibustion therapy, i. e., the reducing therapy should be used to treat the excess diseases as contrasted with "treating deficiency with tonification".

失眠 insomnia

又称不寐。指经常入睡困难,或易醒,甚至彻夜不眠。本症多由阴血亏损、中气不足,心脾两虚或痰饮内停等多种原因使心神不安所致。治宜滋阴养血、平肝降火、化痰和胃。取穴：神门、三阴交、太溪、太冲、丰隆。

Inability to fall asleep or stay asleep, due to irritability resulting from deficiency of yin-blood, insufficiency of middle qi, asthenia of the heart and the spleen or retention of phlegm. Treatment principle：Nourish yin and blood, calm and suppress liver-fire, resolve phlegm and regulate the stomach. Point selection：Shenmen(HT7), Sanyinjiao(SP6), Taixi (KI3), Taichong (LR3), Fenglong (ST40).

失眠穴 Shimian point

经外奇穴名。位于足底部，当足底中线与内、外踝连线的交点。主治：失眠，足底痛等。治疗常用直刺或温灸。

Name of extra points. Located at the crossing point of the sole midline and the line between the medial and the external ankles. Indications：Insomnia, sole pain, etc., with perpendicular acupuncture or warm moxibustion.

失音 dysphonia

又称喑，即发音困难。若突然失音，多因外感风寒、风热所致，属实证；若慢性失音发作，多因肺肾受伤、阴精亏损所致，属虚证。治宜通络开窍。取穴：哑门、廉泉、通里。

Difficult in speaking. If with sudden onset due to exposure to wind-cold evil or wind-heat evil, it generally belongs to sthenia syndrome；if with chronic relapses due to the impairment of the lung and kidney or the consumption of yin-essence, it generally belongs to asthenia syndrome. Treatment principle：Remove obstruction in the meridians and open orifices. Point selection：Yamen (GV15), Lianquan(CV23), Tongli(HT5).

湿热 damp-heat

①湿与热相结合形成的一种致病因子。②温病的一种。症见发热、头痛、身重而痛、倦怠、腹满、食欲减退、小便短少而黄、舌苔黄腻、脉濡数等。治宜清热利湿。取穴：合谷、足三里、阴陵泉、三阴交。

① A pathogenic factor formed by blending of heat-evil and dampness-evil. ②One of the warm diseases, manifested as fever, headache, pantalgia, fatigue, abdominal distention, anorexia, oliguria with yellowish urine, yellow and greasy fur on the tongue, soft and rapid pulse, etc. Treatment principle：Clear heat and promote diuresis. Point selection：Hegu (LI4), Zusanli (ST36), Yinlingquan (SP9), Sanyinjiao(SP6).

湿阻中焦 dampness-evil stagnated in the middle jiao

湿邪滞留脾胃的病理。症见头重，倦怠，腹胀，食欲不振，口渴喜热饮，小便短赤，舌苔厚白，脉缓等。治宜健脾利湿。取穴：足三里、三阴交、阴陵泉、脾俞。

A morbid condition due to retention of dampness-evil in the spleen and stomach; manifested as heavy sensation of the head, fatigue, abdominal distension, poor appetite, thirst and desire for hot drink, oliguria with deep-colored urine, thick and whitish fur on the tongue, slow pulse, etc. Treatment principle: Tonify the spleen and promote dieresis. Point selection: Zusanli (ST36), Sanyinjiao (SP6), Yinlingquan (SP9), Pishu (BL20).

十二刺 twelve needling methods

指古代应用的十二种刺法,即偶刺、报刺、恢刺、齐刺、扬刺、直针刺、输刺、短刺、浮刺、阴刺、傍针刺、赞刺。

They are twelve ancient acupuncture techniques, i. e., coupled needling, successive trigger needling, relaxing needling, triple Needling, centro-square needling, perpendicular needling, shupoint needling, short needling, superficial needling, yin needling, perpendicular and lateral needling, repeated shallow need-ling.

十二地支 twelve earthly branches

中国古代用以计时序的一种手段,也称十二支,现中国阴历仍用十二支与天干相配纪年。

The means of marking the time and the order in ancient China, also called twelve branches. The Chinese lunar calendar is now still expressed by the combination of the twelve earthly branches and the ten heavenly stems to record years.

十二节 twelve joints

①中国农历表示气候变化的标志日期。②人有四肢,每肢三节,共十二节,即双侧肩、肘、腕、股、膝、踝关节。

①In Chinese lunar calendar there are twelve dates in a year to designate the change of climate. ②In the human body there are also twelve joints which are evenly distributed in the four extremities, i. e., bilateral joint of shoulder, elbow, wrist, hip, knee and ankle.

十二禁 twelve acupuncture contraindications

指针刺前后的一些禁忌情况,如房事、醉酒、愤怒、劳累、饥渴等。

Acupuncture is prohibited in some cases such as right before or after sexual intercourse, alcohol intoxication, anger, overtired, hunger and thirst.

十二经标本 origins and terminals of the twelve meridians

经络部位名。手足六经各有本部和标部。本指根本,为经气所起;标指末梢,为经气所止。

Name of meridian parts. There are the origins and terminals in the six hand meridians and the six foot meridians. Origins mean the sources of the meridians while the terminals mean the ends of the meridians where the meridian qi stops.

十二经别 twelve divergent meridians

是十二经脉别出的正经,分别起于四肢,循行于内脏深部,上出于颈项浅部。能加强十二经脉中表里经的联系,补正经循行之不足。

Branches departed from the twelve regular meridians. They start from limbs, run in the deep part of the internal organs and come up to the superficial part of the neck. The branches strengthen the ralations between the externally-internally related meridians to make up the shortage of the regular meridians.

十二经动脉 arteries of the twelve meridians

指在十二经循行过程中有脉搏应手的动脉部位,也就是身体浅表的一些动脉血管。

The arteries along the course of the twelve meridians where the pulse can be easily felt. Those arteries are located superficially.

十二经筋 twelve muscle regions

是在十二经脉循行部位上分布的体表肌肉系统的总称。

A collective name for the muscular system which is distributed along the courses of the twelve meridians.

十二经脉 twelve meridians

经络分类名。为经络中的主体部分。每一经脉,内部隶属于一定的脏腑,外部分布于四肢、躯干和头面。分手足三阴、手足三阳经脉。

Name of meridian classification. The twelve meridians are the main parts of the meridian system. Each meridian belongs to specific zang or fu-organ in the interior and is distributed on the limbs, the trunk and the head in the exterior. They are classified into three yin meridians and three yang meridians of hand and foot.

十二经之海 the convergence of the twelve meridians

指冲脉,是十二经脉会合的海洋。

Referring the Thoroughfare Vessel. It is the sea where the twelve meridians flow into.

十二井穴、十二井 twelve Jing-Well points

十二井穴的总称。十二井穴位于四肢末端,即少商(肺)、中冲(心包)、少冲(心)、商阳(大肠)、关冲(三焦)、少泽(小肠)、隐白(脾)、大敦(肝)、涌泉(肾)、厉兑(胃)、足窍阴(胆)、至阴(膀胱)。临床治疗发热、昏迷、休克等症。

The general name of the twelve Jing-Well points located at the ends of the four extremities, namely Shaoshang (LU11), Zhongchong (PC9), Shaochong (HT9), Shangyang (LI1), Guanchong (TE1), Shaoze (SI1), Yinbai (SP1), Dadun (LR1), Yongquan (KI1), Lidui (ST45), Zuqiaoyin (GB44), Zhiyin (BL67). All those points are clinically used to treat fever, coma, shock, etc.

十二皮部 twelve cutaneous regions

十二经脉在体表皮肤部位的反映区。

The reflex zones of the twelve meridians on the defined skin areas.

十二原穴、十二原 twelve Yuan-primary points

十二经均有原穴,合称十二原,即太渊(肺)、合谷(大肠)、冲阳(胃)、太白(脾)、神门(心)、腕骨(小肠)、京骨(膀胱)、太溪(肾)、大陵(心包)、阳池(三焦)、丘墟(胆)、太冲(肝)。

The twelve meridians each have their own Yuan-Primary point, namely Taiyuan (LU9), Hegu (LI4), Chongyang (ST42), Taibai (SP3), Shenmen (HT7), Wangu

(SI4)，Jinggu (BL64)，Taixi (KI3)，Daling (PC7)，Yangchi (TE4)，Qiuxu (GB40) and Taichong (LR3).

十干 ten stems

即天干，用于记载时序，也用于时间配穴法中。

Ten heavenly stems. They are used to record the time and the order, and also used for time combination points selection in acupuncture.

十六郄穴 sixteen Xi-Cleft points

在经脉上位于气血汇集的空隙处的十六个穴位，即孔最、会宗、郄门、养老、阴郄、梁丘、温溜、外丘、金门、跗阳、地机、交信、中都、阳交、水泉、筑宾。

Sixteen points located in the clefts where qi and blood collect. They are Kongzui (LU6)，Huizong (TE7)，Ximen (PC4)，Yanglao (SI6)，Yinxi (HT6)，Liangqiu (ST34)，Wenliu (LI7)，Waiqiu (GB36)，Jinmen (BL63)，Fuyang (BL59)，Diji (SP8)，Jiaoxin (KI8)，Zhongdu (LR6)，Yangjiao (GB35)，Shuiquan (KI5)，Zhubin (KI9).

十七椎 Shiqizhui (EX-B8)

经外奇穴名。定位：在第五腰椎棘突下。主治：腰腿痛，下肢瘫痪，月经不调，痛经等。操作：直刺，0.5～1 寸。

Name of an extra point. Location：Below the spinous process of the 5th lumbar vertebra. Indications：Lumbar and thigh pain，paralysis of the lower limbs，irregular menstruation，dysmenorrhea，etc. Method：Puncture perpendicularly 0.5-1 cun.

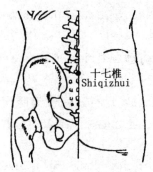

十四经 fourteen meridians

指十二经脉加上任、督二脉。

The Conception Vessel and the Governor Vessel are added to the twelve meridians，total fourteen Meridians.

十四经穴 fourteen-meridian points

指十二经脉及任、督二脉上的腧穴，总计约 361 个，其中单穴 52 个，两侧双穴 309 个。

All the points on the twelve meridians，plus the Governor Vessel and the Conception Vessel，the number of which is about 361 including 52 single points and 309 bilateral double points.

十五络脉 fifteen collateral meridians

指全身十五条最大的络脉。十四经各有一条大的络脉，脾脏区域另有一条大络。

The fifteen largest collateral meridians. Each of the fourteen meridians has a collateral meridian，plus the extra large collateral meridian of the splenic region.

十五络穴 fifteen callateral points

十五络脉在十四经脉和脾脏区域的起始穴位。

The start points where the fifteen collaterals branching out from the fourteen meridians and the splenic region.

十宣 Shixuan (EX-UE11)

经外奇穴名。定位:在手十指尖端,距指甲游离缘 0.1 寸处。主治:中风、昏迷、癫痫、高热、咽喉肿痛、小儿惊风、指端麻木等。操作:浅刺 0.1 寸,或三棱针点刺出血;可灸。

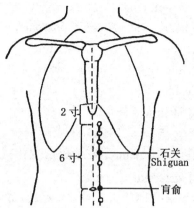

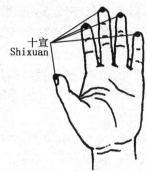

the center of the umbilicus, and 0.5 cun lateral to the anterior midline. Indications:Vomiting, abdominal pain, constipation, postpartum abdominal pain, sterility, etc. Method:Puncture perpendicularly 1-1.5 cun. Moxibustion is applicable.

石门 Shimen(CV5)

经穴名。属任脉,三焦的募穴。定位:在下腹部,当脐中下 2 寸。主治:腹痛泄泻,水肿,疝气,小便不利,遗尿,经闭,带下,崩漏,产后出血等。操作:直刺 0.5～1.5 寸;可灸。

Name of extra points. Location:On the tips of the ten fingers, about 0.1 cun from the free edge of the nails. Indications:Apoplexy, coma, epilepsy, high fever, sore throat, infantile convulsion, numbness of the finger tips, etc. Method:Puncture shallowly 0.1 cun or prick with a three-edged needle to cause bleeding. Moxibustion is applicable.

石宫 Shigong

阴都穴别名。

The other name of Yindu(KI19).

石关 Shiguan(KI18)

经穴名。属足少阴肾经。定位:在上腹部,当脐中上 3 寸,前正中线旁开 0.5 寸。主治:呕吐,腹痛,便秘,产后腹痛,不孕等。操作:直刺 1～1.5 寸;可灸。

Name of an acupoint. It belongs to the Kidney Meridian of Foot-Shaoyin. Location:On the upper abdomen, 3 cun above

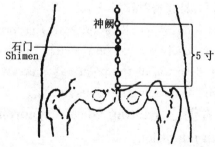

Name of an acupoint. It belongs to the Conception Vessel. Front-Mu point of sanjiao. Location:On the lower abdomen, 2 cun below the center of the umbilicus. Indications:Abdominal pain, diarrhea, edema, hernia, dysuria, enuresis, amenorrhea, leukorrhea, metrorrhagia and metrostaxis, postpartum hemorrhage, etc. Method: Puncture perpendicularly 0.5-1.5 cun. Moxibustion is applicable.

石阙 Shique

石关穴别名。

The other name of Shiguan(KI18).

时病 seasonal diseases

多指季节性的常见病、多发病,如春季的春温、风温等,夏季的泄泻、痢疾、中暑等,秋季的疟疾、秋燥等,冬季的伤寒、冬温等。

It refers to the diseases which are common and prevalent in a particular season, e.g., spring fever and wind fever in spring; diarrhea, dysentery and sunstroke in summer; malaria and the autumn dryness; cold damage and winter warmth.

实按灸 pressing moxibustion

将艾条点燃后,隔布或隔纸按在穴位上灸,与"悬起灸"相对。

A kind of moxibustion with the moxa stick closely pressed on the cloth or paper placed on top of the point, as contrasted with "suspending moxibustion".

实者泻之 treating sthenia syndrome with purgation

属邪实的疾病,宜用泻法以祛其邪气。临床上一般宜按病邪的性质及其所在的部位而采用不同的泻法。如属热结大肠,宜寒下;属寒积,宜温下等。

A therapeutic principle for treating the case with sthenic evils. Different types of purgation are applied according to the character and the location of the evil, e.g., the accumulation of heat-evil in the large intestine should be purged with cold-nature herbs, while the cold-evil with warm-nature herbs.

实证 sthenia syndrome

病邪亢盛而正气亦不虚,正邪斗争剧烈,或脏腑功能障碍引起气血郁结、痰饮内停、食积等所致的一种证候。症见高热、口渴、烦躁、谵语、腹胀腹痛而拒按、便秘、尿少而深黄、舌红、苔黄而干糙、脉实有力等。

A syndrome occurring in a hard struggling between relatively strong vital qi and evil or dysfunction of the viscera leading to the stagnation of qi and blood, phlegm-retention, indigestion, etc.; manifested as high fever, thirst, irritability, delirium, abdominal distension, pain and tenderness, constipation, oliguria with deep-colored urine, red tongue with rough, dry and yellowish fur, solid and strong pulse, etc.

食窦 Shidou(SP17)

经穴名。属足太阴脾经。定位:在胸外侧部,当第五肋间隙,距前正中线6寸。主治:胸胁胀痛等。操作:平刺或斜刺0.5～0.8寸;可灸。

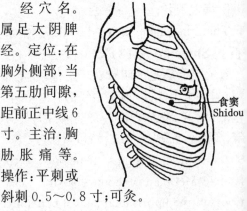

食窦 Shidou

Name of an acupoint. It belongs to the Spleen Meridian of Foot-Taiyin. Location: On the lateral side of the chest, and in the 5th intercostal space, 6 cun lateral to the anterior midline. Indications: Fullness and pain in the chest and hypochondriac regions, etc. Method: Puncture horizontally or obliquely 0. 5-0. 8 cun. Moxibustion is applicable.

食宫 Shigong

阴都别名。

The other name of Yindu(KI19).

食关 Shiguan

经外奇穴名。中脘穴旁开 1. 5 寸。直刺或灸治消化系统疾病。

Name of an extra point. Located 1. 5 cun lateral to Zhongwan (CV12). Perpendicular acupuncture or moxibustion is adopted to cure digestive system diseases.

食管 Shiguan

耳穴名。定位：在耳轮脚下方前 2/3 处。主治：食道炎，吞咽困难等。

Name of an ear point. Location: At the anterior 2/3 of the inferior helix crus. Indications: Esophagitis, dysphagia, etc.

食积 dyspepsia

因脾胃运化失常，食物积滞不化所致的一种疾病。症见胸脘满闷、腹痛拒按或有痞块、大便秘结、纳食减少、嗳腐吞酸、舌苔厚腻等。治宜消积导滞、调理脾胃。取穴：脾俞、胃俞、足三里、四缝、中脘。

A disease caused by indigestion resulting from the functional disorder of the spleen and stomach; manifested as fullness of the chest and upper abdomen, abdominal pain and tenderness, or palpable mass, constipation, poor appetite, eructation with fetid odor, acid regurgitation, thick and greasy fue on the tongue, etc. Treatment principle: Promote digestion and remove stagnation, and regulate the function of the spleen and stomach. Point selection: Pishu(BL20), Weishu(BL21), Zusanli (ST36), Sifeng (EX-UE10), Zhongwan(CV12).

视区 visual zone

自枕外粗隆平齐旁开 1cm 处，向上与正中线平行做 4cm 长的直线即是本区。主治：皮质性失盲症。

Make a 4cm line parallel to the posterior midline from the point located on the horizontal line passing the external occipital protuberance and 1 cm to the anteropesterior midline. It is used for treating visual disorders of cortical origin.

是动病 meridian diseases

①经脉经气变动引起所连络脏腑的病证。②经脉循行路线上的病证。

①Diseases of a certain organ induced by disorders in its corresponding meridian; ②Diseases located on the pathway of a certain meridian.

手厥阴心包经 the Pericardium Meridian of Hand-Jueyin

十二正经之一。它的循行路线是：在体内，属心包，络三焦，并与横膈膜相连；在体表，起于侧心包，经腋下、上肢屈侧正中线，止于手中指指尖。本经患病，主要有心烦、心痛、心悸、精神病、面黄、目赤等，以及本经循行部位的局部症状。

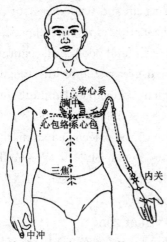

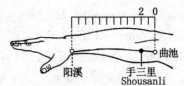

One of the twelve regular meridians. Its circulating path is as following: Inside the body, it is related to the pericardium and connected with sanjiao and the diaphragm; on the body surface, it runs from the lateral aspect of the pericardium, along the axilla, the median of the flexor surface of the upper limb, and terminates at the tip of the middle finger. When this meridian is diseased, there appear symptoms such as dysphoria, precardial ache, palpitation, mental disorder, yellowish complexion, redness of the eyes, etc., as well as the local symptoms of the parts along its pathway.

手三里 Shousanli (LI10)

经穴名。属手阳明大肠经。定位：在前臂掌面桡侧，当阳溪与曲池连线上，肘横纹下 2 寸。主治：齿痛颊肿，上肢不遂，腹痛腹泻，肩背痛等。操作：直刺 0.5～1 寸；可灸。

Name of an acupoint. It belongs to the Large Intestine Meridian of Hand-Yangming. Location: On the radial side of the dorsal side of the forearm and on the line connecting Yangxi (LI5) and Quchi (LI11), 2 cun below the cubital crease. Indications: Toothache, swelling of the cheeks, motor impairment of the upper limbs, abdominal pain, diarrhea, pain in the shoulder and back, etc. Method: Puncture perpendicularly 0.5-1 cun. Moxibustion is applicable.

手三阳经 three yang meridians of the hand

指手部的三条阳经，即手阳明大肠经、手太阳小肠经、手少阳三焦经。

The Large Intestine Meridians of Hand-Yangming, the Small Intestine Meridian of Hand-Taiyang, and the Sanjiao Meridian of Hand-Shaoyang.

手三阴经 three yin meridians of the hand

指手部的三条阴经，即手太阴肺经、手少阴心经、手厥阴心包经。

The Lung Meridian of Hand-Taiyin, the Heart Meridian of Hand-Shaoyin, and the Pericardium Meridian of Hand-Jueyin.

手少阳三焦经 the Sanjiao Meridian of Hand-Shaoyang

十二正经之一。它的循行路线是：在体内，属三焦，络心包络，并与耳、眼相连；在体表，起于无名指端，沿上肢伸侧正中线，经过肩部、侧头部、耳部、止于眼部。本经患病，主要有耳病、咽喉病、眼痛、颊肿、出汗等，以及本经循行部位的局部症状。

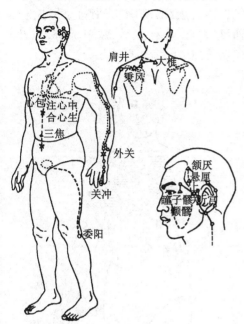

One of the twelve regular meridians. Its circulating path is as following: Inside the body, it is related to sanjiao and connected with the pericardium, ears and eyes; on the body surface, it runs form the tip of the ring finger, along the median of the extensor surface of the upper limb, lateral side of the neck, lateral aspect of head and ear, terminates at the eyes. When this meridian is diseased, there appear symptoms such as ear disease, throat disease, pain of the eyes, swelling of the cheeks, perspiration, etc., as well as the local symptoms of the parts along its pathway.

手少阴心经 the Heart Meridian of Hand-Shaoyin

十二正经之一。循行路线：在体内，属心，络小肠，并与咽部及眼相连；在体表，由腋下部，沿上肢屈侧后面向下，止于小指端。本经患病，主要有心痛、口渴、咽干、目黄、胸痛等，以及本经循行部位的局部症状。

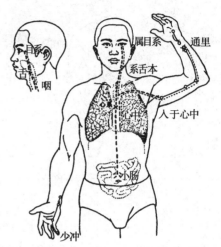

One of the twelve regular meridians. Its circulating path is as following: Inside the body, it is related to the heart and connected with the small intestine, throat, and the eyes; on the body surface, it arises from the axilla, runs downward along the posterior aspect of the flexor surface of the upper limb, and terminates at the tip of the little finger. When this meridian is diseased, there appear symptoms such as cardiac pain, thirst, dryness of the throat, yellowish sclera, chest pain, etc., as well as the local symptoms of the parts along its pathway.

手太阳小肠经 the Small Intestine Meridian of Hand-Taiyang

十二正经之一。循行路线：在体内，属小肠，络心，并与胃、眼和内耳相连；在体表,由手小指端,经过上肢伸侧后面、肩胛部、侧颈部、颜面、眼部,止于耳部。本经患病,主要有耳聋、目黄、面颊和下颌部肿胀而使颈部不能回旋,咽喉病等病症,以及在本经循行部位的局部症状。

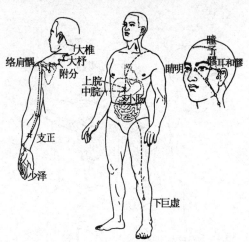

One of the twelve regular meridians. Its circulating path is as following: Inside the body, it is related to the small intestine and connected with the heart, stomach, eyes and internal ears; on the body surface, it runs from the tip of the small finger, along the posterior aspect of the extensor surface of the upper limb, scapula, lateral aspect of the neck, face, and eyes, and terminates at the ears. When this meridian is diseased, there appear symptoms such as deafness, yellowish sclera, swelling of the cheeks and mandible leading to stiffness of the neck, sore throat, etc., as well as the local symptoms of the parts along its pathway.

手太阴肺经 the Lung Meridian of Hand-Taiyin

十二正经之一。循行路线:在体内,属肺,络大肠,并与胃、喉相连;在体表,由胸部外上方沿上肢屈侧前面向下,止于拇指端。本经患病,主要有咳嗽、咯血、喘息短气、口渴、烦躁、胸满、肩背痛、手心发热、伤风、自汗、小便频数、尿黄赤等,以及本经循行部位的局部症状。

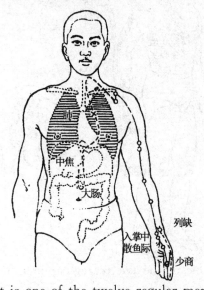

It is one of the twelve regular meridians. Its circulating path is as following: Inside the body, it is related to the lungs and connected with the large intestine, and communicates with the stomach and throat; on the body surface, it runs from the laterosuperior aspect of the chest, along the flexor aspect of the upper limb and ends at the tip of the thumb. When this meridian is diseased, the main symptoms are cough, hemoptysis, dyspnea and shortness of breath, thirst, restlessness, fullness in the chest, pain of the shoulders and upper back, heat in the palms, mild common cold, spontaneous sweating, frequent urination and deep-colored urine, as well as local symptoms of the parts along the path of this meridian.

手五里 Shouwuli(LI13)

经穴名。属手阳明大肠经。定位：在臂外侧，当曲池与肩髃连线上，曲池上 3 寸处。主治：肘臂挛痛，瘰疬等。操作：直刺 0.5～1 寸；可灸。

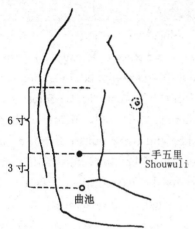

Name of an acupoint. It belongs to the Large Intestine Meridian of Hand-Yangming. Location: On the lateral side of the upper arm and on the line connecting Quchi (LI11) and Jianyu(LI15), 3 cun above Quchi(LI11). Indications:Contracture and pain of the elbow and arm, scrofula, etc. Method: Puncture perpendicularly 0.5-1 cun. Moxibustion is applicable.

手阳明大肠经 the Large Intestine Meridian of Hand-Yangming

十二正经之一。循行路线：在体内，属大肠，络肺；在体表，由示指端经过上肢伸面桡侧、肩部、颈部、颊部，止于对侧鼻孔旁。在本经患病，主要有泄泻、痢疾、肠鸣、恶寒战栗、目黄、口干、鼻衄、鼻塞、咽喉炎、牙痛、颈部肿大等，以及本经循行部位的局部症状。

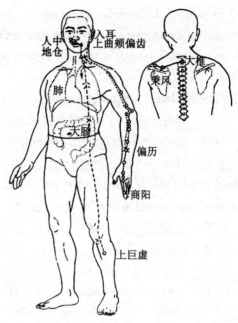

It is one of the twelve regular meridians. Its circulating route is as following: In the deep part of the body, it is related to the large intestine and connected with the lungs; on the body surface, it runs from the tip of the index finger, along the extensor aspect of the radial side of the upper limb, to the shoulder, neck and cheek, and ends at the side of the contralateral nostril. The diseases of the meridian manifest chiefly as diarrhea, dysentery, borborygmus, aversion to cold and shivering, yellowish sclera, dryness of the mouth, epistaxis, stuffiness of the nose, sore throat, toothache, swelling of the neck, etc., as well as local symptoms and signs of the parts along the pathway of the meridian.

手针 hand acupuncture

指针刺手部所特有的一些穴位(多在指间关节或掌指关节处)，以治疗疾病的方法。

To needle the specific acupoints of the hand (mainly located on the interphalangeal or metacarpophalangeal joints) for therapeutic purposes.

手针麻醉　hand acupuncture anesthesia

选用手部的穴位进行针刺麻醉的方法。

To administer acupuncture anesthesia by puncturing the acupoints on the hand.

手之三阳手外头　three yang meridians of the hand travel from hand to head

指手之三阳经的体表循行路线均是从手部沿手臂外侧到头部。

The circulating routes of the three yang meridians of the hand are from the hand along the lateral aspect of the upper limb to the head.

手之三阴胸内手　three yin meridians of the hand travel from chest to hand

指手三阴经的体表循行路线均是从胸部沿着手臂内侧到手部。

The circulating routes of the three yin meridians of the hand are from the chest along the medial aspect of the upper limb to the hand.

手指麻木　numbness of fingers

多因气虚而兼有湿痰、瘀血阻滞所致的一种症状。治宜通经活络。取穴：内关、水沟、极泉、少海、委中、三阴交。

A symptom usually caused by deficiency of qi with retention of phlegm-damp and blood stasis. Treatment principle：Clear and activate the meridians and collaterals. Point selection：Neiguan(PC6), Shuigou(GV26), Jiquan(HT1), Shaohai(HT3), Weizhong(BL40), Sanyinjiao (SP6).

手足厥冷　cold hands and feet

四肢肘膝以下厥冷的症状。由阳气衰微，阴寒内盛所致者，常伴有怕冷、下利清谷、脉沉微等；由热邪阻遏、阳气不能通达四肢所致者，常伴有胸腹烦热、口渴等。治宜回阳救逆。取穴：百会、气海（针刺）、神阙（灸）。

Coldness of the extremities below the elbows and knees. If caused by the deficiency of yang-qi and overabundance of yin-cold, it is usually accompanied with intolerance of cold, lienteric diarrhea, sunken and weak pulse; If caused by the retention of heat-evil and yang-qi fails to flow to the extremities, it is usually accompanied by feverishness in the chest and abdomen, thirst, etc. Treatment principle：Restore yang and rescue patient from collapse. Point selection：Baihui(GV20), Qihai(CV6), moxibustion on Shenque (CV8).

手足心热　heat in the palms and soles

因阴虚生内热或火热内郁所致的手足心发热感。治宜滋阴清热。取穴：照海、三阴交、合谷、太溪。

A symptom caused by endogenous heat due to yin deficiency or the stagnation of fire-heat evil inside the body. Treatment principle：Nourish yin to clear heat. Point selection：Zhaohai(KI6), Sanyinjiao(SP6), Hegu(LI4), Taixi(KI3).

守气　maintain needling sensation

指针刺得气后需适当行针，不使已得之气消失。

After getting the sensation during acupuncture, needles should be properly manipulated to keep the obtained needling sensation.

疏风泻热 disperse wind and clear heat

即解表清热。用具有疏散在表风邪和清热作用的药物治疗外感风邪兼有里热病证的方法。适用于头痛、鼻塞、咳嗽、咽痛、口渴,舌质红,苔薄黄,脉浮数的患者。

A treatment for the exogenous wind-evil accompanied with heat syndrome in the interior by the application of herbs of eliminating the wind-evil in the superficies and clearing away the heat-evil effects, applicable to cases manifested as stuffy nose, cough, sore throat, thirst, reddish tongue with thin and yellowish fur, floating and rapid pulse, etc.

疏肝 soothing the liver

又称疏肝理气、舒肝、泄肝。常用于肝气郁结。症见胁肋胀痛、胸闷不舒或恶心、呕吐酸水、食欲不振、腹痛腹泻,舌苔薄,脉弦等。

A treatment for the stagnation of liver-qi, applicable to cases with manifestations as distending pain over the hypochondrium, oppressive feeling over the chest, nausea, acid regurgitation, loss of appetite, abdominal pain, diarrhea, thin fur on the tongue, wiry pulse, etc.

疏通经络 dredging the meridian

用行气活血及具有温通作用的药物组成方剂,以治疗因气血凝滞致经络阻塞的一种方法。

A treatment for the obstruction of meridians resulting from the stagnation of qi and blood, by the application of prescriptions composed of herbs with the action of promoting qi and blood circulation and with warming and dispersing effects.

输刺 shu-point needling

①九刺法之一。指刺四肢部的井、荥、输、经、合等穴位和背部的背俞穴。②十二刺的一种,用于治疗气盛而有热的病症。其方法是将针直入直出地进行深刺,取穴宜少。③五刺法的一种,用于治疗骨痹,刺法是将针直入直出,深入至骨。这是古代用于治疗肾病的一种针法。

①One of the Nine Needling techniques. Puncturing the acupoints such as Jing-well points, Xing-Spring points, Shu-Stream points, Jing-River points, He-sea points, etc., and the Back-Shu points. ②One of the Twelve Needling techniques to treat diseases with excessive qi and heat. The technique is to thrust the needle deeply and perpendicularly. Only a few acupoints should be selected. ③One of the Five Needling techniques for treating osteal pain. The technique is to thrust the needle deeply and perpendicularly to the bone. This is an ancient Chinese acupuncture technique to treat renal diseases.

输脉 Shu meridian

指背部联系脏腑的经脉,即足太阳经。

The meridian which connects the zang-fu organs on the back, i. e., the Meridian of Foot-Taiyang.

输尿管 Shuniaoguan

耳穴名。在肾与膀胱两穴之间。主治：输尿管结石绞痛。

Name of an ear point. Located between Shen and Pangguang. It is used for treating stone and colic pain of ureter.

输穴 point；Shu-Stream points

①指腧穴。②五输穴之一。位于手足部，十二经脉各一个，经气在此如细小水流逐渐输注汇聚至更大的水流一样。阴经的输穴与其原穴同，而阳经则不同。

①A general name of all the acupoints. ②One of the five Shu points. Located at the hands and feet，each belongs to one meridian，and the qi pours and gathers at this point just like small streams meet together and pour into bigger river. The Shu-Stream points are the same as the Yuan-Primary points in yin meridians but different from the Yuan-Primary points in yang meridians.

暑 summer-heat

六淫之一。暑为阳邪，多在夏季致病。感受暑邪后表现为高热、口渴、多汗、心烦、体倦、脉洪等。

One of the six evils，yang in nature，usually pathogenetic in summer time，and causing the syndrome manifested as high fever，thirst，profuse sweating，restlessness，fatigue，surging pulse，etc.

鼠粪灸 mouse feces moxibustion

将干燥鼠粪点燃，灸脐中，可强身延年。

A kind of moxibustion with mouse feces on the navel，which can make body strong and prolong life.

鼠尾 Shuwei

经外奇穴名。位于足跟骨上缘处，灸治瘰疬。

Name of an extra point. Located at the upper margin of the heel bone. Moxibustion is used to cure scrofula.

束骨 Shugu(BL65)

经穴名。属足太阳膀胱经，本经输穴。定位：在足外侧，足小趾本节的后方，赤白肉际处。主治：癫狂，头痛，项强，目眩，下肢及背痛等。操作：直刺0.3～0.5寸；可灸。

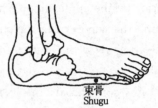

束骨
Shugu

The acupoint，Shu-Steam point of the Bladder Meridian of Foot-Taiyang. Location：On the lateral side of the foot，posterior to the root segment of the little toe，on the dorso-ventral boundary of the foot. Indications：Mania，headache，neck rigidity，blurred vision，pain in the lower extremities，backache，etc. Method：Puncture perpendicularly 0.3-0.5 cun. Moxibustion is applicable.

俞府 Shufu（KI27）

经穴名。属足少阴肾经。定位：在胸部，当锁骨下端，前正中线旁开2寸。主治：咳嗽，气喘，胸痛等。操作：斜刺或平刺0.5～0.8寸；可灸。

Name of an acupoint. It belongs to the Kidney Meridian of Foot-Shaoyin. Location：On the chest，below the lower bor-

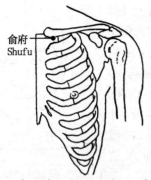

der of the clavicle, 2 cun lateral to the anterior midline. Indications: Cough, asthma, chest pain, etc. Method: Puncture obliquely or horizontally 0. 5-0. 8 cun. Moxibustion is applicable.

俞募配穴法 Shu-Mu points combination

配穴法之一。指以病变脏腑所属之背俞穴与募穴相配合应用。

One of the points combining methods, i. e. , combination of the Front-Mu points and Back-Shu points, both pertaining to the diseased zang-fu organs.

率谷 Shuaigu(GB8)

经穴名。属足少阳胆经。定位:在头部,当耳尖直上入发际 1. 5 寸,角孙穴直上方。主治:偏头痛,眩晕,呕吐,小儿惊风等。操作:平刺 0. 5~0. 8 寸;可灸。

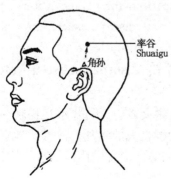

Name of an acupoint. It belongs to the Gallbladder Meridian of Foot-Shaoyang. Location: On the head, directly above the ear apex, 1. 5 cun above the hairline, directly above Jiaosun(TE20). Indications: Migraine, vertigo, vomiting, infantile convulsion etc. Method: Puncture horizontally 0. 5-0. 8 cun. Moxibustion is applicable.

水不涵木 water failing to nourish wood

肾阴不足,不能滋养肝脏而引起肝阴不足、虚风内动的病理。常见眩晕、耳鸣、遗精、口干,甚至出现抽搐等。治宜补益肝肾、熄风。取穴:太溪、肾俞、曲泉、百会。

A morbid condition of the deficiency of liver-yin with the hyperactivity of asthenic wind resulting from the inability of kidney-yin to nourish the liver; manifested as dizziness, tinnitus, nocturnal emission, dry mouth, even convulsion. Treatment principle: Tonify the liver and kindey to clear the pathogenic wind. Point selection: Taixi (KI3), Shenshu (BL23), Ququan(LR8), Baihui(GV20).

水道 Shuidao(ST28)

经穴名。属足阳明胃经。定位:在下腹部,当脐中下 3 寸,距前正中线 2 寸。主治:小腹胀满,小便不利,水肿,疝气,痛经,不孕等。

Name of an acupoint. It belongs to the Stomach Meridian of Foot-Yangming. Location: On the lower abdomen, 3 cun below the center of the umbilicus and 2 cun lateral to the anterior midline. Indi-

---

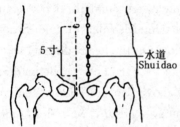

5寸

水道
Shuidao

cations: Lower abdominal distension, dysuria, edema, hernia, dysmenorrhea, infertility, etc.

水分 Shuifen(CV9)

经穴名。属任脉。定位：在上腹部，前正中线上，当脐中上 1 寸。主治：腹痛，肠鸣，水肿，小便不利，泄泻等。操作：直刺 0.8～1.2 寸；可灸。

Name of an acupuncture. It belongs to the Conception Vessel. Location: On the upper abdomen, on the anterior midline, 1 cun above the center of the umbilicus. Indications: Abdominal pain, borborygmus, edema, dysuria, diarrhea, etc. Method: Puncture perpendicularly 0. 8-1. 2 cun. Moxibustion is applicable.

水沟 Shuigou(GV26)

经穴名。属督脉。定位：在面部，当人

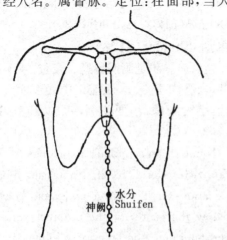

水分
Shuifen
神阙

中沟的上 1/3 与中 1/3 交点处。主治：癫狂痫，痓病，小儿惊风，昏迷，中风昏厥，牙关紧闭，口眼歪斜，面肿，腰脊强痛等。操作：向上斜刺 0.3～0.5 寸。

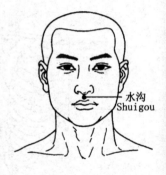

水沟
Shuigou

Name of an acupoint. It belongs to the Governor Vessel. Location: On the face, at the junction of the upper 1/3 and middle 1/3 of the philtrum. Indications: Mental disorders, epilepsy, hysteria, infantile convulsion, coma, apoplexy fainting, trismus, deviation of mouth and eyes, puffiness of the face, pain and stiffness of the lower back, etc. Method: Puncture obliquely upward 0. 3-0. 5 cun.

水谷之海 the sea of food and drink

指胃。

It refers to the stomach.

水罐法 water cupping therapy

竹罐用水煮沸后进行拔罐的一种治疗方法，适用于风寒湿痹、痈肿等疾病。

A method of cupping with a hot bamboo cup from the boiling water, applicable to the diseases such as wind-cold-damp bi, carbuncle, etc.

水火不济 disorder between water and fire

肾的水火或心火与肾水互相制约、互相协调功能丧失的病理。常表现为心烦、失眠、遗精等。治宜滋阴清热。取穴：肾俞、太溪、照海、三阴交。

A morbid condition caused by the inco-ordination between kidney-water and kidney-fire or kidney-water and heart-fire; manifested as restlessness, insomnia, nocturnal emission, etc. Treatment principle: Nourish kindey-yin to clear the heat. Point selection: Shenshu (BL23), Taixi(KI3), Zhaohai(KI6), Sanyinjiao (SP6).

水火相济 water and fire coordinate each other

肾的水火或心火与肾水互相制约、互相协调，以维持心、肾的正常活动。

Coordination between kidney-water and kidney-fire, or kidney-water and heart-fire, a physiological function necessary for the maintainence of normal activities of the organs.

水灸 watery moxibustion

指用大蒜涂擦体表以治病的方法。除大蒜外，也可对症加入其他药物。

A kind of therapy with garlic rubbed the body surface, other herbs can be added according to the diseases.

水泉 Shuiquan(KI5)

经穴名。属足少阴肾经，本经郄穴。定位：在足内侧，内踝后下方，当太溪之下1寸。主治：月经不调，痛经，经闭，阴挺，小便不利，目视昏花等。操作：直刺0.3～0.5寸；可灸。

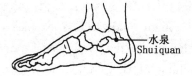

The acupoint, Xi-Cleft point of the Kidney Meridian of Foot-Shaoyin. Location: On the medial side of the foot, posterior and inferior to the medial malleolus, 1 cun directly below Taixi(KI3). Indications: Irregular menstruation, dysmenorrhea, amenorrhea, prolapse of uterus, dysuria, blurred vision. Method: Puncture perpendicularly 0.3-0.5 cun. Moxibustion is applicable.

水突 Shuitu(ST10)

经穴名。属足阳明胃经。定位：在颈部，胸锁乳突肌的前缘，当人迎与气舍连线的中点。主治：咽喉肿痛，气喘，咳嗽等。操作：直刺0.3～0.5寸；可灸。

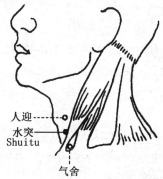

Name of an acupoint. It belongs to the Stomach Meridian of Foot-Yangming. Location: On the neck, on the anterior border of the sternocleidomasoid muscle, at the midpoint of the line connecting Renying(ST9) and Qishe(ST11). Indications: Sore throat, asthma, cough, etc. Method: Puncture perpendicularly 0.3-0.5 cun. Moxibustion is applicable.

水原 Shuiyuan

水泉穴别名。

The other name of Shuiquan(KI5).

水针疗法 point injection therapathy

指将药液、生理盐水或葡萄糖溶液注射于穴位内或病痛的局部以治疗疾病的方法。

The therapeutic method of injecting the medicinal fluid, normal saline, or glucose solution into the point or the affected area.

水肿 edema

体内水湿潴留而致全身浮肿的一种病证。多与肾、脾、肺、三焦、膀胱等脏腑功能失调有关。

A condition of anasarca caused by the retention of fluid in the body, usually due to the dysfunction of the kidney, spleen, lung, sanjiao and bladder.

数脉 rapid pulse

脉搏急速,每分钟超过 90 次,主热证。数而有力为实热,数而无力为虚热。

A pulse condition with more than 90 beats per minute, indicating a heat-syndrome. The rapid and strong pulse indicates sthenia heat syndrome, while the rapid and weak indicates asthenia heat syndrome.

丝竹空 Sizhukong (TE23)

经穴名。属手少阳三焦经。定位:在面部,当眉梢凹陷处。主治:头痛,目赤肿痛,视物不清,眼睑瞤动,齿痛,面瘫等。操作:沿皮刺 0.5～1 寸;禁灸。

Name of an acupoint. It belongs to the Meridian of Hand-Shaoyang. Location: On the face, in the depression of the lateral end of the eyebrow. Indications: Headache, redness, swelling and pain of the eyes, blurred vision, twitching of the eyelids, toothache, facial paralysis, etc.

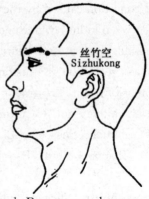

丝竹空 Sizhukong

Method: Puncture subcutaneously 0.5-1 cun. Moxibustion is prohibited.

四白 Sibai (ST2)

经穴名。属足阳明胃经。定位:在面部,瞳孔直下,当眶下孔凹陷处。主治:目赤痒痛,面瘫,眼球瞤动等。操作:直刺 0.2～0.3 寸;不宜灸。

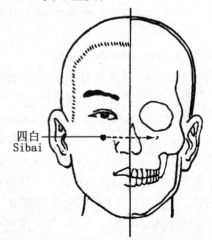

四白 Sibai

Name of an acupoint. It belongs to Stomach Meridian of Foot-Yangming. Location: On the face, directly below the pupil, in the depression of the infraorbital foramen. Indications: Redness, pain and itching of the eyes, facial paralysis, twitching of the eyelids, etc. Method: Puncture perpendicularly 0.3-0.5 cun.

Moxibustion is not advisable.

四渎 Sidu(TE9)

经穴名。属手少阳三焦经。定位：在前臂背侧，当阳池与肘尖的连线上，肘尖下5寸，尺骨与桡骨之间。主治：耳聋，齿痛，偏头痛，暴喑，前臂痛等。操作：直刺0.5～1寸；可灸。

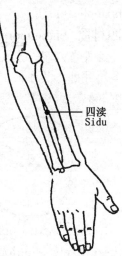

四渎
Sidu

Name of an acupoint. It belongs to the Sanjiao Meridian of Hand-Shaoyang. Location：On the dorsal side of the forearm and on the line connecting Yangchi (TE4) and the tip of the olecrannon, 5 cun inferior to the tip of the olecrannon, between the radius and ulna. Indications：Deafness, toothache, migraine, sudden hoarseness of voice, pain in the forearm, etc. Method：Puncture perpendicularly 0.5-1 cun. Moxibustion is applicable.

四缝 Sifeng (EX-UE10)

经外奇穴名。在第二、三、四、五指掌面，近端指关节横纹中点。主治：小儿疳积，百日咳。

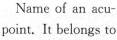

四缝
Sifeng

Name of extra points. Location：On the palmar side, in the midpoint of the transverse crease of the proximal in-terphalangeal joints of the index, middle, ring and little finger. Indications：Malnutrition and indigestion syndrome in children, whooping cough, etc.

四根三结 four roots and three terminals

是对十二经脉根结部位的概括，即十二经脉是以四肢末端的井穴为根，以头、胸、腹三部为结。

A generalization of the roots and terminals of the twelve regular meridians which all originate from the Jing-Well points at the end of the four extremities and all terminate in the head, thorax and abdomen.

四关 four important parts or points

①指两肘和两膝。②指两肘、两腋、两髀、两腘。③指太冲、合谷的组穴。主治寒热痛痹。

① Two elbows and two knees. ②Two elbows, two axillas , two hips and two hollows of the knee. ③Combined points of Taichong (LR3) and Hegu (LI4), mainly used to cure arthralgia caused by cold or heat.

四海 four seas

即髓海、血海、气海、水谷之海的总称。髓之海为脑，血之海为冲脉，气之海为膻中，水谷之海为胃。

The collective name of medulla sea, blood sea, qi sea, and food and drink sea. Brain is the sea of medulla, Throughfare Vessel is the sea of blood, Danzhong (part around Danzhong point) is the sea of qi, and the stomach is the sea of food and drink.

四花 Sihua

经外奇穴名。相当于膈俞与肝俞的 4 个组穴。主治：劳瘵，咳嗽，哮喘，虚弱消瘦等。艾炷灸。

Name of extra-points corresponding to the four combined points of Geshu (BL17) and Ganshu (BL18). Indications：Pulmonary tuberculosis, cough, asthma, weakness and emaciation, etc., by moxa cone moxibustion.

四经 four channels

指肝、心、肺、肾四经脉，因其与四时相应。

It refers to the Liver, Heart, Lung and Kidney Meridians which match the four seasons of the year.

四满 Siman (KI14)

经穴名。属足少阴肾经。定位：在下腹部，当脐中下 2 寸，距前正中线旁开 0.5 寸。主治：腹胀腹痛，泄泻，遗精，月经不调，痛经，产后腹痛等。操作：直刺 1～1.5 寸；可灸。

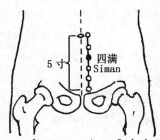

Name of an acupoint. It belongs to the Kidney Meridian of Foot-Shaoyin. Location：On the lower abdomen，2 cun below the centre of the umbilicus and 0.5 cun lateral to the anterior midline. Indications：Abdominal pain and distension, diarrhea, nocturnal emission, irregular menstruation, dysmenorrhea, postpartum abdominal pain, etc. Method：Puncture perpendicularly 1-1.5 cun. Moxibustion is applicable.

四神聪 Sishencong (EX-HN1)

经外奇穴名。定位：在百会穴前后左右各 1 寸处。共 4 穴。主治：头痛，眩晕，失眠，健忘，癫痫等。

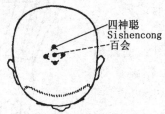

Name of extra points. Location：1 cun respectively anterior, posterior, and lateral to Baihui (GV20). Four points in all. Indications：Headache, vertigo, insomnia, poor memory, epilepsy, etc.

四时 four seasons

即春、夏、秋、冬四季，其中夏季的第三个月（农历六月）称为长夏。

A general term for spring, summer, autumn and winter. The third month of summer(June in lunar calandar) is called "long summer".

四诊 four diagnostic methods

四种诊病方法。即望诊、闻诊、问诊和切诊。

Referring to inspection, listening smelling, inquiry and palpation and pulse taking.

四肢拘急 spasm of the four limbs

四肢筋肉拘挛，难以伸屈的一种症状。多因寒邪侵袭经脉或热灼阴液，使筋脉失养所致。治宜泻热救阴、平肝熄风。取穴：风府、大椎、曲池、涌泉、太冲、十二井。

A disorder with difficulty in movement of the extremities and tendons resulting from the attack of cold-evil to the meridians or the consumption of yin-fluid by heat-evil. Treatment principle:Purge heat to rescue yin, calm the liver to stop wind. Point selection:Fengfu(GV16), Dazhui(GV14), Quchi(LI11), Yongquan (KI1), Taichong(LR3), the Jing-Well points of the twelve regular meridians.

四肢麻木 numbness of the four limbs

手足麻木,不知痛痒,多由气虚风痰侵入经络,营卫流通受阻引起。治宜通经活络。取穴:内关、水沟、极泉、少海、委中、三阴交。

A symptom usually due to wind-phlegm attacking the meridians and blocking nutrient qi and defense qi resulting from deficiency of qi. Treatment principle:Clear and activate the meridians and collaterals. Point selection:Neiguan(PC6), Shuigou(GV26), Jiquan(HT1), Shaohai (HT3), Weizhong (BL40), Sanyinjiao (SP6).

四肢无力 myasthenia of the four limbs

指手足软弱无力的症状。多见于痿证、痹证等。治宜通经活络、补脾益气。取穴:肩髃、合谷、阳溪、髀关、梁丘、足三里、解溪、肾俞、气海、三阴交。

A symptom commonly seen in flaccidity syndrome, bi syndrome, etc. Treatment principle:Clear and activate the meridians and collaterals, invigorate the spleen and replenish qi. Point selection:

Jianyu(LI15), Hegu(LI4), Yangxi (LI5), Biguan(ST31), Liangqiu(ST34), Zusanli(ST36), Jiexi(ST41), Shenshu (BL23), Qihai(CV6), Sanyinjiao(SP6).

四周取穴 nearby point selection

即邻近取穴。

Selecting points near the diseased region.

四总穴 four important points

即足三里、委中、列缺、合谷四个常用要穴。

It refers to ZuSanli (ST36), Weizhong (BL40), Lieque (LU7), and Hegu (LI4), which are the most important and widely used points.

素髎 Suliao(GV25)

经穴名。属督脉。定位:在面部,当鼻尖的正中央。主治:昏迷,鼻塞,衄衊,酒渣鼻等。操作:向上斜刺0.3~0.5寸;禁灸。

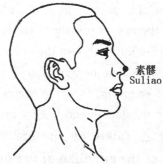

Name of an acupoint. It belongs to the Governor Vessel. Location:On the face, at the centre of the nose apex. Indications:Loss of consciousness, nasal obstruction, clear nasal discharge and epistaxis, rosacea, etc. Method:Puncture obliquely upward 0.3-0.5 cun. Moxibustion is prohibited.

素问 *Plain Questions*

《黄帝内经》中的一部分,该书为最早的中医学著作。

A part of *Huangdi's Canon of Medicine* which is the most ancient work in traditional Chinese medicine.

蒜泥 pounded garlic

冷灸发泡剂之一。将大蒜捣烂敷于鱼际治喉痹,敷于足心治噤口痢。

One of the cold, blistering moxibustion herbs, which is applied to the thenar to cure sore throat and applied to the center of the sole to cure fasting dysentery.

随变而调气 regulating qi in accordance with the changing of diseases

针灸治疗的原则。意指病情的变化是无穷无尽的,灸刺的方法必须根据不断变化的病情而变化,以达到调气即治愈的目的。

A principle of acupuncture and moxibustion therapy, i. e. , the changes of the diseases are infinitely, so the acupuncture and moxibustion therapy should also be modified according to the changes of diseases to regulate qi and to cure diseases.

随而济之 following the moving direction of the meridian qi to reinforce

为针刺补法要领。即针刺时针尖要顺着经气运行的方向运针为补,与"迎而夺之"相对。

A rule of reinforcing, i. e. , the manipulations should be performed with the needle point moves along the direction of the movement of qi in the channel, as contrasted with " against the channel movement to reduce".

随年壮 age-depending moxibustion

灸法用语。即患者年几岁,灸几壮。

A term used in moxibustion, i. e. , the number of cones burnt in moxibustion is the same as the patient's age.

随症取穴 points selection according to symptoms

取穴法之一。即根据疾病的症候而选取有关的穴位。

One of the point-selecting methods, i. e. , select the point relevant to the signs and symptoms of the disease.

髓 marrow

奇恒之腑之一。包括骨髓和脊髓,由肾的精气和饮食营养物质所化生,有营养骨骼和脑的作用。

One of the extraordinary fu-organs, including the bone marrow and spinal marrow, derived from the kidney essence and the nutrients of food. It nourishes the bones and the brain.

髓海 sea of marrow

指脑。

It refers to the brain.

髓会 influential point of marrow

指悬钟穴,又名绝骨,八会穴之一。

It refers to Xuanzhong (GB39), also known as Juegu. It is one of the eight influential points.

髓中 Suizhong

四满穴别名。

The other name of Siman (KI14).

孙络 minute collaterals

指极小的络脉分支。

The minute branches of the collaterals.

孙思邈　Sun Simiao

唐代著名医学家（581—682）。著有《备急千金要方》和《千金翼方》，是唐代宝贵的医学资料。

An renowned physician（581-682）of the Tang Dynasty，compiler of *Essential Prescriptions Worth Thousand Gold for emergency* and *Supplement to Prescriptions Worth Thousand Gold for emergency*，which are valuable information about Chinese medicine in the Tang Dynasty.

所生病　meridian diseases due to related organs

经脉病候用语。指某一经脉有异常变动时就出现有关病症，而此经脉的穴位即能主治这种病症。

A term of meridian diseases manifestation，i. e.，the abnormal changes of a certain meridian will cause the relative disease which can be cured by selecting the points from this meridian.

锁骨　Suogu

耳穴名。定位：在与屏轮切迹相平的耳舟处。主治：肩关节周围炎。

Name of an ear point. Location：On the scapha，at the same level with helix-fragic notch. Indication：Peripheral arthritis of the shoulder.

T

胎动不安 fetal restlessness

孕妇自觉胎儿频频躁动,伴有腹痛下坠感,腰酸,甚则阴道少量出血,多由气血虚弱,肾气不足或血热、外伤等因素,使冲任不固,不能摄血养胎所致。治宜补气养血、调和冲任。取穴:足三里、三阴交、肾俞、脾俞、百会。

A condition usually accompanied with abdominal pain, bearing-down sensation, lumbago, or even with minor vaginal bleeding; due to unconsolidation of the Troughfare Vessel and the Conception Vessel with failure to nourish the fetus resulting from the deficiency of qi and blood, insufficiency of kidney-qi, or blood-heat, trauma, etc. Treatment principle: Strengthen the qi and nourish the blood, regulate the Throughfare Vessel and the Conception Vessel. Point selection: Zusanli (ST36), Sanyinjiao (SP6), Shenshu(BL23), Pishu(BL20), Baihui(GV20).

胎位不正 abnormal position of fetus

妊娠后因气滞或临产惊恐,影响胞胎转运所致。治宜疏气导滞,矫正胎位。方法:用艾条灸两侧至阴穴,每天 1~2 次,每次 15 分钟,至胎位转正为止。

A condition due to stagnation of qi during pregnancy or frightening during the course of labour. Treatment principle: Promote the flow of qi, remove the stag- nation and correct the position of the fe- tus. Method: Apply moxa stick moxibus- tion to bilateral Zhiyin(BL67)points for 15 minutes, once or twice a day until the position of the fetus is normal.

胎衣不下 retention of placenta

即胞衣不下。指胎儿娩出后,胎盘超过半小时仍未能排出。多因分娩后气血大虚,无力继续排出所致。治宜行气活血、温经祛瘀。取穴:中极、气海、合谷、三阴交、独阴。

Failure to expel the placenta more than half an hour after childbirth, due to ute- rine inertia resulting from over consump- tion of qi and blood during labour. Treat- ment principle: Promote the flow of qi and blood and remove the blood stasis by warming the meridians. Point selection: Zhongji (CV3), Qihai (CV6), Hegu (LI4), Sanyinjiao (SP6), Duyin (EX- LE11).

太白 Taibai (SP3)

经穴名。属足太阴脾经,本经输、原穴。定位:在足内侧缘,当足大趾本节后下方赤白肉际凹陷处。主治:胃痛,腹胀,便秘,痢疾,呕吐,泄泻,肠鸣,脚气,体重节痛等。操作:直刺 0.3~0.5 寸;可灸。

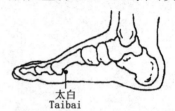

太白
Taibai

The acupoint, Shu-stream point and Yuan-Primary point of the Spleen Meri- dian of Foot-Taiyin. Location: On the medial border of the foot, in the depression of the dorso-ventral boundary of the foot, posterior and inferior to the 1st metatarsophalangeal joint. Indications: Gastralgia, abdominal distension, constipation, dysentery, vomiting, diarrhea, borborygmus, beriberi, feeling of heaviness, joints pain, etc. Method: Puncture perpendicularly 0.3-0.5 cun. Moxibustion is applicable.

太仓 Taicang

①指胃部。②中脘穴别名。

①It refers to the stomach. ②The other name of Zhongwan (CV12).

太冲 Taichong (LR3)

经穴名。属足
厥阴肝经,本经
输、原穴。定位:
足背侧,当第1、
2 跖骨结合部之
前凹陷中。主
治:头痛,眩晕,
失眠,目赤肿痛,
小儿惊风,口歪,
胁痛,崩漏,疝

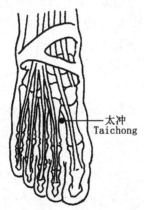

气,小便不利,癫痫等。操作:直刺0.5~1寸;可灸。

The acupoint, Shu-Stream and Yuan-Primary point of the Liver Meridian of Foot-Jueyin. Location: On the dorsum of the foot, in the depression distal to the 1st and 2nd metatarsal bones. Indication: Headache, vertigo, insomnia, redness, swelling and pain of the eyes, infantile convulsion, deviation of the mouth, pain in the hypochondriac region, uterine bleeding, hernia, dysu-ria, epilepsy, etc. Method: Puncture perpendicularly 0.5-1 cun. Moxibustion is applicable.

太冲脉 Taichong Meridian

冲脉的别称。它的功能正常对于调节月经、妊娠以及胎儿的发育很重要。

The other name of the Throughfare Ve-ssel. Its normal function is necessary for the regulation of menstruation, pregnancy and growth of the fetus.

太平圣惠方 Taiping Holy Prescriptions for Universal Relief

书名。宋代王怀隐等编,共 100 卷。其中包括针灸方面的内容。

Name of the book compiled by Wang Huaiyin in the Song Dynasty, totally 100 volumes, including some materials of acupuncture and moxibustion.

太泉 Taiquan

太渊穴别名。

The other name of Taiyuan (LU9).

太溪 Taixi (KI3)

经穴名。属足少阴肾经,本经原穴、输穴。定位:在足内侧,当内踝尖与跟腱之间的凹陷中。主治:咽喉肿痛,齿痛,耳鸣耳聋,头晕,吐血,气喘,口渴,月经不调,失眠,遗精,阳痿等。操作:直刺0.5~1寸;可灸。

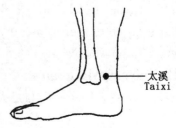

The acupoint, Shu-Stream and Yuan-Primary point of the Kidney Meridian of Foot-Shaoyin. Location: On the medial malleolus, in the depression between the tip of the medial malleolus and achilles tendon. Indications: Sore throat, toothache, deafness, tinnitus, dizziness, spitting of blood, asthma, thirst, irregular menstruation, insomnia, nocturnal emission, impotence, etc. Method: Puncture perpendicularly 0.5-1cun. Moxibustion is applicable.

太阳 Taiyang (EX-HN5)

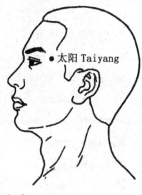

①经外奇穴名。定位:在眉梢与目外眦之间向后约1寸凹陷中。主治:头痛,目疾,口眼歪斜等。②瞳子髎穴的别名。③经脉名之一,有阳气旺盛之意。

①Name of an extra point. Location: In the depression about 1 cun posterior to the midpoint between the lateral end of the eyebrow and the outer canthus. Indications: Headache, eye diseases, deviation of eyes and mouth, etc. ②Another name of Tongziliao(GB1). ③A collective name for a group of meridians. It means the yang-qi is flourishing.

太阳经 Taiyang Meridian

三阳经之一,手太阳小肠经与足太阳膀胱经的合称。

One of the three yang meridians, a joint name for the Small Intestine Meridian of Hand-Taiyang and the Bladder Meridian of Foot-Taiyang.

太阳为开 the Taiyang Meridians are open

指太阳经位于身体"三阳"经的最表层部位,感受外邪后常先发病。

The Taiyang Meridians are the most superficial ones of the three yang meridians, and often the first ones to be affected by exogenous pathogen.

太阳为六经之藩篱 Taiyang Meridians are the fence of the six meridians

指太阳经位于身体之最表层,像竹篱笆一样起着保护机体的作用。

Taiyang Meridians are the most superficial part of the body, playing a role in protecting the body like a fence.

太医 imperial physician

中国古代专门为帝王和宫廷服务的医生。

Physicians in ancient China appointed for giving medical service to the Emperor and the imperial court.

太医丞 assistant officer of imperial medical affairs

太医令的副手。

A medical official as the assistant of the minister of imperial medical affairs.

太医令 minister of imperial medical affairs

中国古代主管医事行政的长官。

A high official in charge of administration of medical affairs in ancient China.

太医局 Imperial Medical Service

宋代官方主管医疗和医学教育的机构。

An official organization in charge of medical affairs and medical education in the Song Dynasty.

太医署 Imperial Medical Academy

中国古代官方的医疗、医学教育机构。始建于南北朝时期,至隋唐臻于完备。

An official organization of medical therapeutics and education in ancient China, established in the Northern and Southern Dynasties and became perfect in the Sui and Tang Dynasties.

太医院 Imperial Academy of Medicine

金代开始设立的医疗机构,专为帝王和皇室服务。元、明、清各代均设有太医院。

A medical organization offering medical service to emperor and royal family, first set up in the Jin Dynasty. Later, in the Yuan, Ming and Qing Dynasties, similar organizations were also established.

太乙 Taiyi (ST23)

经穴名。属足阳明胃经。定位:在上腹部,当脐中上 2 寸,距前正中线 2 寸。主治:胃痛,消化不良,心烦不宁,癫狂等。操作:直刺 0.8～1.2 寸;可灸。

Name of an acupoint. It belongs to Stomach Meridian of Foot-Yangming. Location: On the upper abdomen, 2 cun above the centre of the umbilicus and 2 cun lateral to the anterior midline. Indications: Gastric pain, indigestion, irritability, mania, etc. Method: Puncture perpendicularly 0.8-1.2 cun.

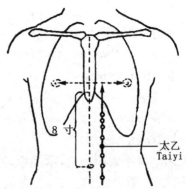

Moxibustion is applicable.

太乙神针 taiyi miraculous moxa roll

①艾灸的一种,艾条中掺有某些中药,将一端点燃,隔布数层按于穴位上。②书名。清代邱时敏编。

① One kind of moxa stick moxibustion. The stick is mixed with some Chinese medicinal herbs and is lighted at one end to be put directly on the point with a cloth partition. ②Name of the book compiled by Qiu Shimin in the Qing Dynasty.

太阴 Taiyin

经脉名称之一。有阴气旺盛之意。

A collective name for a group of meridians. It means that the yin-qi is flourishing.

太阴经 Taiyin Meridian

手太阴肺经与足太阴脾经的合称。

A joint name of the Lung Meridian of Hand-Taiyin and the Spleen Meridian of Foot-Taiyin.

太阴络 Taiyinluo

漏谷穴别名。

The other name of Lougu (SP7).

太阴为开 the Taiyin Meridians are open

指太阴经位于身体三阴经的最表层部

位。

The Taiyin Meridians are the most superficial ones of the three yin meridians.

太阴阳 Taiyinyang

液门穴别名。

The other name of Yemen (TE2).

太渊 Taiyuan (LU9)

经穴名。属手太阴肺经,本经输、原穴。八会穴之一,脉会太渊。定位:在腕掌侧横纹桡侧,桡动脉搏动处。主治:咳嗽,哮喘,心悸,胸痛,腕臂疼痛等。操作:直刺0.3~0.5寸;可灸。

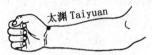

太渊 Taiyuan

The acupoint,Shu-Stream and Yuan-Primary point of the Lung Meridian of Hand-Taiyin. One of the eight influential points. Location:At the radial end of the transverse crease of the wrist where the pulsation of the radial atery is felt. Indications:Cough, asthma, palpitation, pain in chest, wrist and arm, etc. Method:Puncture perpendicularly 0.3-0.5 cun. Moxibustion is applicable.

瘫痪 paralysis of limbs

指四肢不用的疾患。多由肝肾亏虚,气血不足,复因邪气侵袭经络所致。常见于脑血管意外以及某些神经系统疾病。治宜通经活络、补益肝肾。取穴:肩髃、曲池、合谷、阳溪、髀关、梁丘、足三里、解溪、肝俞、肾俞。

Inability to move the extremities due to insufficiency of qi and blood causing by deficiency of liver and kidneys, in addition to the attack of meridians by pathogens, usually seen in the cerebrovascular accident and certain diseases of the nervous system. Treatment principle:Clear and activate the meridians, tonify liver and kidneys. Point selection:Jianyu (LI15),Quchi(LI11),Hegu(LI4),Yangxi(LI5), Biguan (ST31), Liangqiu (ST34), Zusanli(ST36), Jiexi(ST41), Ganshu(BL18),Shenshu(BL23).

弹法 plucking manipulation; 弹针 plucking the needle

针刺辅助手法。①指针刺前用手弹动皮肤。②指针刺后弹动针柄,以增强针感。

Supplementary manipulations in acupuncture. It means:①Plucking the skin before insertion. ②Plucking the needle handle after insertion to increase the needling sensations.

弹筋 plucking the muscle

推拿手法之一,指医生提起肌肉后迅速放手的方法。

A technique of massage repeatedly performed by pulling up the muscle and immediately releasing it.

痰 phlegm

脏腑病理变化的产物,包括呼吸道分泌的痰液。痰的形成多与肺、脾二脏功能失常有关,火热煎熬津液也可成痰。痰也是致病因素之一,常可导致多种疾病的发生发展,如喘咳、眩晕、胸痹、癫痫、惊风、昏厥、瘰疬、骨及关节结核等。

A product of pathological activities of the viscera, including the sputum secreted by the respiratory tract. It is usually formed by the dysfunction of the lungs and the spleen, and occasionally by fire-heat pathogens consuming the body fluid. Moreover, phlegm is also one of the pathogenic factors which is responsible for the occurrence and development of various disorders, such as asthmatic cough, dizziness, chest pain, epilepsy, convulsion, syncope, scrofula, tuberculosis of bones and joints, etc.

痰湿　phlegm-dampness

指因脾不健运、湿浊内停日久而产生的痰。症见阵发性咳嗽,痰多稀白,胸闷,恶心,喘咳,食欲减退,舌胖苔滑腻等。治宜健脾化痰。取穴:脾俞、足三里、丰隆、阴陵泉。

A pathogenic factor produced by prolonged retention of damp pathogens in the body as a result of the hypofunction of the spleen. It may cause a syndrome manifested as paroxysmal and productive cough with watery, whitish sputum, feeling of oppression over the chest, nausea, asthma, poor appetite, enlarged tongue with smooth and greasy fur, etc. Treatment principle: Strengthen spleen and resolve phlegm. Point selection: Pishu(BL20), Zusanli(ST36), Fenglong (ST40), Yinlingquan(SP9).

痰饮　phlegm and fluid retention

①体内过量水液停留或渗注于某局部所致的疾病。多与肺、脾、肾功能失调有关。②指饮邪留于肠胃的疾病。症见饮食减少,消瘦,肠鸣便溏,或伴心悸气短,区吐涎沫等。

①A disease resulting from local retention or permeate of body fluid, mostly attributable to the functional disorders of the lungs, spleen and kidneys. ②Specially referring to the disease resulting from the retention of fluid in the intestine and stomach, manifested as poor appetite, emaciation, borborygmus, diarrhea, or accompanied with palpitation, shortness of breath, salivation, etc.

唐代四科　four medical departments in the Tang Dynasty

唐代医学教育分为四个专业:医科、针科、按摩科和咒禁科。

In the Tang Dynasty traditional Chinese medicine education was divided into four specialities: Medicine, acupuncture, massage, and charms and incantations.

陶道　Taodao (GV13)

经穴名。属督脉。定位:在背部,当后正中线上,第一胸椎棘突下凹陷中。主治:脊强,头痛,疟疾,热病等。操作:直刺0.5~1寸;可灸。

Name of an acupoint. It belongs to the Governor Vessel. Location: On the back, on the posterior midline, in the depression below the spinous process of the 1st thoracic vertebra. Indications: Stiffness of the back, headache, malaria, febrile diseases, etc. Method: Puncture perpendicularly 0.5-1 cun. Moxibustion is applicable.

陶针　pottery needle

古代针具,用废旧陶瓷片洗净敲碎制成,按其锋芒大小分别使用,粗者用于重刺放血,细者可用于小儿。一般多取中者。针刺部位常取背正中线、夹脊穴及腹正中线、夹脐旁线等。

An ancient acupuncture needle. The needles are made of fragments of waste or used pottery which have been cleaned. Their uses vary according to the sizes of the cutting edges. The big ones are used for pricking heavily to cause bleeding, the small ones for children, the medium-sized ones for general use. The needling region are usually the posterior midline, Jiaji(EX-B2) points, the anterior midline and the lines lateral to the umbilicus,etc.

提插补泻 lifting-thrusting reinforcing-reducing method

针下得气后将针上下提插,先浅后深,重插轻提为"补"法;反之,先深后浅,重提轻插为"泻"法。

After the generation of the needling sensation, the needle is gently lifted and heavily thrusted first superficially and then deeply. This is "reinforcing". While heavily lifted and gently thrusted first deeply and then superficially. This is "reducing".

提法 lifting method

针刺十四法之一。即慢慢提针为泻,与插针为补相对应。

One of the fourteen acupuncture methods, i. e., slowing lifting the needle to reduce by contrast with the reinforcing method of thrusting.

体位 body position

指针灸时患者的体位。多采取坐位或卧位。

The body position of the patient during acupuncture or moxibustion. The sitting position and lying position are mostly adopted.

体针 body needling; 体针疗法 body acupuncture therapy

泛指用于身体各部经脉、穴位的针刺方法。

It generally refers to the acupuncture of the human body by puncturing the points along the meridians.

天部 sky level

也称天才,指人体皮下浅部。

Also called Tiancai, namely the shallow subcutaneous part of the human body.

天池 Tianchi (PC1)

经穴名。属手厥阴心包经。定位:在胸部,当第四肋间隙,乳头外 1 寸,前正中线旁开 5 寸。

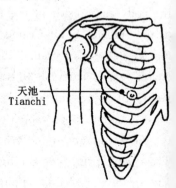

主治:胸闷,胁痛,腋下肿痛等。操作:向外斜刺 0.3～0.5 寸;可灸。

Name of an acupoint. It belongs to the Pericar-dium Meridian of Hand-Jueyin. Location:On the chest, in the 4th intercostal space, 1 cun lateral to the nipple and 5 cun lateral to the anterior midline. Indications:Suffocating sensation in th chest, pain in the hypochondriac region, swelling and pain of the axillary region, etc. Method: Puncture obliquely 0. 3-0. 5 cun. Moxibustion is applicable.

天冲 Tianchong (GB9)

经穴名。属足少阳胆经。定位:在头部,当耳根后缘直上入发际 2 寸,率谷后 0.5 寸处。主治:头痛,癫痫,齿龈肿痛等。操作:平刺 0.5～0.8 寸;可灸。

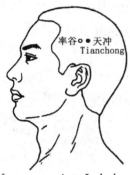

Name of an acupoint. It belongs to the Gallbladder Meridian of Foot-Shaoyang. Location: On the head, directly above the posterior border of the ear root, 2 cun above the hairline and 0. 5 cun posterior to Shuaigu(GB8). Indications: Headache, epilepsy, swelling and pain of the gums, etc. Method: Puncture horizontally 0. 5-0. 8 cun. Moxibustion is applicable.

天窗 Tianchuang (SI16)

经穴名。属手太阳小肠经。定位:在颈外侧部,胸锁乳突肌的后缘,扶突后,与喉结相平。主治:咽痛,暴喑,耳聋,耳鸣,颈项强痛等。操作:直刺 0.5～1 寸;可灸。

Name of an acupoint. It belongs to the Small Intestine Meridian of Hand-Taiyang. Location: On the lateral side of the neck, posterior to the sternocleidomastiod

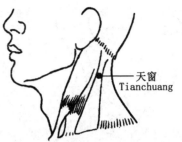

muscle and Futu(LI18), at the same the level with the laryngeal protuberance. Indications: Sore throat, sudden aphonia, deafness, tinnitus, stiffness and pain of the neck, etc. Method: Puncture perpendicularly 0. 5-1 cun. Moxibustion is applicable.

天聪 Tiancong

经外奇穴名。定位:位于头部中线,入前发际的距离为鼻尖至发际的距离的 1/2。主治:头痛,腰背强直等。治疗常用沿皮刺或灸。

Name of an extra point. Location: On the head midline, the distance from the point to the anterior hairline being half the distance from the nose tip to the anterior hairline. Main indications are headache, lumbar and back stiffness, etc. , by subcutaneous acupuncture or moxibustion.

天鼎 Tianding (LI17)

经穴名。属手阳明大肠经。定位:在颈外侧部,胸锁乳突肌的后缘,喉结旁,扶突穴与缺盆连线中点。主治:暴喑,咽喉肿痛,瘰疬,瘿气等。操作:直刺 0.3～0.5 寸;可灸。

Name of an acupoint. It belongs to the Large Intestine Meridian of Hand-Yangming. Location: On the lateral side of the neck, posterior to the sternocleidomastiod

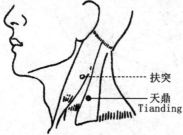

扶突
天鼎
Tianding

muscle and beside the larngeal protuberance, at the midpoint of the line connecting Futu(LI18)and Quepen(ST12). Indications: Sudden aphonia, sore throat, scrofula, goiter, etc. Method: Puncture perpendicularly 0. 3-0. 5 cun. Moxibustion is applicable.

天府 Tianfu (LU3)

经穴名。属手太阴肺经。定位：在臂内侧面，肱二头肌桡侧，腋前纹头下 3 寸处。主治：气喘，鼻衄，臑痛等。操作：直刺 0.5～1寸;可灸。

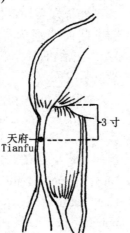

天府
Tianfu

3寸

Name of an acupoint. It belongs to the Lung Meridian of Hand-Taiyin. Location: On the medial side of the upper arm and on the radial border of the biceps brachii, 3 cun below the anterior end of the axilary fold. Indications: Asthma, epistaxis, pain in medial aspect of the upper arm, etc. Method: Puncture perpendicularly 0. 5-1 cun. Moxibustion is applicable.

天盖 Tiangai

缺盆穴别名。

The other name of Quepen (ST12).

天干 heavenly stems

即十天干，为记载时、序用语，与十二地支相配后，用于时间配穴法。

Also called ten heavenly stems. It's a terms used to record time and order, which are combined with the twelve earthly branches in acupuncture or moxibustion to select points.

天会 Tianhui

天池穴别名。

The other name of Tianchi (PC1).

天井 Tianjing (TE10)

经穴名。属手少阳三焦经，本经合穴。定位：在臂外侧，屈肘时，当肘尖直上 1 寸凹陷处。主治：偏头痛，肩臂项痛，痫病，瘰疬，瘿气等。操作：直刺 0.5～1 寸;可灸。

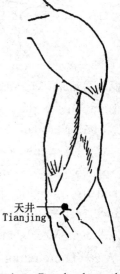

天井
Tianjing

The acupoint, He-Sea point of the Sanjiao Meridian of Hand-Shaoyang. Location: On the lateral side of the upper arm, in the depression 1 cun above the tip of the olecranon when the elbow is flexed. Indications: Migraine, pain in the neck, shoulder and arm, epilepsy, scrofula, goiter, etc. Method: Puncture perpendicularly 0. 5-1 cun. Moxibustion is applicable.

天灸 Tianjiu (natural moxibustion)

指将某些中药点涂于穴位以治病的方法。现代医家指穴位敷药发泡法。

A kind of therapy by applying certain Chinese medicinal substances on the points. Modern physicians refer to this as blistering method by applying stimulate medicines onto the points.

天癸 tiangui

①来源于肾精,是调节人体生长和生殖功能,维持妇女月经和胎孕所必须的物质。②即月经。

① A substance originating from the kidney essence necessary for the regulation of growth, reproduction, menstruation and pregnancy. ②Menstruation.

天髎 Tianliao (TE15)

经穴名。属手少阳三焦经。定位:在肩胛部,肩井与曲垣的中间,当肩胛骨上角处。主治:肩肘痛,项强等。操作:直刺0.5~1寸;可灸。

Name of an acupoint. It belongs to the Sanjiao Meridian of Hand-Shaoyang. Location：On the scapula, at the midpoint between Jianjing (GB21) and Quyuan (SI13), at the superior angle of scapula. Indications：Pain in the shoulders and elbows, stiffness of the neck, etc. Method: Puncture perpendicularly 0. 5-1 cun. Moxibustion is applicable.

天满 Tianman

百会穴别名。

The other name of Baihui (GV20).

天瞿 Tianqu

天突穴别名。

The other name of Tiantu (CV22).

天泉 Tianquan (PC2)

经穴名。属手厥阴心包经。定位:在臂内侧,当腋前纹头下2寸,肱二头肌的长短头之间。主治:心痛,胸胁胀满,咳嗽,胸背、上肢内侧痛等。操作:直刺0.5~1寸;可灸。

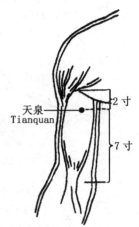

Name of an acupoint. It belongs to the Pericardium Meridian of Hand-Jueyin. Location：On the medial side of the arm, 2 cun below the anterior end of the axillary fold, between the long and short heads of the biceps brachii. Indications：Cardiac pain, fullness in chest and hypochondrium, cough, chest pain, backache, pain in the medial side of upper limbs, etc. Method：Puncture perpendicularly 0. 5-1 cun. Moxibustion is applicable.

天人相应 correspondence between nature and human body

指人体的组织结构、生理现象以及疾病同自然界的对应关系。

Referring to the corresponding relation between the human body (bodily structure, physiological phenomenon, pathological changes, etc.) and the nature.

天容 Tianrong (SI17)

经穴名。属手太阳小肠经。定位:在颈外侧,当下颌角的后方,胸锁乳突肌的前缘凹陷中。主治：耳聋，耳鸣，咽喉肿痛，颊肿，咽中如梗，瘿气等。操作：直刺0.5～1寸；可灸。

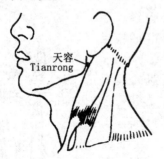

天容
Tianrong

Name of an acupoint. It belongs to the Small Intestine Meridian of Hand-Taiyang. Location：On the lateral side of the neck, posterior to the andibular angle, in the depression of the anterior border of the sternocleidomastoid muscle. Indications：Deafness, tinnitus, sore throat, swelling of the cheeks, globus hysteriocus, goiter, etc. Method：Puncture perpendicularly 0. 5-1 cun. Moxibustion is applicable.

天枢 Tianshu (ST25)

经穴名。属足阳明胃经，大肠募穴。定位：在腹中部，距脐中2寸。主治：腹痛腹胀，肠鸣，绕脐痛，便秘，泄泻，痢疾，月经不调，水肿等。操作：直刺0.8～1.2寸；可灸。

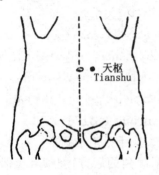

天枢
Tianshu

The acupoint, Front-Mu point of the large intestine, belongs to the Stomach Meridian of Foot-Yangming. Location：On the middle abdomen, 2 cun lateral to the centre of the umbilicus. Indications：Abdominal pain and distension, borborygmus, pain around the umbilicus, constipation, diarrhea, dysentery, irregular menstruation, edema, etc. Method：Puncture perpendicularly 0. 8-1. 2 cun. Moxibustion is applicable.

天庭 tianting

额部中央的部位。

The middle part of the forehead.

天突 Tiantu (CV22)

经穴名。属任脉。定位：在颈部，当前正中线上，胸骨上窝中央。主治：气喘，咳嗽，咽喉肿痛，咽干，呃逆，暴喑，噎膈，瘿气等。操作：直刺0.1～0.5寸；可灸。

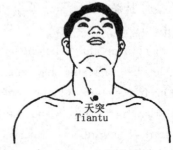

天突
Tiantu

Name of an acupoint. It belongs to the Conception Vessel. Location：On the neck, on the anterior midline, at the centre of the superasternal fossa. Indications：Asthma, cough, sore throat, dry throat, hiccup, sudden aphonia, dysphagia, goiter, etc. Method：Puncture perpendicularly 0. 1-0. 5 cun. Moxibustion is applicable.

天温 Tianwen

天泉穴别名。

The other name of Tianquan (PC2).

天五会 Tianwuhui

人迎穴别名。

The other name of Renying (ST9).

天溪 Tianxi (SP18)

经穴名。属足太阴脾经。定位：在胸外侧，当第四肋间隙，距前正中线 6 寸。主治：胸胁满痛，咳嗽，乳痈，乳汁少等。操作：直刺 0.5～1 寸；可灸。

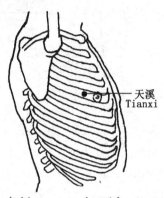

Name of an acupoint. It belongs to the Spleen Meridian of Foot-Taiyin. Location：On the lateral side of the chest, in the 4th intercostal space, 6 cun lateral to the anterior midline. Indications：Fullness and pain in the chest and hypochondrium, cough, acute mastitis, insufficient lactation, etc. Method：Puncture perpendicularly 0.5-1 cun. Moxibustion is applicable.

天星十二穴 twelve sky-star points

十二个经验特效穴，即足三里、内庭、曲池、合谷、委中、承山、太冲、昆仑、环跳、阳陵泉、通里及列缺。

Twelve especially effective empirical points, i. e. , Zusanli (ST36), Neiting (ST44), Quchi (LI11), Hegu (LI4), Weizhong (BL40), Chengshan (BL57), Taichong (LR3), Kunlun (BL60), Huantiao (GB30), Yanglingquan (GB34), Tongli (HT5), and Lieque (LU7).

天血 Tianxue

通天穴别名。

The other name of Tongtian (BL7).

天医 heavenly treament

古代针灸忌宜说之一。按日时的干支推算天医所在，为治病的吉利时日（最佳时间）。

One of the theories of acupuncture and moxibustion indications or contraindications in ancient China. The time when Tianyi exists could be calculated using the heavenly stems and earthly branches of the date and hour. And that time would be the favorable time for curing diseases.

天牖 Tianyou (TE16)

经穴名。属手少阳三焦经。定位：在颈侧部，当乳突的后方直下，平下颌角，胸锁乳突肌的后缘。主治：头痛，项强，面肿，视物不清，暴聋。操作：直刺 0.5～1 寸；可灸。

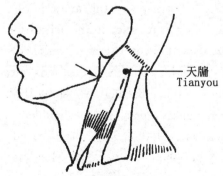

Name of an acupoint. It belongs to the Sanjiao Meridian of Hand-Shaoyang. Location：On the lateral side of the neck, directly below the posterior border of the mastoid process, at the same level with the mandibular angle, and on the posterior border of the sternocleidomastoid muscle. Indications: Headache, neck rigidity, facial swelling, blurred vision, sudden deafness, etc. Method: Puncture perpendicularly 0. 5-1 cun. Moxibustion is applicable.

天柱 Tianzhu (BL10)

经穴名。属足太阳膀胱经。定位：在后颈部，斜方肌外缘，后发际凹陷中，约后发际正中旁开 1.3 寸。主治：头痛，鼻塞，咽喉肿痛，颈强，肩背痛等。操作：直刺或斜刺 0.5～1 寸；可灸。

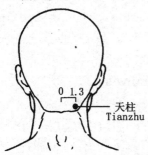

Name of an acupoint. It belongs to the Bladder Meridian of Foot-Taiyang. Location: On the nape, on the lateral border of the trapezius muscle, in the depression of and about 1. 3 cun lateral to the middle of the posterior hairline. Indications: Headache, nasal obstruction, sore throat, neck rigidity, pain in the shoulders and back, etc. Method: Puncture perpendicularly or obliquely 0. 5-1 cun. Moxibustion is applicable.

天宗 Tianzong (SI11)

经穴名。属手太阳小肠经。定位：在肩胛部，当冈上窝中央凹陷处，与第四胸椎相平。主治：肩胛痛，肘臂后外侧痛，气喘等。操作：直刺或斜刺 0.5～1 寸；可灸。

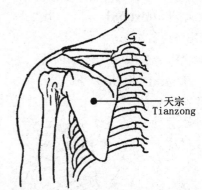

Name of an acupoint. It belongs to the Small Intestine Meridian of Hand-Taiyang. Location: On the scapula, in the depression of the centre of the supraspinous fossa, at the same level with the 4th thoracic vertebra. Indications: Pain in the scapular region, pain in the posterolateral aspect of the elbow and arm, asthma, etc. Method: Puncture perpendicularly or obliquely 0. 5-1 cun. Moxibustion is applicable.

挑治疗法 pricking therapy

指在患者一定部位的皮肤上，用粗针挑断皮下白色纤维状物以进行治疗的方法。

The therapeutic technique to break the white fibrous substance under the skin at a particular location with a big needle.

挑痔法 pricking method to cure hemorrhoids

挑治法的一种。即以针挑刺腰骶部的疹点或穴位以治痔疾的方法。

One of the pricking therapies, i. e., poke and prick the rashes or acupoints with needles on the lumbosacral part to cure hemorrhoids.

条口 Tiaokou (ST38)

经穴名。属足阳明胃经。定位：犊鼻下8寸，距胫骨前缘一横指。主治：腿膝酸痛，下肢痿痹，肩痛，腹痛等。操作：直刺1～1.5寸；可灸。

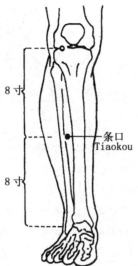

Name of an acupoint. It belongs to the Stomach Meridian of Foot-Yangming. Location：8 cun below Dubi(ST35)，one finger breadth from the anterior border of the tibia. Indications：Numbness, soreness and pain of the knee and leg, weakness and motor impairment of the lower limbs, shoulder pain, abdominal pain, etc. Method：Puncture perpendicularly 1-1. 5 cun. Moxibustion is applicable.

调和肝脾 harmonize liver and spleen

治疗肝气犯脾、肝脾不和的方法。症见胁胀或痛、肠鸣、大便稀薄、食欲不振、性情急躁、舌苔薄白、脉弦细。

A treatment for the excessive liver-qi over-restrains the spleen and incoordination between liver and spleen, applicable to the case manifested as distending or pain over the hypochondrium, borborygmus, discharge of loose stools, poor appetite, irritability, thin and whitish fur on the tongue, stringy and thin pulse, etc.

调和肝胃 harmonize liver and stomach

使用疏通调和的药物治疗肝气犯胃、肝胃不和的方法。适用于胁肋胀痛、胃脘胀闷疼痛、食欲减退、嗳气吞酸、呕吐者。

A treatment for the invading of the stomach by excessive liver-qi and incoordination between the liver and stomach by the application of drugs with dispersing and regulating effects, applicable to the case manifested as distending pain over the hypochondrium and the epigastrium, poor appetite, eructation, acid regurgitation, vomiting, etc.

调经 regulating menstruation

治疗月经病方法的总称。包括月经不调、痛经、经闭、经量不正常等的治法。临床上常按患者的气血变化及寒热虚实不同进行处理。对原发性月经病一般以调经为主，而对继发性月经病则以治疗原发病为主。

A treatment for menopathy including menoxenia, dysmenorrhea, amenorrhea, scanty or profuse mentruation, etc. Clinically, the management varies according to the condition of qi and blood, and the manifestation of the case, such as cold or heat, deficiency or excessive. The treatment of primary menopathy should aim at the regulation of menstruation, while that of secondary menopathy should aim at the treatment of the primary disease.

调气 regulating qi

指通过针刺补泻，调节人体的生理机

能,增强抗病能力,改善病理状态的方法。

To regulate physiological functions of the body, to reinforce its resistance against diseases, and to improve the pathological state through reinforcing and reducing in acupuncture therapy.

听宫 Tinggong (SI19)

经穴名。属手太阳小肠经。定位:在面部,耳屏前,下颌骨髁突的后方,张口时呈凹陷处。主治:耳聋,耳鸣,牙痛等。操作:张口取穴,直刺 0.5～1 寸;可灸。

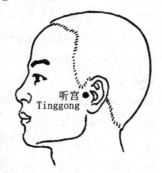

Name of an acupoint. It belongs to the Small Intestine Meridian of Hand-Taiyang. Location: On the face, anterior to the tragus and posterior to the mandibular condyliod process, in the depression formed by opening the mouth. Indications: Deafness, tinnitus, toothache, etc. Method: Ask the patient to open his/her mouth, puncture perpendicularly 0. 5-1 cun. Moxibustion is applicable.

听会 Tinghui (GB2)

经穴名。属足少阳胆经。定位:在面部,当耳屏间切迹的前方,下颌骨髁突的后缘,张口有凹陷处。主治:耳聋耳鸣,牙痛,下颌功能障碍,痄腮,面瘫等。操作:张口取穴,直刺 0.5～1 寸;可灸。

Name of an acupoint. It belongs to the Gallbladder Meridian of Foot-Shaoyang. Location: On the face, anterior to the in-

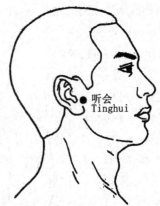

tertragic notch, in the depression formed by opening mouth and posterior to the condyliod process of the mandible. Indications: Deafness, tinnitus, toothache, motor impairment of the mandibular joint, mumps, facial paralysis, etc. Method: Ask the patient to open his/her mouth, puncture perpendicularly 0. 5-1 cun. Moxibustion is applicable.

亭头 Tingtou

经外奇穴名。定位:脐中直下 4.5 寸,旁开一横指处。直刺主治子宫脱垂。

Name of an extra point. Location: 4. 5 cun directly below the center of the navel and one transverse finger to that above measured point, perpendicular acupuncture is used to cure the uterine prolapse.

艇角 Tingjiao

耳穴名。定位:在耳甲艇前上角。主治:前列腺炎,尿道炎等。

Name of an ear point. Location: At the anterosuperior corner of cymba conchae. Indications: Prostatitis, urethritis, etc.

艇中 Tingzhong

耳穴名。定位:在耳甲艇中央。主治:

低热,腹胀腹痛,腮腺炎,胆道蛔虫病等。

Name of an ear point. Location: In the center of cymab conchae. Indications: Low grade fever, abdominal distension and pain, parotitis, biliary ascariasis, etc.

通谷 Tonggu

经穴名。有二:一属肾经,在腹;一属膀胱经,在足。为便于区分,前者称腹通谷,后者称足通谷。

Name of acupoints. They are: One belongs to the Kidney Meridian on the abdomen; the other belongs to the Bladder Meridian on the foot. In order to distinguish them, the former is named Futonggu (KI20), the other is named Zutonggu (BL66).

通关 Tongguan

阴都穴别名。

The other name of Yindu (KI19).

通间 Tongjian

三阳络别名。

The other name of Sanyangluo(TE8).

通经 promoting menstruation

治疗闭经(病理性闭经),使月经通畅的方法。临床上常按虚实的不同,采用补气血或行气活血的方法。前者适用于气血两虚引起的闭经,后者适用于气滞血瘀引起的闭经。

A treatment for suppressed menstruation by tonifying qi and blood for the deficiency type, and by activating qi and blood circulation for the excessive type.

通里 Tongli (HT5)

经穴名。属手少阴心经,本经络穴。定位:在前臂掌侧,当尺侧腕屈肌腱的桡侧缘,腕横纹上 1 寸。主治:心悸,头晕,目

中不了了,咽痛,暴喑,舌强不语,腕肘痛等。操作:直刺 0.3～0.5 寸;可灸。

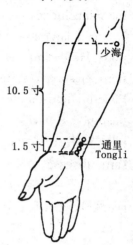

The acupoint, Luo-Connecting point, belongs to the Heart Meridian of Hand-Shaoyin. Location: On the palmar side of the forearm and on the radial side of the tendon of the ulnar flexor musle of the wrist, 1 cun above the transverse crease of the wrist. Indications: Palpitation, dizziness, blurred vision, sore throat, sudden loss of voice, aphasia with stiff tongue, pain in the wrist and elbow, etc. Method: Puncture perpendicularly 0.3-0.5 cun. Moxibustion is applicable.

通天 Tongtian (BL7)

经穴名。属足太阳膀胱经。定位:在头部,当前发际正中直上 4 寸,旁开 1.5 寸。主治:头痛,眩晕,鼻塞,鼻衄,鼻渊等。操作:平刺 0.3～0.5 寸;可灸。

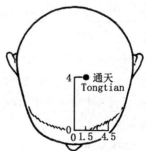

Name of an acupoint. It belongs to the

Bladder Meridian of Foot-Taiyang. Location: On the head, 4 cun directly above the midpoint of the anterior hairline and 1.5 cun lateral to the midline. Indications: Headache, vertigo, nasal obstruction, epistaxis, sinusitis, etc. Method: Puncture horizontally 0.3-0.5 cun. Moxibustion is applicable.

同病异治 different treatment for the same disease

针对同一疾病,因不同个体、地点、时间、病机、疾病类型等而采取不同的治疗方法。

The treatment of the same disease may vary with the individual, place, time and pathogenesis and type of the disease.

同名经 meridians with the same name

同名为太阴、少阴、厥阴、阳明、太阳或少阳的一对手经和足经。

Six pairs of meridians on the upper and lower extremities with same names, e. g., meridians of Taiyin of hand and of foot, meridians of Shaoyin of hand and of foot.

同名经配穴法 point-combining method in identically named meridians

配穴法之一。指手足同名称的经脉所属穴位可以配合使用。

One of the point-combining methods, i. e., the points in the identically named meridians of hand and foot can be combined together.

同身寸 body cun

指以患者本人手指为标准来测量穴位的一种测量单位。①以中指的中节两侧横纹间为1寸。②以拇指第一指节的宽度为1寸。③以手指第2～5指并拢的最大横径为3寸。

Using the patient's finger as a measuring unit to locate points. ① Take the width of the crease of the 2nd interphalangeal joints of the middle finger as 1 cun. ② Take the width of the 1st interphalangeal joint of the thumb as 1 cun. ③ Take the maximum width of the four fingers as 3 cun when they close together.

铜人 bronze figure

供教学所用的铜铸人体经脉腧穴模型。最早的铜人为北宋针灸家王惟一所铸造。

A human figure made of bronze for teaching purpose, which is marked with meridians and acupoints. The first one was cast by Wang Weiyi, an acupuncture expert in the Northern Song Dynasty.

铜人腧穴针灸图经 Illustrated Manual of Acupuncture Points of the Bronze Figure

宋代王惟一撰。该书列举并订正经脉的循行和腧穴。

A book written by Wang Weiyi, in which the author enumerated and corrected the previously mistaken location of meridians and acupoints.

瞳子髎 Tongziliao (GB1)

经穴名。属足少阳胆经。定位:在面部,目外眦旁,当眶外侧缘处。主治:头痛,目赤痛,失明,流泪,口眼歪斜等。操作:沿皮刺0.3～0.5寸;可灸。

Name of an acupoint. It belongs to the

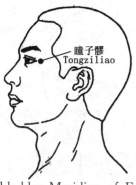

瞳子髎
Tongziliao

Gallbladder Meridian of Foot-Shaoyang. Location：On the face，lateral to the outer canthus，on the lateral border of the orbit. Indications：Headache，redness and pain of the eyes，blindness，lacrimation，devation of eyes and mouth，etc. Method：Puncture subcutaneously 0. 3-0. 5 cun. Moxibustion is applicable.

痛经 dysmenorrhea

指妇女在经期或经期前后，出现周期性小腹疼痛或痛引腰骶，甚则剧痛难忍，伴有恶心、呕吐的病症。多因气滞、血瘀、寒湿凝滞、气血虚弱或肝肾亏损引起。治宜疏肝理气、活血化瘀、补气养血止痛。取穴：气海、太冲、三阴交、阴陵泉、膈俞、血海、地机、次髎、足三里、关元。

The disease usually due to stagnation of qi，blood stasis or cold-damp pathogens，deficiency of qi and blood，or deficiency of the liver and kidneys. Treatment principle：Relieve the depressed liver and regulate the flow of qi，invigorate blood circulation to remove blood stasis，benefit qi and nourish blood to alleviate pain. Point selection：Qihai（CV6），Taichong（LR3），Sanyinjiao（SP6），Yinlingquan（SP9），Geshu（BL17），Xuehai（SP10），Diji（SP8），Ciliao（BL32），Zusanli（ST36），Guanyuan（CV4）.

头第二侧线 second lateral head line

经穴定位线，为头临泣至风池间的连线，足少阳胆经经此。

Point-locating line，i. e. the line between Toulinqi（GB15） and Fengchi（GB20）. The Gallbladder Meridian of Foot-Shaoyang passes along it.

头第一侧线 first lateral head line

经穴定位线，为曲差至天柱间的连线，足太阳膀胱经经此。

Point-locating line，i. e.，the line between Qucha（BL4） and Tianzhu（BL10）. The Bladder Meridian of Foot-Taiyang passes along it.

头风 Toufeng

经外奇穴名。位于大腿外侧。直立垂手贴股，拇、示指指蹼缘中点下是穴。治疗常用直刺或灸治头风、眩晕。

Name of an extra point. Located at the lateral side of the thigh，under the midpoint of the thumb-index web margin when standing upright and putting the two hands closely to the thigh，perpendicular acupuncture or moxibustion can be used to cure head wind and giddiness.

头临泣 Toulinqi (GB15)

经穴名。属足少阳胆经。定位：在头部，当瞳孔直上入前发际 0.5 寸，神庭与头维连线的中点处。主治：头痛，呕吐，流泪，目外眦痛，鼻塞，鼻渊等。操作：平刺 0.5～0.8 寸；可灸。

Name of an acupoint. It belongs to the Gallbladder Meridian of Foot-Shaoyang.

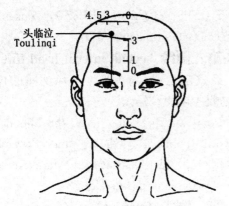

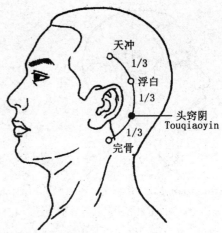

Location:On the head, directly above the pupil and 0.5 cun above the anterior hairline, at the midpoint of the line connecting Shenting(GV24)and Touwei(ST8). Indications:Headache, vomiting, lacrimation, pain in the outer canthus, nasal obstruction, sinusitis, etc. Method: Puncture horizontally 0.5-0.8 cun. Moxibustion is applicable.

头窍阴 Touqiaoyin (GB11)

经穴名。属足少阳胆经。定位:在头部,当耳后乳突的后上方,天冲与完骨连线的中 1/3 与下 1/3 交点处。主治:头项痛,耳鸣,耳聋,耳痛等。操作:平刺 0.5~0.8 寸;可灸。

Name of an acupoint. It belongs to the Gallbladder Meridian of Foot-Shaoyang. Location:On the head, posterior and superior to the mastiod process, at the junction of the middle one third and lower one third of the curved line connecting Tianchong(GB9) and Wangu(GB12). Indications:Pain in the head and neck, deafness, tinnitus, earache, etc. Method:Puncture horizontally 0.5-0.8 cun. Moxibustion is applicable.

头痛 headache

以头部(整个或局部)疼痛为主症的一种病证。凡外感六淫或脏腑内伤均能引起头痛。治宜疏风、化痰、通络止痛。取穴:风池、太阳、合谷、大椎、外关。

Pain in the head (local or general) caused by the attack of the six-pathogens or the disorders of internal organs. Treatment principle:Expel the wind, resolve phlegm,remove obstruction in the meridians and collaterals to relieve pain. Point selection:Fengchi(GB20), Taiyang(EX-HN5), Hegu (LI4), Dazhui (GV14), Waiguan(TE5).

头维 Touwei (ST8)

经穴名。属足阳明胃经。定位:在头侧部,当额角发际上 0.5 寸,头正中线旁 4.5 寸。主治:头痛,目眩等。操作:沿皮刺 0.5~1 寸;可灸。

Name of an acupoint. It belongs to the Stomach Meridian of Foot-Yangming. Location:On the lateral side of the head, 0.5 cun above the anterior hairline at the corner of the forehead,and 4.5 cun lateral

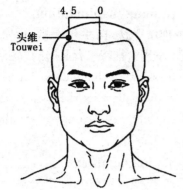

头维
Touwei

4.5　0

to the midline of the head. Indications：
Headache，blurred vision，etc. Method：
Puncture Subcutaneously 0.5-1 cun.
Moxibustion is applicable.

头项强痛 rigidity and pain in the nape and head

指头及颈项疼痛，伴后颈部肌肉牵引不
舒的症状，多因外感六淫，遏阻经脉所致。
治宜调气活血、舒筋散寒。取穴：风池、天
柱、后溪、悬钟。

A symptom caused by the attack of the
six pathogens and the stagnation of the
meridians. Treatment principle：Promote
the flow of qi and blood circulation，relax
muscles and dispel cold. Point selection：
Fengchi(GB20)，Tianzhu(BL10)，Houxi
(SI3)，Xuanzhong(GB39).

头针 scalp acupuncture

针刺头部与大脑皮质各区相应的头皮
投射区以治疗疾病的方法。

To puncture certain points on the scalp
which reflect the corresponding areas of the
cerebral cortex for therapeutic purposes.

头针麻醉 scalp acupuncture anesthesia

选用头部的穴位进行针刺麻醉的方法。

To administer acupuncture anesthesia
by puncturing the points on the scalp.

头重 heaviness of head

自觉头部重坠如裹的症状，多因外感湿
邪或湿痰内阻所致。治宜化痰降浊、通络
止痛。取穴：中脘、丰隆、百会、印堂、丝竹
空。

A symptom of tightly bound feeling o-
ver the head，caused by the attack of
exo-genous damp pathogen or the retention of phlegm. Treatment principle：Re-
solve phlegm and lower turbidity，remove
obstruction in the meridians and collaterals to relieve pain. Point selection：
Zhongwan（CV12），Fenglong（ST40），
Baihui（GV20），Yintang（GV29），
Sizhukong(TE23).

透天凉 heaven-penetrating cooling method

指将针直接刺入一定深度后，按照深、
中、浅的顺序三退一进，反复操作，使患者
出现凉感的方法。

After the needle is inserted into a certain depth，it is repeatedly lifted thrice
according to the deep，medium and superficial sequences and thrusted once so
as to make the patient feel cool.

透针 piercing needling

指用长针同时穿透两个或两个以上穴
位，或两条以上经脉的一种针法。

An acupuncture technique to insert a
long needle through two or more points
or meridians at the same time.

吐纳法 deep respiration exercise

利用深呼吸和有意控制意念，使神思安
定，以进行保健和治病的一种方法。

A method of breathing exercise for health care and treatment of certain diseases by tranquilizing oneself with deep respiration and self-control of ones mind.

吐血 spitting blood

指血从口中吐出的症状。血可出自呼吸道及上消化道。多因郁怒、伤酒、伤食、劳倦等因素导致脏腑热盛、阴虚火旺或气虚脾寒引起。治宜清肝和胃、泻火止血，或益气摄血。取穴：中脘、郄门、内庭、行间、脾俞、足三里。

A condition resulting from the bleeding of the respiratory or upper digestive tract, due to overabundance of heat-pathogen in the viscera, yin deficiency with hyperactivity of fire-pathogen, or deficiency of qi with spleen-cold after a rage, overdrinking, overeating, or overstrain, etc. Treatment principle: Remove heat from the liver and harmonize the stomach, purge fire and stop bleeding, or replenish qi to control blood. Point selection: Zhongwan (CV12), Ximen (PC4), Neiting (ST44), Xingjian (LR2), Pishu (BL20), Zusanli(ST36).

推而纳之 pushing and thrusting acupuncture

为针刺补法要领。与泻法"动而伸之"相对。即得气后将针推进按纳为补法。

An important rule of reinforcing acupuncture, i. e. , after having the sensation, the needle is pushed and thrust deeper to reinforce, as contrasted with the rule of reducing acupuncture called "pulling and lifting acupuncture".

推法 pushing manipulation

一种推拿手法，医生用手指（通常为拇指）或手掌用力推挤患者肌肉的方法。

A massage technique performed by pushing and squeezing the patient's muscles forcefully with a finger (usually the thumb) or palm.

推罐 sliding cupping

在需要拔罐的部位和罐边先涂上凡士林或其他油类，将火罐拔好后，于皮肤上水平行上下左右移动的治疗方法。

The therapeutic technique to administer cupping by first smearing vaselin or the like on the affected area and the edge of the cup, after applying the cup, sliding it on the skin in different directions.

退法 withdrawing method

出针时先将针提至浅部稍作停留，再拔出体外。

It implies that during the withdrawal of the needle, it should be lifted up to the shallow part of the point, retained there for a while and finally pulled out of the body.

退针 backing up of the needle

针刺手法之一。即针入体内后，逐渐由深至浅向外退的方法。

One of the acupuncture techniques, i. e. , gradually withdraw the inserted needle from the deeper layer to the superficial layer.

臀 Tun; buttocks

①耳穴名。在对耳轮下脚的后 1/3 处。主治相应部位的疼痛。②位于腰下方，骶骨两侧的部分，相当于臀大肌突起部位。

①Name of an ear point. Located at the posterior 1/3 of the inferior antihelix crus. It is used for treating pain at the corresponding area. ②The part located below the loins, at both sides of the sacrum, corresponding to the prominences formed by the gluteus maximus.

脱肛 rectal prolapse

直肠或直肠黏膜脱出肛门的一种证候。多因气虚下陷或湿热下注大肠所致,多见于老人、小儿。治宜清泻湿热、益气提升。取穴:长强、大肠俞、承山、百会、气海。

A disease caused by the deficiency and depression of qi or the attack of damp-heat pathogen to the large intestine; mostly seen in children and the aged. Treatment principle: Remove pathogenic damp-heat, supplement qi to uprise the rectum. Point selection: Changqiang (GV1), Dachangshu(BL25), Chengshan (BL57),Baihui(GV20), Qihai(CV6).

脱证 collapse syndrome

由于气血阴阳严重耗损、重要脏腑功能衰竭所致,以汗出如珠,四肢厥冷,二便失禁,精神萎靡,甚至神昏、脉微欲绝为主要临床表现的证候。治宜回阳固脱、调节阴阳。取穴:素髎、关元、涌泉、足三里、气海、太溪。

A syndrome due to exhaustion of qi, blood, yin and yang, and failure of important organs, manifested as profuse sweating, deadly cold limbs, incontinence of urine and feces, listlessness, even fading pulse and coma. Treatment principle: Recuperate depleted yang, and rescue the patient from collapse, regulate yin and yang. Point selection: Suliao (GV25), Guanyuan (CV4), Yongquan (KI1), Zusanli (ST36), Qihai (CV6), Taixi(KI3).

W

外鼻 Waibi

耳穴名。在耳屏外侧面正中稍前。主治：鼻塞，鼻疮，鼻炎等。

Name of an ear point. It is in the center of the lateral aspect of tragus. Indications: Nasal obstruction, nose furuncles, rhinitis, etc.

外耳 Waier

耳穴名。又称耳、屏上。位于屏上切迹前方近耳轮部。主治：耳疾，眩晕等。

Name of an ear point. Er, or Pingshang is its another name. It is on the supratragic notch close to helix. Indications: Ear diseases, vertigo, etc.

外耳门 orifice of the external auditory meatus

解剖名称。在耳甲腔内，被耳屏遮盖着的孔窍。

Terminologia anatomica. The opening in the cavity of auricular concha shielded by the tragus.

外府 outer organs

指六腑，与中府（五脏）相对。

It refers to the six fu-organs as contrasted with the central organs (the five zang-organs).

外感 exogenous disease

感受风、寒、暑、湿、燥、火、疫疠等外邪侵犯所致的疾病。

The diseases which are due to attack of exogenous evils such as wind, cold, summer-heat, dampness, dryness, fire, pestilence, etc.

外勾 Waigou

伏兔穴别名。

The other name of Futu (ST32).

外关 Waiguan (TE15)

经穴名。属手少阳三焦经，本经络穴，八脉交会穴之一，通于阳维脉。定位：在前臂背侧，当阳池与肘尖的连线上，腕背横纹上2寸，尺骨与桡骨之间。主治：热病，头痛，颊痛，耳聋，耳鸣，胁痛，臂肘屈伸不利，手指疼痛，手颤等。操作：直刺0.5～1寸；可灸。

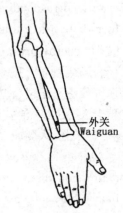
外关
Waiguan

The acupoint, Luo-Connecting point, of the Sanjiao Meridian of Hand-Shaoyang. One of the eight confluence points, communicate with the Yang Link Vesssl. Location: On the dorsal side of the forearm, on the line connecting Yangchi (TE4) and the tip of the olecranon, 2 cun above the transverse crease of the dorsal carpus, between the ulna and radius. Indications: Febrile diseases, headache, pain in the cheeks, deafness, tinnitus, pain in the hypochondriac region, motor impairment of the elbows and arms, pain of the fingers, hand tremor, etc. Method: Puncture perpendicularly 0.5-1 cun. Moxibustion is applicable.

外踝 lateral malleolus

又名核骨，即腓骨下端向外的骨突。为

足太阳膀胱经与足少阳胆经所过之部位。

Also known as bony nodule, where the Bladder Meridian of Foot-Taiyang and Gallbladder Meridian of Foot-Shaoyang pass thorough.

外金津玉液 Waijinjinyuye

经外奇穴名。定位：位于廉泉穴直上1.5寸，旁开各0.3寸处。主治：中风不语，流涎，舌肌麻痹，口腔炎等。向舌根方向斜刺0.5～1寸。

Name of an extra point. Location：1.5 cun directly above Lianquan (CV23), and 0.3 cun lateral to the midline. Indications：Aphasia due to apoplexy, salivation, lingual muscular paresis, stomatitis, etc. Method：Slanting acupuncture 0.5-1 cun toward the root of the tongue.

外经 external meridian

经脉的体表部分。

The part of the meridian in the superficial part of the body.

外劳宫 Wailaogong (EX-UE8)

经外奇穴名。近称项强穴。定位：位于手背二、三掌骨之间，与劳宫穴相对处。

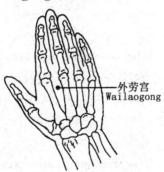
外劳宫 Wailaogong

主治：消化不良，腹泻，小儿急、慢惊风，指掌麻痒等。治疗上常用直刺或灸治。

Name of an extra point, recently known as Xiangqiang. Location：On the dorsal side of the hand, between the 2nd and 3rd metacarpal bones, just opposite to Laogong (PC8). Indications：Indigestion, diarrhea, acute and chronic infantile convulsion, numbness and itchiness of the fingers and palms, etc., using perpendicular acupuncture or moxibustion.

外陵 Wailing (ST26)

经穴名。属足阳明胃经。定位：在下腹部，当脐中下1寸，距前正中线2寸。主治：腹痛，疝气，痛经等。操作：直刺1～1.5寸；可灸。

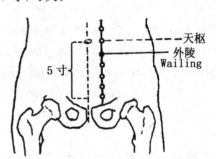
天枢
外陵 Wailing
5寸

Name of an acupoint. It belongs to the Stomach Meridian of Foot-Yangming. Location：On the lower abdomen, 1 cun below the centre of the umbilicus and 2 cun lateral to the anterior midline. Indications：Abdominal pain, hernia, dysmenorrhea, etc. Method：Puncture perpendicularly 1-1.5 cun. Moxibustion is applicable.

外丘 Waiqiu (GB36)

经穴名。属足少阳胆经，本经郄穴。定位：在小腿外侧，当外踝尖上7寸，腓骨前缘，平阳交。主治：胸胁项腿痛，猘犬伤毒不出等。操作：直刺0.5～1寸；可灸。

The acupoint, Xi-Cleft point, belongs to the Gallbladder Meridian of Foot-Shaoyin. Location：On the lateral side of

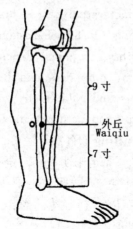

9寸

外丘
Waiqiu

7寸

the leg, 7 cun above the tip of the lateral malleolus, at the same level as Yangjiao (GB35). Indications: Pain in the chest, hypochondriac region, neck, and thigh, rabies, etc. Method: Puncture perpendicularly 0.5-1 cun. Moxibustion is applicable.

外生殖器 Waishengzhiqi

耳穴名。在与对耳轮下脚上缘相对的耳轮处。主治：外生殖器炎症，会阴湿疹，阳痿。

Name of an ear point. It is on the helix opposite to the upper border of the inferior crura of antihelix. Indications: Inflammation of external genital organs, eczema of the perineum, impotence.

外台秘要 *Medical Secrets of An Official*

医书名。唐代王焘编著，其中第39卷载述灸法和经穴。

Name of the medical book written by Wang Tao in the Tang Dynasty. The 39th volume of the book deals with the moxibustion and acupoints.

外膝眼 Waixiyan

与内膝眼相对，合称膝眼。外膝眼与犊鼻穴同位。

Opposite to Neixiyan(EX-LE4), at the same site as Dubi (ST35).

外眼角 outer canthus; temporal canthus

又名外眦。即上下眼睑在颞侧连结部，是足少阳胆经的起点处，也是瞳子髎穴所在部位。

The angle at the outer or temporal end of the fissure between the eyelids, where the Meridian of Foot-Shaoyang begins and Tongziliao(GB1) is located.

外因 exogenous pathogenic factors

①泛指各种外来的致病因素。②古代三因分类法的一类病因，即风、寒、暑、湿、燥、火等六淫邪气。

①Generally referring to all the factors which are exogenous in origin. ②One of the three kinds of pathogenic factors in accordance with the classification in ancient times, including the six pathogens, i.e., wind, cold, summer-heat, dampness, dryness, and fire.

外治法 external therapy

泛指除口、眼药外，施于体表或从体外进行治疗的方法，如针灸、膏贴、熏洗、按摩等法。

The treatments other than oral and ocular used of drugs, such as acupuncture, plaster, steam bath, massage, etc.

外痔 external hemorrhoids

位于肛门齿线以下的痔疮。治宜清热化瘀。取穴：次髎、长强、会阳、二白。

Located right at the opening of the anal dentate line. Treatment principle：Clear heat and resolve stasis. Point selection：Ciliao(BL32)，Changqiang(GV1)，Huiyang(BL35)，Erbai(EX-UE2).

弯针 bending needle

指针法操作时，刺入体内的针产生弯曲的异常情况。

An unusual situation that the needle inserted into the body is bent.

完骨 Wangu (GB12)

① 经穴名。属足少阳胆经。定位：在头部，当耳后乳突的后下方凹陷处。主治：头痛，失眠，颊肿，耳后痛，口眼歪斜，齿痛等。操作：

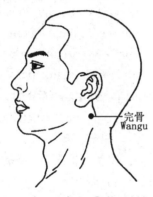

向下斜刺 0.5～0.8 寸；可灸。②指颞骨乳突部。

①Name of an acupoint. It belongs to the Gallbladder Meridian of Foot-Shaoyang. Location：On the head，in the depression posterior and inferior to the mastoid process. Indications：Headache，insomnia，swelling of the cheeks，retro-auricular pain，deviation of eyes and mouth，toothache，etc. Method：Puncture obliquely downward 0. 3-0. 5 cun. Moxibustion is applicable. ②The mastoid process of the temporal bone.

腕 Wan

耳穴名。在肘、指穴之间。主治腕部疼痛。

Name of an ear point. It is at the midway between Zhou and Zhi. It is used for treating pain in wrist region.

腕骨 Wangu (SI4)

经穴名。属手太阳小肠经,本经原穴。定位：在手掌尺侧，当第五掌骨基底与钩骨之间的凹陷中，赤白肉际处。主治：热病无汗，头痛项强，指挛腕痛，黄疸。操作：直刺 0.3～0.5 寸；可灸。

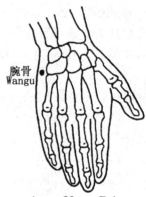

The acupoint, Yuan-Primary point, belongs to the Small Intestine Meridian of Hand-Taiyang. Location：On the ulnar border of the hand，in the depression between the 5th metacarpal bone and the hamate bone， on the dorso-ventral boundary of the hand. Indications：Febrile diseases without sweating， headache，rigidity of the neck，contracture of the fingers，pain in the wrist，jaundice，etc. Method：Puncture perpendicularly 0. 3-0. 5 cun. Moxibustion is applicable.

腕踝针 wrist-ankle acupuncture

针刺腕、踝周围特有的穴位以治疗疾病的方法。

To puncture points particular to the

wrists and ankles for therapeutic purposes.

王焘　Wang Tao

唐代医家。在弘文馆任职期间,采集诸家医方,编成《外台秘要》。

A medical scholar in Tang Dynasty. As an official of the Hongwen State Library, he collected prescriptions from all sources and compiled *Medical Secrets of an Official*.

王惟一　Wang Weiyi

宋代著名针灸学家。编有《铜人腧穴针灸图经》,主持铸造针灸铜人两具供教学用。

A celebrated expert of acupuncture and moxibustion in the Song Dynasty, author of *Illustrated Manual of Acupuncture Points of the Bronze Figure*. He took charge of casting two life-size bronze figures for teaching purpose.

望诊　inspection

四诊之一。运用视觉观察患者的精神状态、体态、舌质和舌苔的变化,大小便和其他排泄物、分泌物的变化等。

One of the four methods of physical examination by observing the patient's mental status, posture, appearances of the tongue body and tongue fur, the changes of urine, feces and other excretions and secretions, etc.

微脉　faint pulse

细小无力,指感搏动微弱的一种脉象。多因阴阳气血均虚所致。常见于休克、虚脱的患者。

A pulse condition with thin and weak beats which are only palpable faintly, usually caused by deficiency of yin, yang, qi and blood. Commonly seen in the patients suffering from shock and collapse.

维胞　Weibao

经外奇穴名。位于髂前上棘内下方之凹陷处,平关元穴。沿腹股沟韧带斜刺或温灸治子宫脱垂、肠疝、肠功能紊乱等。

Name of an extra point. Location: At the depression medial and inferior to the anterior superior iliac spine, level to Guanyuan (CV4). Puncture obliquely along the inguinal ligament or moxibustion is used to cure uterus prolapse, intestinal hernia and dysfunction, etc.

维道　Weidao (GB28)

经穴名。属足少阳胆经。定位:在侧腹部,当髂前上棘的前下方,五枢穴前下0.5寸。主治:带下,下腹痛,疝气,阴挺等。操作:直刺0.5～1寸;可灸。

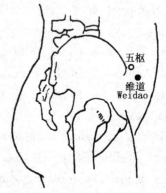

Name of an acupoint. It belongs to the Gallbladder Meridian of Foot-Shaoyang. Location: On the lateral side of the abdomen, anterior and inferior to the anterior superior iliac spine, 0.5 cun anterior and inferior to Wushu (GB27). Indications:

Leukorrhea, lower abdominal pain, hernia, uterine prolapse, etc. Method: Puncture perpendicularly 0.5-1 cun. Moxibustion is applicable.

维宫 Weigong

经外奇穴名。定位：维道穴下 1 寸处。沿腹股沟韧带斜刺或温灸主治子宫下垂。

Name of an extra point. Location: 1 cun below Weidao (GB28). Puncture obliquely along the inguinal ligament or warm moxibustion is used to cure uterus prolapse.

维会 Weihui

指百会或神阙穴。

It refers to Baihui (GV20) or Shenque (CV8).

维脉 Link Vessels

奇经八脉中阴维脉与阳维脉的总称。

A collective term of the Yin Link and Yang Link Vessels, two of the Eight Extra Meridians.

尾翠 Weicui

经外奇穴名。定位：位于尾骨尖直上 3 寸。主治：小儿疳瘰，消瘦，消化不良，腹痛下痢，脱肛等。治疗常用沿皮刺或灸治。

Name of an extra point. Location: 3 cun directly above the coccygeal tip. Subcutaneous acupuncture or moxibustion is used to treat infantile malnutrition, emaciation, indigestion, abdominal pain and dysentery, rectal prolapse, etc.

委阳 Weiyang (BL39)

经穴名。属足太阳膀胱经，三焦下合穴。定位：在腘横纹外侧端，当股二头肌

肌腱的内侧处。主治：腰脊强痛，小腹胀满，水肿，小便不利，腿足挛痛。操作：直刺 0.5～1 寸；可灸。

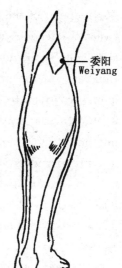

The acupoint, lower He-Sea point of sanjiao, belongs to the Bladder Meridian of Foot-Taiyang. Location: At the lateral end of the popliteal crease, medial to the tendon of the biceps femoris. Indications: Stiffness and pain of the lower back, distension and fullness of the lower abdomen, edema, dysuria, cramp of the legs and feet, etc. Method: Puncture perpendicularly 0.5-1 cun. Moxibustion is applicable.

委中 Weizhong (BL40)

经穴名。属足太阳膀胱经，本经合穴。定位：在腘横纹中点，当股二头肌肌腱与半腱肌肌腱的中间。主治：腰痛，髋关节伸屈不利，腘筋挛急，下肢痿痹，偏瘫，腹痛，呕吐，泄泻，丹毒等。操作：直刺 0.5～1 寸；可灸。

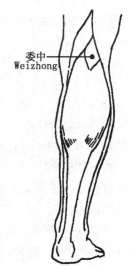

The acupoint, He-Sea point, belongs to the Bladder Meridian of Foot-Taiyang. Location: At the midpoint of the popliteal creases, between the tendons of the biceps femoris and the semitendinosus. Indications: Lumbago, motor impairment of the hip joints, contracture of the tendon in the popliteal fossa, muscular atrophy, pain, numbness and motor impairment of the lower extremities, hemiplegia, abdominal pain, vomiting, diarrhea, erysipelas, etc. Method: Puncture perpendicularly 0.5-1 cun. Moxibustion is applicable.

痏 Wei

①指针刺后所留下的针眼。泻法时扩大针眼而不使闭合，补法时闭合针眼。②指针刺的次数单位。③穴位名。指少泽、关冲、商阳和少商、中冲、少冲。

①The hole left after acupuncture. For reducing purpose, the hole should be left opened or enlarged; while for reinforcing, the hole should be left closed. ②The counting unit of acupuncture therapy. ③A general term for six pairs of acupoints, i. e., Shaoze (SI1), Guanchong (TE1), Shangyang (LI1), Shaoshang (LU11), Zhongchong (PC9) and Shaochong (HT9).

痿证 flaccidity syndrome

指肢体软弱无力，渐致肌肉萎缩而不能随意运动的证候，尤以下肢为甚。因肺热伤津或湿热浸淫，或肝肾亏虚、精血不足而筋失濡养所致。治宜通经活络、补脾益气、清热生津。取穴：肩髃、曲池、合谷、阳溪、髀关、梁丘、足三里、解溪、阴陵泉。

A syndrome marked by weakness, limited movement and muscular atrophy of the limbs, especially the lower limbs; due to failure of nourishing the muscle resulting from the consumption of body fluid by heat in the lung, overwhelming of damp-heat pathogen, or deficiency of liver and kidney leading to insufficiency of essence and blood. Treatment principle: Dredge and activate the meridians and collaterals, tonify the spleen and replenish qi, clear heat and promote production of fluid. Point selection: Jianyu (LI15), Quchi(LI11), Hegu(LI4), Yangxi(LI5), Biguan (ST31), Liangqiu (ST34), Zusanli(ST36), Jiexi(ST41), Yinlingquan(SP9).

卫气 defensive qi

阳气的一种。由水谷精微和自然清气所化生，行于脉外，其性剽悍，运行迅疾滑利，具有护卫肌表，抗御外邪，温养脏腑、肌肉、皮毛及开阖汗孔等功能。

One kind of yang-qi, derived from the food essence and clear qi from the nature. It flows quickly outside of the vessels. It functions to protect the skin, defend the body against exogenous pathogenic factors, warm and nourish zang-fu organs, muscles, skin and hair, and control the opening and closing of skin pores.

胃 stomach; Wei

①六腑之一。有受纳和消化食物的作用。中医学的胃与现代医学的胃的概念大致相同，但有时则为胃肠的总称。②耳穴名。在耳轮脚消失处。主治：胃痛，呕吐，消化不良，胃炎，胃十二指肠溃疡，失眠，牙痛等。

① One of the six fu-organs，which serves to receive and digest food. In TCM the term expresses more or less the same concept as that in western medicine，but sometimes refers to the gastrointestinal tract. ② The name of the ear point located in area where helix crus terminates. Indications：Gastralgia，vomiting，indigestion，gastritis，gastroduodenal ulcer，insomnia，toothache，etc.

胃病　stomach disorder

泛指胃的病变。由于饮食不节、饥饱失调、冷热不适，或胃气虚弱、胃阴不足影响受纳和消化所致。常表现为脘腹胀满疼痛、呕吐恶心、嗳气纳减等症。

A general term applied to all gastric trouble with absorptive and digestive disturbances of the stomach，caused by improper diet，unbalanced hunger and satiety，inadaptability to hot and cold food or drink，or by deficiency of stomach-qi，or insufficiency of stomach-yin；usually manifested as epigastric and abdominal distending pain，vomiting，nausea，eructation，poor appetite，etc.

胃仓　Weicang (BL50)

经穴名。属足太阳膀胱经。定位：在背部，当第十二胸椎棘突下，旁开 3 寸。主治：胃脘痛，腹胀，小儿消化不良等。操作：斜刺 0.5～0.8 寸；可灸。

Name of an acupoint. It belongs to the Bladder Meridian of Foot-Taiyang. Location：On the back，below the spinous process of the 12th thoracic vertebra，3 cun lateral to the posterior midline. Indi-

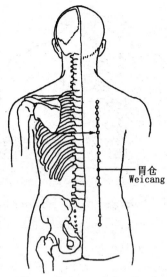

胃仓
Weicang

cations：Gastralgia，abdominal distension，infantile indigestion. Method：Puncture obliquely 0.5-0.8 cun. Moxibustion is applicable.

胃区　gastric zone

以瞳孔直上的发际处为起点，向后与正中线平行做 2cm 长的直线即为本区。主治：急、慢性胃炎及消化性溃疡所致的疼痛。

Draw a line upward from the midpoint of the hairline directly above the pupil，parallel to the anterior midline，the gastric zone is 2 cun upward from the hairline on this line. Indications：Pain caused by acute and chronic gastritis and peptic ulcer.

胃俞　Weishu (BL21)

经穴名。属足太阳膀胱经，胃的背俞穴。定位：在背部，当第十二胸椎棘突下，旁开 1.5 寸。主治：胸胁胃脘痛，腹胀，肠鸣，泄泻，呕吐，恶心等。操作：直刺 0.5～1 寸；可灸。

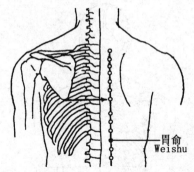

胃俞
Weishu

The acupoint, Back-Shu point of the stomach, belongs to the Bladder Meridian of Foot-Taiyang. Location: On the back, below the spinous process of the 12th thoracic vertebra, 1. 5 cun lateral to the posterior midline. Indications: Pain in the chest, hypochondriac and epigastric regions, abdominal distension, borborygmus, diarrhea, vomiting, nausea, etc. Method: Puncture perpendicularly 0. 5-1 cun. Moxibustion is applicable.

胃脘痛 gastralgia

指在胃脘部近心窝处的疼痛。多因饮食失常,饥饱劳倦,脾胃虚寒,情志郁结等所致。治宜疏肝理气、温胃散寒、消食导滞止痛。取穴:中脘、足三里、内关、太冲、阳陵泉、脾俞、胃俞、公孙、梁丘。

Pain over the epigastrium due to immoderate eating and drinking, over fatigue, deficiency cold of the spleen and stomach, emotional depression, etc. Treatment principle: Disperse the depressed liver-qi, warm the stomach and dispel cold, promote digestion and remove stagnation to alleviate pain. Point selection: Zhongwan (CV12), Zusanli (ST36), Neiguan (PC6), Taichong (LR3), Yang-lingquan (GB34), Pishu (BL20), Weishu (BL21), Gongsun (SP4), Liangqiu (ST34).

胃脘下俞 Weiwanxiashu

经外奇穴名。定位:在第八胸椎棘突下,旁开 1. 5 寸处。主治:消渴,呕吐,腹痛,胸胁疼痛等。

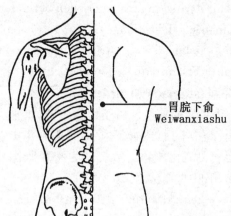

胃脘下俞
Weiwanxiashu

Name of an extra point. Location: 1. 5 cun lateral to the lower border of the spinous process of the 8th thoracic vertebra. Indications: Consumptive thirst, vomiting, abdominal pain, pain in the chest and hypochondriac region, etc.

胃系 stomach system

指食管。

It refers to the esophagus.

胃之大络 the large collateral of stomach

指胃区域的一条大络脉。

The large collateral of the stomach region.

温经祛寒 warm the meridians to dissipate cold

即温通经络、祛散寒邪的方法。适用于寒邪凝滞经络、气血运行受阻者,症见关节疼痛,痛有定处,日轻夜重,或月经不调等。

A treatment applicable to the case with stagnation of cold-pathogen in the meridians and impediment of qi and blood circulation, manifested as localized arthralgia with aggravation at night, or menoxenia, etc.

温灸器　moxa burner

金属制的筒形灸具。直径3～4cm,高4～5cm,周围及底部有数十个小孔,用以散热。用时将点燃的艾绒贮筒内,置于施灸部位上,往复移动使产生温热感。宜用于孕妇、儿童及畏灸者。

A metal container used to hold moxa floss with a dimension of about 3-4 cm in diameter, and 4-5 cm in length, and numerous small openings around and at the bottom of the instrument to permit emission of heat from the floss. During the procedure, the instrument with its contents of smolder moxa is moved about over the area to be treated to produce a sensation of warmth. It is suitable for pregnant patients, children and individuals apprehensive of conventional moxibustion therapy.

温和灸　Gentle moxibustion

指将艾条点燃的一端与穴位保持一定距离,使患者感觉热度适中,以不过分灼热为度的灸法。

To administer moxibustion by keeping the burning end of the moxa stick at a certain distance from the point to make the patient feel warm but not hot.

温溜　Wenliu（LI7）

经穴名。属手阳明大肠经,本经郄穴。定位:屈肘,在前臂背面桡侧,当阳溪与曲池连线上,腕横纹上5寸。主治:头痛,面肿,咽喉肿痛,肠鸣,腹痛,肩臂酸痛。操作:直刺0.5～1寸;可灸。

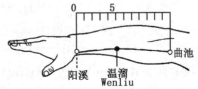

The acupoint, Xi-Cleft point, belongs to the Large Intestine Meridian of Hand-Yangming. Location: With the elbow flexed, on the radial side of the dorsal side of the forearm, on the line connecting Yangxi(LI5) and Quchi(LI11), 5 cun above the crease of the wrist. Indications: Headache, swelling of face, sore throat, borborygmus, abdominal pain, aching of the shoulders and arms, etc. Method: Puncture perpendicularly 0. 5-1 cun. Moxibustion is applicable.

温肾　warming the kidney

又称补肾阳,是治疗肾阳虚证的方法。适用于肾阳不足者,症见腰膝酸冷、软弱无力、阳痿、小便频数、舌淡苔白、脉沉弱等。

A treatment for deficiency of kidney-yang, applicable to the case manifested as soreness and coldness of loins and knees, general weakness, impotence, frequent micturition, pale tongue with whitish fur, sunken and weak pulse, etc.

温胃健中　warming the stomach and strengthening the middle

是一种治疗方法,适用于胃气虚寒者,症见上腹部隐痛而食后疼痛减轻、吐清水、大便泄泻、舌淡苔白、脉细等。

A treatment for deficiency cold of the stomach-qi, applicable to the case manifested as dull aching in the upper abdomen which is relieved after eating, vomiting of watery fluid, diarrhea, pale tongue with whitish fur, thin pulse, etc.

温阳利湿 warming yang for diuresis

又称化气利水,是一种治疗因阳气被水寒之邪阻遏而致的小便不利的方法。常将温阳化气药与健脾利水药同用,使小便通畅。

A kind of treatment for dysuria due to suppression of yang-qi by water-cold pathogen, by the application of drugs with founctions of warming yang and transforming qi, strengthening the spleen and eliminating the accumulation fluid to promote diuresis.

温针 warm needling

指针刺时,将艾绒缠绕于针柄并燃烧的一种治疗方法。

An acupuncture technique, i. e. , burning the moxa floss on the handle of the needle after inserting it into the body.

温针灸 needle warming through moxibustion

灸法的一种。针刺留针时,在针柄周围裹以点燃的艾绒,通常一次燃烧 1~3 团。这种方法可以增强针刺效果,用于治疗阴寒积聚、风寒湿痹等病症。

A type of moxibustion, i. e. , attaching burning moxa floss to an inserted needle during retention. Usually 1-3 stubs burned during a single treatment. This method enhances the effect of needling and is suitable for treating diseases caused by pathogenic cold, e. g. , rheumatoid arthritis.

温中祛寒 warm the middle and dissipate cold

温法之一。治疗脾胃阳虚,阴寒内盛的方法。适用于脾胃虚寒者,症见食不消化、呕吐清水、大便清稀、舌淡苔白、脉沉细等。

A treatment for the deficiency of spleen-yang and stomach-yang with overabundance of yin-cold in the body, applicable to the case with deficiency cold of the spleen and stomach, manifested as indigestion, vomiting of watery fluid, clear and loose stools, pale tongue with whitish fur, deep and thin pulse, etc.

闻诊 listening and smelling examination

四诊之一。通过听觉和嗅觉器官来了解患者的语言、呼吸、咳嗽、呻吟以及分泌物、排泄物的气味变化,以判断病情。

One of the four methods of physical examination for the diagnosis of diseases by means of the doctor's auditory and olfactory organs, i. e. , to listen to the patient's voice during speaking, breathing, coughing and moaning, and to smell the odour of the secretion and excretion.

问诊 Inquiry

四诊之一,即询问患者的现病史、既往史、月经史、生育史、生活习惯、饮食嗜好,以及年龄、籍贯、职业、住址等与了解病情有关的情况,是判断病情、明确诊断的重要方法之一。

One of the four methods of physical examination for the diagnosis of diseases, i. e. , to ask the patient about his/her present illness, past history, menstruation and childbirth history, living and diet habits, as well as age, native place, occupation, address and other related information.

卧位 lying position

针灸时的一种体位,包括仰卧、侧卧和俯卧。

A kind of body position during acupuncture and moxibustion, including the supine position, lateral position and prone position.

卧针 lying needle

行针时将针退至皮下,使针倾斜,以做沿皮刺或留针。

During the acupuncture, the needle is lifted beneath the skin and slanted in order to perform the subcutaneous acupuncture or to retain the needle.

屋翳 Wuyi (ST15)

经穴名。属足阳明胃经。定位:在胸部,当第二肋间隙,距前正中线 4 寸。主治:胸胁胀痛,咳嗽,气喘,乳痈等。操作:直刺 0.2～0.3 寸;可灸。

Name of an acupoint. It belongs to the Stomach Meridian of Foot-Yangming. Location: On the chest, in the 2nd interostal space, 4 cun lateral to the anterior midline. Indications: Fullness and pain in the chest and hypochondriac region, cough, asthma, acute mastitis,

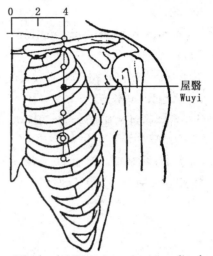

屋翳
Wuyi

etc. Method: Puncture perpendicularly 0. 2-0. 3 cun. Moxibustion is applicable.

无瘢痕灸 moxibustion without scarring

指灸后不留瘢痕的灸法。

A kind of moxibustion which does not cause scarring after the therapy.

无汗 anhidrosis

肌表腠理为暑湿所闭,或外感时风寒束闭于表;或阴血、津液不足,化汗无源;或阳气亏虚,蒸腾气化无权所致的一种无汗症状。

A symptom with absence of perspiration due to the skin pores closed by summerheat-damp or due to wind-cold pathogen attacking the superficies, or due to yin, blood and body fluid deficiency failing to be transformed into sweating, or yang-qi deficiency failing to steam and transform.

无名 Wuming

经外奇穴名。即二椎下。

Name of the extra point, i. e., Erzhuixia.

无热灸 non-heated moxibustion

即敷药发泡法。

Blistering method by applying drugs.

五处 Wuchu (BL5)

经穴名。属足太阳膀胱经。定位：在头部，当前发际正中直上1寸，旁开1.5寸。主治：头痛，视物不清，惊厥抽搐等。操作：斜刺0.3～0.5寸；可灸。

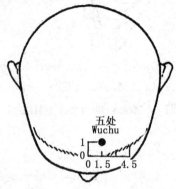

Name of an acupoint. It belongs to the Bladder Meridian of Foot-Taiyang. Location：On the head, 1 cun directly above the midpoint of the anterior hairline and 1.5 cun lateral to the head midline. Indications：Headache, blurred vision, convulsion, etc. Method：Puncture obliquely 0.3-0.5 cun. Moxibustion is applicable.

五刺 five needling techniques

指适用于与五脏有关病变的五种古代针法，即半刺、豹文刺、关刺、合谷刺、输刺。

They are the five ancient acupuncture techniques according to the pathological changes of the five zang-organs, i. e., extreme shallow needling, leopard-spot needling, joint needling, hegu needling, and shu-point needling.

五大 five large parts of the human body

指两手、两足及头。又称五体。

Two hands, two feet, and the head form the five large parts of the human body, also called five body parts.

五夺 five extreme losses

指脱形、亡血、大汗亡阳、大泄亡阴、产后暴崩等五种元气大虚的病情。此五种病情，针刺皆不可用泻法。

Great emaciation, great hemorrhage, hyperhidrosis leads to over depletion of yang, severe diarrhea leads to over depletion of yin and puerperal metrorrhagia are the five conditions severely losing primordial qi, in which reducing method of acupuncture is prohibited.

五更泄 predawn diarrhea

于黎明前泄泻的病证。多因肾阳虚衰所致，也有因食积、酒积、肝火而引起者。治宜温肾健脾、固涩止泻。取穴：肾俞、关元、气海、命门、中脘、脾俞、足三里、天枢。

A disease mostly caused by deficiency of kidney-yang, or by dyspepsia, alcoholism, and liver-fire. Treatment principle：Warm the kindey to tonify yang and strengthen the spleen, arrest diarrhea. Point selection：Shenshu (BL23), Guanyuan(CV4), Qihai(CV6), Mingmen (GV4), Zhongwan (CV12), Pishu (BL20), Zusanli(ST36), Tianshu(ST25).

五官 five facial features

指鼻、眼、口、舌、耳等五个器官，与五脏

有密切关系。

The five facial features, i. e., nose, eye, lip, tongue and ear, which bear a close relationship to the five zang-organs.

五虎 Wuhu

奇穴名。定位：位于手背侧第二、四掌骨小头高点之处，握拳取之，灸治。

Name of extra points. Location：On the dorsal side of the hand, on the prominences of the 2nd and 4th metacarpal bones. Have the points on the fist during moxibustion.

五里 Wuli

经穴名。有二：①即手五里与足五里。②劳宫穴别名。

Name of acupoints, there are two of them：① Shouwuli (LI13) and Zuwuli (LR10). ② It also refers to Laogong (PC8).

五门十变 five matches and ten derivations

子午流注针法用语。五门，指十天干隔五相合；十变，指十天干相结合后的变化，两两相合生五行，又称五运。时间取穴时可以"夫妻互用"。

A term used in the acupuncture method of qi movement in accordance with the time-passing. Five matches mean that anyone of the ten heavenly stems can match the every sixth one; ten derivations mean the changement caused by the five matches. This kind of matching can derive the five elements, also called five movements. In the point-selecting method by time-passing, the "husband" time and "wife" time can replace each other.

五禽戏 five mimic-animal boxing

模仿虎、鹿、熊、猿、鸟等五种禽兽动作的体育保健操，为三国时期名医华佗所设计。

Physical fitness exercise conducted by imitating the motions of tiger, deer, bear, monkey, and bird, devised by the famous doctor Huatuo in the Three Kingdoms.

五枢 Wushu (GB27)

经穴名。属足少阳胆经。定位：在侧腹部，当髂前上棘的前方，横平脐下 3 寸处。主治：带下，少腹痛，腰痛，疝气，便秘等。操作：直刺 1～1.5 寸；可灸。

Name of an acupoint. It belongs to the Gallbladder Meridian of Foot-Shaoyang. Location：On the lateral side of the abdomen, anterior to the anterior superior iliac spine, 3 cun below the level of the umbilicus. Indications：Leukorrhea, lower ab-

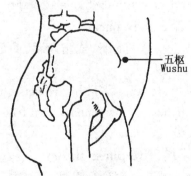

dominal pain, lumbago, hernia, constipation, etc. Method：Puncture perpendicularly 1-1.5 cun. Moxibustion is applicable.

五输穴 the five Shu points

是十二经分布于四肢肘膝关节以下的具有特殊治疗意义的常用穴位的总称。属五脏的为"井、荥、输、经、合"五输穴；属六腑的为"井、荥、输、原、经、合"六输穴。

A collective term for the commonly used points of the twelve regular meridians with special therapeutic significance on the limbs distal to the elbows and the knees. The five Shu points for the five zang-organs are Jing-Well, Xing-Spring, Shu-Stream, Jing-River, and He-Sea. The six Shu points for six fu-organs are Jing-Well, Xing-Spring, Shu-Stream, Yuan-Primary, Jing-River, and He-Sea.

五态之人 five-typed people

古代根据阴阳学说把人分为五种类型。现代中医指因人施治，即根据患者体质的不同采用不同的针灸方法。

In ancient China people were classified into five types according to the yin-yang theory. The treatment must be regulated in accordance with each one's condition.

五体 five body parts

指皮、肉、脉、筋、骨；或指两手、两足及头，也称五大。

They are skin, flesh, vessels, tendons, bones; or two hands, two feet and the head (Wuda).

五行学说 five-phase theory

中国古代哲学理论。阐明五行(木、火、土、金、水)的物质属性及其相互关系。中医学用它来说明脏腑器官的属性、相互之间的关系、生理现象和病理变化，并用以指导疾病的诊断和治疗。

A theory on philosophy in ancient China, classifying the material characters and the mutual relationships of the five elements (wood, fire, earth, metal, water). In TCM, the five-phase theory is chiefly used for explaining the properties of zang-fu organs of the human body, their mutual relations, physiological phenomena and pathological changes. It is also served as a guide for diagnosing and treating diseases.

五运六气 five evolutive phases and six climatic factors

五运即木、火、土、金、水的运行。六气指风、寒、暑、湿、燥、火六气的变化。在医学中，五运六气这一理论主要用来解释气候变化与疾病发生的关系。

An ancient theory dealing with the motion of the five elements (wood, fire, earth, metal and water) and the changes of the six kinds of weather (wind, cold, summer-heat, dampness, dryness, fire). In TCM, it is chiefly applied to interpret the relationship between the weather changes and the development of the diseases.

五脏 five zang-organs

是心、肝、脾、肺、肾五个脏器的合称。它虽然有一定的解剖概念，但不能与解剖学中的各脏器完全等同，而应把它看作是一个功能单位。

A general name of the heart, liver, spleen, lung and kidney, each of them is considered as a functional unit. The terms for five zang-organs in TCM do not completely match those used in western medicine.

五脏六腑之海 **the convergence of the five zang-organs and the six fu-organs**

①指冲脉,因其总领诸经,调节五脏六腑的气血灌注,故名。②指胃。因其受纳水谷,为各脏腑精气之源,故名。

①Referring to the Thoroughfare Vessel control all the meridians and regulates qi and blood of five zang-organs and six fu-organs. ②Referring to the stomach, since the stomach receives food and supplies essential qi to the various zang-fu organs.

五主 **five dominations**

肺、脾、心、肝、肾,分别主皮、肉、脉、筋、骨,称五主。

Lungs, spleen, heart, liver and kidneys dominate respectively skin, flesh, vessels, tendons and bones, which are called five dominations.

舞蹈震颤控制区 **chorea and tremor controlling area**

自运动区向前平移 1.5 cm 处。主治:对侧四肢不自主的震颤和运动。

It is parallel to and 1.5 cm in front of the motor zone. Indications: Involuntary movement and tremor of the extremities on the opposite side.

X

吸门 inspiring portal

指会厌,七冲门之一。

The epiglottis, one of the seven important portals of the digestive system.

溪谷 intermuscular septum

部位名。指肢体与躯干相互接触的肌肉之间的缝隙或凹陷部位。大的凹陷称谷,小的凹陷或缝隙称溪。

Name of body parts. Referring to the fissure or depression between the muscles at the junction of the limbs and the trunk. The bigger depression of the muscles is called "valley", while the narrow one is called "stream".

膝 knee;Xi

①大、小腿接合的部位,古人称之为筋之府。②耳穴名。在对耳轮上脚的中部。主治:膝关节炎,膝关节扭伤。

①Articulation of the thigh and leg, also called "residence of tendons" in ancient times. ②Name of an ear point. Location:In the middle part of the superior crura of antihelix. Indications:Sprain and arthritis of the knee joints.

膝关 Xiguan (LR7)

经穴名。属足厥阴肝经。定位:在小腿内侧,当胫骨内上髁的后下方,阴陵泉后1寸,腓肠肌内侧头的上部。主治:膝痛。操作:直刺1～1.5寸;可灸。

Name of an acupoint. It belongs to the Liver Meridian of Foot-Jueyin. Location:

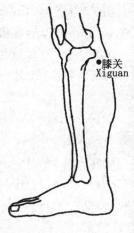

●膝关
Xiguan

On the medial side of the leg,posterior and inferior to the medial epicondyle of the tibia,1 cun posterior to Yinlingquan(SP9), at the upper end of the medial head of the gastrocnemius muscle. Indications: Knee pain. Method:Puncture perpendicularly 1-1.5 cun. Moxibustion is applicable.

膝旁 Xipang

经外奇穴名。定位:位于腘窝横纹内、外侧两端。直刺或灸治腰痛、脚酸不能久立。

Name of extra points. Location:At the ends of the popliteal crease. Perpendicular acupuncture or moxibustion is used to cure lumbago, soreness of lower limbs which unable to stand for a long time, etc.

膝上 Xishang

经外奇穴名。定位:位于髌骨上缘两侧凹陷处。直刺或灸治膝关节炎。

Name of extra points. Location:At the medial and lateral depressions of the upper margin of the patella. Perpendicular acupuncture or moxibustion is used to cure the knee arthritis.

膝痛 knee pain

指膝部肌肉、经脉及骨节间作痛。多因肝肾虚、风寒湿气外袭所致。治宜疏通经络、祛邪止痛。取穴:阳池、肾俞、关元、足三里、犊鼻、梁丘、阳陵泉、膝阳关。

A disorder usually due to asthenia o:

liver and kidney, and exposure to the wind, cold, and dampness-evils. Treatment principle: Dredge the meridians and collaterals, eliminate the pathogenic factors to alleviate pain. Point selection: Yangchi (TE4), Shenshu (BL23), Guanyuan(CV4), Zusanli(ST36), Dubi (ST35), Liangqiu(ST34), Yanglingquan (GB34), Xiyangguan(GB33).

膝外 Xiwai

经外奇穴名。定位:位于腘窝横纹外侧端,直刺或灸治膝关节炎、下肢溃疡等。

Name of extra points. Location: At the lateral end of the popliteal crease. Vertical acupuncture or moxibustion is used for knee arthritis, ulcerations of the legs, etc.

膝下 Xixia

经外奇穴名。定位:位于髌骨下缘韧带处。灸治关节炎、关节损伤及下肢痛。

Name of extra points. Location: At the ligament directly below the patella. Moxibustion is used to cure arthritis, joint injuries, lower limb pain, etc.

膝眼 Xiyan

经外奇穴名。定位:在髌韧带两侧凹陷中。主治膝痛,下肢无力等。

Name of extra points. Location: The pair of points are respectively in the two depressions medial and

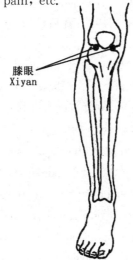

lateral to the patellar ligament. Indications: Knee pain, weakness of the lower extremities, etc.

膝阳关 Xiyangguan (GB33)

经穴名。属足少阳胆经。定位:在膝外侧,当阳陵泉上3寸,股骨外上髁上方的凹陷处。主治:膝肿痛,腘筋挛急,腿麻等。操作:直刺 1～1.5寸;可灸。

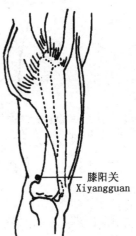

Name of an acupoint. It belongs to the Gallbladder Meridian of Foot-Shaoyang. Location: On the lateral side of the knee, 3 cun above Yanglingquan(GB34), in the depression above the external epicondyle of the femur. Indications: Swelling and pain in the knees, contracture of the tendons in popliteal fossa, numbness of the legs, etc. Method: Puncture perpendicularly 1-1.5 cun. Moxibustion is applicable.

郄门 Ximen (PC4)

经穴名。属手厥阴心包经,本经郄穴。定位:在前臂掌侧,当曲泽与大陵的连线上,腕横纹上5寸,掌长肌腱与桡侧腕屈肌腱之间。主治:心痛,心悸,鼻衄,呕血,疔疮,痫证等。操作:直刺0.5～1寸;可灸。

The acupoint, Xi-Cleft point of the Pericardium Meridian of Hand-Jueyin. Location: On the palmar side of the forearm and

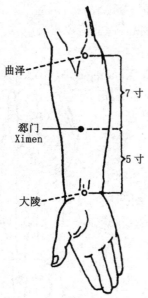

曲泽
郄门 Ximen
大陵
7寸
5寸

on the line connecting Quze(PC3) and Da-ling(PC7), 5 cun above the crease of the wrist, between the tendon of palmaris longus and flexox carpi radialis. Indications:Cardiac pain, palpitation, epistaxis, hematemesis, furuncle, epilepsy, etc. Method:Puncture perpendicularly 0.5-1 cun. Moxibustion is applicable.

郄下 Xixia

经外奇穴名。定位:位于委中直下5寸,又称承筋穴。

Name of an extra point. Location:5 cun directly below Weizhong (BL40), also known as Chengjin(BL56).

郄穴 Xi-Cleft point

是各经经气深聚的部位。十二经脉及阴跷、阳跷、阴维、阳维脉各有一个郄穴,共16个郄穴。多用于治疗急性病证及本经所属脏腑的顽固性病证。

A kind of specific points where the meri-dian qi infuses. There are all together 16 Xi-Cleft points, one on each of the twelve regu-lar meridians, the Yin Heel Vessel, Yang Link Vessel. They are often employed to treat emergent diseases or stubborn diseases involving their correspon-ding meridians and zang-fu organs.

郄阳 Xiyang

委阳穴别名。

The other name of Weiyang (BL39).

细脉 thin pulse

脉体细小如线,软弱无力,应指明显。多见于气血两虚,诸虚劳损,以及湿证。

It refers to a fine, feeble and clearly per-ceptible pulse, usually indicating deficiency of qi and blood, and impairments due to de-ficiency conditions or dampness syndrome.

侠白 Xiabai (LU4)

经穴名。属手太阴肺经。定位:在臂内侧面,肱二头肌桡侧缘,腋前纹头下4寸,或肘横纹上5寸。主治:咳嗽,胸闷,臑痛等。操作:直刺0.5~1寸;可灸。

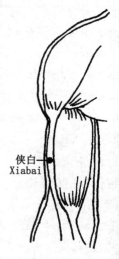

侠白 Xiabai

Name of an acu-point. It belongs to the Lung Meridian of Hand-Taiyin. Loca-tion:On the medial side of the upper arm, on the radial border of the biceps brachii, 4 cun below the anterior end of the axillary fold, or 5 cun above the cubital crease. Indi-cations: Cough, fullness in the chest, pain in the medial aspect of the upper arm, etc.

Method: Puncture perpendicularly 0. 5-1 cun. Moxibustion is applicable.

侠溪 Xiaxi (GB43)

经穴名。属足少阳胆经,本经荥穴。定位:在足背外侧,当第四、五趾间,趾蹼缘后赤白肉际处。主治:头痛头晕,目外眦痛,耳鸣耳聋,颊肿,胁痛,热病等。操作:直刺0.3～0.5寸;可灸。

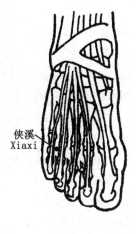

侠溪 Xiaxi

The acupoint, Xing-Spring point, belongs to the Gallbladder Meridian of Foot-Shaoyang. Location: On the lateral side of the dorsum of foot, between the 4th and 5th toes, at the junction of dorso-ventral boundary, posterior and proximal to the margin of the web. Indications: Headache, dizziness, pain of the outer canthus, tinnitus, deafness, swelling of the cheeks, pain in the hypochondriac region, febrile diseases, etc. Method: Puncture perpendicularly 0. 3-0. 5 cun. Moxibustion is applicable.

下病上取 taking the upper points to cure the lower diseases

取穴法之一。指下部的病症取用上部穴。

One of the methods of selecting points which consists in using the upper part points to cure the lower part diseases.

下耳背 Xiaerbei

耳穴名。主治:皮肤病,坐骨神经痛,背痛等。

Name of an ear point. Indications: Skin diseases, sciatica, back pain.

下耳根 Xiaergen; lower root of auricle

①耳穴名。定位:在耳根的最下缘。主治:低血压,头痛,腹痛,哮喘等。②解剖名称。指耳垂与面部附着处。

①Name of an ear point. Location: At the lowest border of the auricular root. Indications: Hypotension, headache, abdominal pain, asthma, etc. ②Terminologia anatomica. The area where ear lobe attaches to the face.

下关 Xiaguan (ST7)

经脉名。属足阳明胃经。定位:在面部耳前方,当颧弓与下颌切迹所形成的凹陷中。主治:耳聋耳鸣,聤耳,齿痛,面瘫,口眼歪斜。操作:直刺0.5～1寸;可灸。

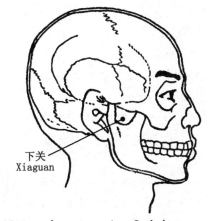

下关 Xiaguan

Name of an acupoint. It belongs to the Stomach Meridian of Foot-Yangming. Location: On the face, anterior to the ear, in the depression between the zygomatic arch and mandibular norch. Indications: Deafness, tinnitus, otorrhea, toothache, facial paralysis, deviation of mouth and eyes, etc.

Method: Puncture perpendicularly 0. 5-1 cun. Moxibustion is applicable.

下合穴 lower He-Sea point

六腑之气下合于下肢足三阳经的六个穴位。主要用于治疗相应的腑病。

A kind of specific points used for treating disease involving corresponding fu-organs. They are six points located on the three yang meridians of foot and associated with the functions of the six fu-organs.

下极 xiaji

①部位名。原意指最低处，一般指鼻根部，两目之间。②横骨穴别名。③指会阴穴，位前后两阴之间。

①Name of a anatomical site. It's proper meaning is the root of the nose between the two eyes. ②The other name of Henggu (KI11). ③The other name of Huiyin (CV1).

下纪 Xiaji

关元穴别名。

The other name of Guanyuan (CV4).

下焦 lower jiao

三焦的下部。即脐以下的空腔部分。从生理功能上说，它包括了大肠、小肠、肾及膀胱。

The lower part of the sanjiao corresponding to the body cavity below the level of the umbilicus. Functionally, it includes the small and large intestines, kidney and bladder.

下巨虚 Xiajuxu (ST39)

经穴名。属足阳明胃经，小肠下合穴。定位：在小腿前外侧，当犊鼻下9寸，距胫骨前缘一横指。主治：小腹痛，腰脊痛引睾丸，乳痈，下肢痿痹等。操作：直刺1～1.5寸；可灸。

Name of an acupoint. It belongs to the Stomach Meridian of Foot-Taiyang. The lower He-Sea point of the small intestine. Location: On the anteriolateral side of the leg, 9 cun below Dubi(ST35), one finger breadth from the anterior of the tibia. Indications: Lower abdominal pain, lower waist pain affects the testis, acute mastitis, numbness and paralysis of the lower extremities, etc. Method: Puncture perpendicularly 1-1. 5 cun. Moxibustion is applicable.

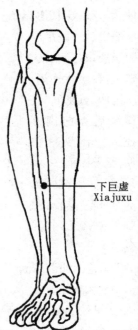

下巨虚
Xiajuxu

下利 diarrhea

指腹泻的症状。治宜健脾益气、升阳止泻。取穴：中脘、章门、脾俞、胃俞、足三里。

A symptom with abnormal frequency and liquidity of fecal discharges. Treatment principle: Strengthen the spleen to replenish qi, raise yang to arrest diarrhea. Point selection: Zhongwan (CV12), Zhangmen(LR3), Pishu(BL20), Weishu (BL21), Zusanli(ST36).

下利清谷 diarrhea with indigested

food in the stool

是以腹泻粪便清稀,夹杂有未消化的食物残渣为特征的证候。多因脾肾阳虚所致。常伴有恶寒肢冷、神倦、脉微等症状。治宜健脾温肾、调理肠胃。取穴:合谷、天枢、上巨虚、肾俞、脾俞。

Diarrhea caused by the deficiency of spleen-yang and kidney-yang, usually accompanied with aversion to cold, cold extremities, lassitude, weak pulse, etc. Treatment principle: Strengthen the spleen and warm the kidney, regulate the intestines and stomach. Point selection: Hegu(LI4), Tianshu(ST25), Shangjuxu(ST37), Shenshu(BL23), Pishu(BL20).

下廉 Xialian (LI8)

经穴名。属手阳明大肠经。定位:在前臂背面桡侧,当阳溪与曲池连线上,肘横纹下4寸。主治:腹痛肠鸣,臂肘酸痛等。操作:直刺0.5～1寸;可灸。

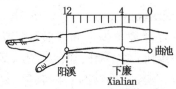

Name of an acupoint. It belongs to the Large Intestine Meridian of Hand-Yangming. Location: On the radial side of the dorsal surface of the forearm, on the line connection Yangxi (LI5) and Quchi (LI11), 4 cun below the cubital crease. Indications: Abdominal pain, borborygmus, aching of the elbow and arm, etc. Method: Puncture perpendicularly 0. 5-1 cun. Moxibustion is applicable.

下髎 Xialiao (BL34)

经穴名。属足太阳膀胱经。定位:在骶部,当中髎内下方,适对第四骶后孔处。主治:腰痛,下腹痛,小便不利,便秘,带下等。操作:直刺1～1.5寸;可灸。

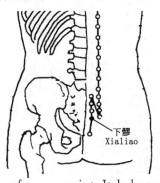

Name of an acupoint. It belongs to the Bladder Meridian of Foot-Taiyang. Location: On the sacrum, medial and inferior to Zhongliao(BL33), just opposite to the 4th posterior sacral foramen. Indications: Lumbago, lower abdominal pain, dysuria, constipation, leukorrhea, etc. Method: Puncture perpendicularly 1-1. 5 cun. Moxibustion is applicable.

下陵 Xialing

足三里穴别名。

The other name of Zusanli(ST36).

下肓 Xiahuang

气海穴别名。

The other name of Qihai(CV6).

下脘 Xiawan (CV10)

经穴名。属任脉。定位:在上腹部,前正中线上,当脐中上2寸。主治:腹痛,胃脘痛,肠鸣,食谷不化,呕吐,泄泻等。操作:直刺0.5～1寸;可灸。

Name of an acupoint. It belongs to the Conception Vessel. Location: On the upper abdomen and on the anterior midline,

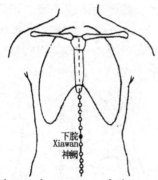

下脘
Xiawan
神阙

2 cun above the centre of the umbilicus. Indications：Abdominal pain， epigastric pain， borborygmus， indigestion， vomiting， diarrhea， etc. Method：Puncture perpendicularly 0.5-1 cun. Moxibustion is applicable.

下消 diabetes involving the lower jiao

以多尿、小便如膏脂样为特征的消渴病。治宜补肾益阴。取穴：肾俞、肝俞、太溪、太冲、复溜。

Diabetes characterized by polyuria and chyluria. Treatment principle：Nourish the kidney to replenish yin. Point selection：Shenshu（BL23），Ganshu（BL18），Taixi（KI3），Taichong（LR3），Fuliu（KI7）.

下腰 Xiayao

经外奇穴名。定位：位于第二骶骨棘突与第三骶骨棘突之间。主治：慢性肠炎、久痢不愈、难产等。灸治。

Name of an extra point. Location：Between the 2nd sacral process and the 3rd sacral process. Indications：Chronic enteritis, chronic dysentery, difficult labour, etc. Moxibustion can be performed.

先补后攻 tonifying before attacking the pathogens

对体质虚弱又有实邪，需用攻下的方法治疗，但因体弱难以接受的患者，宜先用补法增强体质，然后用攻下法。这种先补益后攻邪的方法称先补后攻。

A treatment suited for a debilitated patient when the pathogenic evil is sthenic. In such case，the patient is unendurable to the purgatives，and his/her vital qi should be restored by tonics before the purgatives are applied.

先攻后补 attacking the pathogens before tonifying

患者具有用攻下法的适应证，但使用攻下法之后会出现虚弱的症状，此时应根据具体情况使用补益的方法。这种先攻下后补益的方法称先攻后补。

A treatment suited for the patient becoming debilitated after the application of purgatives. In such case，tonics should be applied after the purgative therapy.

痫证 epilepsy

以阵发性神志丧失和四肢抽搐为主症的一种疾病。多由肝、脾、肾受伤，风痰上逆所致。实证治宜熄风化痰、降火宁神。取穴：身柱、本神、鸠尾、丰隆、太冲。虚证治宜补益心脾、化痰镇痉。取穴：丰隆、足三里、中脘、阳陵泉、筋缩。

A disease characterized by episodic impairment of consciousness and convulsive seizures，mostly due to impairment of the liver，spleen and kidney with adverse rising of wind-phlegm. Treatment principle for excess syndrome：Calm the pathogenic wind and dissipate phlegm；desend pathogenic fire and relieve mental stress.

Point selection:Shenzhu(GV12),Benshen（ GB13 ）， Jiuwei （ CV15 ）， Fenglong（ ST40 ）， Taichong （ LR3 ）. Treatment principle for deficiency syndrome:Invigorate heart and spleen,dissipate phlegm and relieve spasm. Point selection:Fenglong(ST40), Zusanli （ ST36 ）, Zhongwan （CV12）, Yanglingquan（GB34）, Jinsuo（GV8）.

弦脉 stringy pulse

脉体直而长，且有紧张感，按之如按琴弦的一种脉象。多见于高血压、肝胆疾病及痛证患者。

A pulse condition which is straight, long and tense,with a feeling of pressing over a string; usually seen in patients suffering from hypertension, liver and gallbladder diseases and pain syndrome.

陷谷 Xiangu (ST43)

经穴名。属足阳明胃经，本经输穴。定位:在足背，当第二、三跖骨结合部前方凹陷处。主治:面浮身肿，腹痛肠鸣，足背肿痛等。操作:直刺0.5～1寸;可灸。

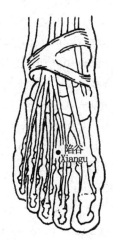

The acupoint, Shu-Stream point, belongs to the Stomach Meridian of Foot-Yangming. Location:On the instep of the foot,in the depression anterior to the commissure of the 2nd and 3rd metatarsal bones. Indications:Facial and general edema, abdominal pain, borborygmus, swelling and pain of the dorsum of the foot，etc. Method:Puncture perpendicularly 0. 5-1 cun. Moxibustion is applicable.

项强 stiff neck

指颈项肌肉筋脉牵强引痛。多由风寒湿邪侵袭太阳经脉，经气不舒所致。也可因失血伤津、筋脉失养所致。治宜调气活血、舒筋散寒。取穴:风池、天柱、后溪、悬钟。

Muscular rigidity and pain over the neck，due to stagnation of Taiyang Meridian qi resulting from the attack of cold-damp pathogen, or due to malnutrition of muscles resulting from hemorrhage and consumption of fluid. Treatment principle:Promote the flow of qi and blood circulation,relax muscles and dispel cold. Point selection:Fengchi(GB20), Tianzhu（ BL10 ）， Houxi （ SI3 ）， Xuanzhong（GB39）.

消泺 Xiaoluo (TE12)

经穴名。属手少阳三焦经。定位:在臂外侧，当清冷渊与臑会连线的中点处。主治:头痛项强，臂痛不举等。操作:直刺0.8～1.2寸;可灸。

Name of an acupoint. It belongs to the Sanjiao Meridian of Hand-Shaoyang. Location:On the lateral side of the arm,at the midpoint of the line joining Qinglingyuan(TE11) and Naohui(TE13). Indications:Headache, neck rigidity, motor impairment and pain of the arms, etc. Method: Puncture perpendicularly 0. 8-1. 2 cun. Moxibustion is applicable.

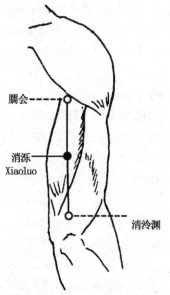

臑会

消泺
Xiaoluo

清冷渊

消食导滞 promoting indigestion and removing food stagnation

消法之一。又称消食化滞或消导,是消除食滞,恢复脾胃功能的一种治疗方法。常用于食积停滞、胸脘痞满、腹胀时痛、嗳腐吞酸、恶食或泄泻、苔黄腻、脉滑等。

A treatment for indigestion and restoring the functions of the spleen and stomach, applicable to the case manifested as dyspepsia, feeling of fullness in the chest and epigastrium, abdominal flatulence and pain, acid regurgitation, anorexia, diarrhea, yellowish and greasy fur on the tongue, slippery pulse, etc.

小便不(失)禁 incontinence of urine

即小便不能随意控制而自行排出。本证以虚寒为多,也有属实热者。前者多因肾与膀胱虚寒所致,后者常由膀胱火邪妄动或肝经郁热内结引起。治宜补益脾肺。取穴:气海、太渊、足三里、三阴交、百会、脾俞、肺俞。

Involuntary discharge of urine, mostly due to deficiency cold syndrome and are attributable to excessive cold of the kidney and bladder; Some appear as excessive heat syndrome, and are attributable to the stirring of fire-pathogen in the bladder or retention of heat-pathogen in the Liver Meridian. Treatment principle: Tonify the spleen and benefit the lung. Point selection: Qihai (CV6), Taiyuan (LU9), Zusanli(ST36), Baihui(GV20), Pishu(BL20), Feishu(BL13).

小便不利 dysuria

指小便量减少,排出困难。多因气化不利、水湿失运或津血耗损所致,常与肺、脾、肾、三焦及膀胱的功能障碍有关。实证治宜清利湿热、益气活血;虚证治宜温补脾肾、益气启闭。取穴:三阴交、阴陵泉、膀胱俞、中极、三焦俞、气海、肾俞。

Difficulty in micturition due to hypofunction of qi, retention of dampness or consumption of fluid and blood, usually referable to the dysfunctions of the lung, spleen, kidney, sanjiao and bladder. Treatment principle for excess sydrome: Clear the damp-heat, benefit qi to activate blood circulation. Treatment principle of deficiency syndrome: Warm and invigorate the spleen and kidney, replenish qi to promote diuresis. Point selection: Sanyinjiao (SP6), Yinlingquan (SP9), Pangguangshu(BL28), Zhongji(CV3), Sanjiaoshu (BL22), Qihai (CV6), Shenshu (BL23).

小便频数 frequent micturition

指排尿次数增多,时欲小便。多因外邪侵袭、脏腑功能失调或虚损所致。膀胱湿热、肝气郁结、中气虚弱、肾阳衰弱、肾阴不足等均可出现本症状。治宜清热利湿、健脾利水。取穴:膀胱俞、阴陵泉、中极、行间、太溪。

A symptom refers to increased frequency and desire of urination due to attack of exogenous pathogens and dysfunction or debility of the internal organs, such as damp-heat in the bladder, stagnation of liver-qi, deficiency of middle qi, weakness of kidney-yang, insufficiency of kidney-yin, etc. Treatment principle:Clear heat and eliminate dampness, strengthen the spleen and remove dampness by diuresis. Point selection:Pangguangshu (BL28), Yinlingquan (SP9), Zhongji(CV3), Xingjian(LR2), Taixi(KI3).

小肠 small intestine; Xiaochang

①六腑之一。上接幽门下连大肠,包括十二指肠、回肠、空肠。有进一步消化食物的作用。②耳穴名。在耳轮脚上方中1/3处。主治:腹痛,消化不良,心悸等。

①One of the six fu-organs, connecting the pylorus and the large intestine, including duodenum, ileum and jejunum, where the food is further digested. ②Name of an ear point. It is in the middle third of the superior aspect of helix crus. Indications:Abdominal pain, indigestion, palpitation.

小肠俞 Xiaochangshu (BL27)

经穴名。属足太阳膀胱经,小肠背俞穴。定位:在骶部,当骶正中嵴旁1.5寸,平第一骶后孔。主治:小腹胀痛,痢疾,梦遗,遗尿,带下,腰痛等。操作:直刺0.8~1.2寸;可灸。

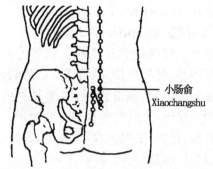
小肠俞
Xiaochangshu

Name of an acupoint. It belongs to the Bladder Meridian of Foot-Taiyang. Back-Shu point of the small intestine. Location:On the sacrum and at the same level with the 1st posterior sacral foramen, 1.5 cun lateral to the median sacral crest. Indications:Lower abdominal pain and distension, dysentery, nocturnal emission, enuresis, leukorrhea, lumbago, etc. Method:Puncture perpendicularly 0.8-1.2 cun. Moxibustion is applicable.

小儿鸡胸穴 Xiaoerjixiong point

经外奇穴名。定位:位于第二、三、四肋间隙,距胸正中线2.5寸处,左右共6穴。主治小儿鸡胸。灸治。

Name of extra points. Location:On the 2nd, 3rd and 4th intercostal spaces, 2.5 cun away from the thoracic midline, altogether 6 points on the left and right. Main indication is infantile pigeon breast by using moxibustion.

小儿食痫穴 Xiaoershixian point

经外奇穴名。定位:位于腹正中线,脐上7.5寸处。灸治癫痫。

Name of an extrapoint. Location: On the abdominal midline, 7.5 cun above the navel. Main indication is epilepsy by using moxibustion.

小儿哮喘 infantile asthma

是小儿呼吸道常见疾病。以阵发性的呼吸困难、呼气延长、喉间哮鸣声为特征。素体脾肾不足、痰湿内盛，复感外邪或与过敏原接触，是引起本病的主要原因。治宜宣肺、化痰、平喘。取穴：列缺、大椎、丰隆、尺泽、肺俞、定喘。

A common respiratory disease in children, marked by paroxysmal dyspnea with bronchial wheezing and prolonged expiration; caused by primary deficiency of spleen and kidney with retention of damp-phlegm, provoked by the attack of exogenous pathogens or the contact with allergens. Treatment principle: Facilitate flow of lung-qi and disperse phlegm to relieve asthma. Point selection: Lieque (LU7), Dazhui (GV14), Fenglong (ST40), Chize (LU5), Feishu (BL13), Dingchuan (EX-B1).

小腹 lower abdomen

腹部脐下部分。

The part of abdomen below the umbilicus.

小腹满 distension of the lower abdomen

多由冷结膀胱所致的症状，也可由癃闭、淋证等多种疾病引起。治宜调畅三焦气机。取穴：三焦俞、偏历、气海、水分、足三里。

A symptom caused by stagnation of cold pathogen in the bladder, or retention of urine, strangury, etc. Treatment principle: Regulate the movement of qi in sanjiao. Point selection: Sanjiaoshu (BL22), Pianli (LI6), Qihai (CV6), Shuifen (CV9), Zusanli (ST36).

小腹痛 pain in the lower abdomen

指下腹部疼痛。多因膀胱湿热、大肠燥结、肾虚或其他疾病（如疝气、痛经、带下、淋证等）引起的症状。治宜补脾温肾、调畅气机。取穴：脾俞、肾俞、章门、关元、太冲。

A symptom caused by the accumulation of damp-heat pathogen in the bladder, dryness of the large intestine, deficiency of kidney, or secondary to other diseases such as hernia, dysmenorrhea, leukorrhea, strangury, etc. Treatment principle: Tonify the spleen and warm the kidney, regulate the movement of qi. Point selection: Pishu (BL20), Shenshu (BL23), Zhangmen (LR13), Guanyuan (CV4), Taichong (LR3).

小骨空 Xiaogukong (EX-UE6)

经外奇穴名。定位：位于小指背侧，近端指关节横纹中点。屈指取之。灸治目疾、耳聋、喉痛、指痛等。

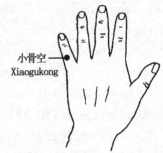

小骨空
Xiaogukong

Name of extra points. Location: On the

dorsal side of the little finger, at the midpoint of the transverse crease of the proximal phalangeal joint of the little finger. Flex the finger while treating. Main indications are eye diseases, deafness, sore throat, fingers pain, etc., using moxibustion.

小海 Xiaohai (SI8)

经穴名。属手太阳小肠经,本经合穴。定位:在肘内侧,当尺骨鹰嘴与肱骨内上髁之间凹陷处。主治:头痛,颊痛,颈背肩臂肘痛,癫痫等。操作:直刺0.3~0.5寸;可灸。

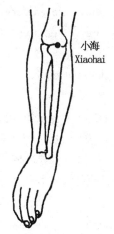

The acupoint, He-Sea point, belongs to the Small Intestine Meridian of Hand-Taiyang. Location: On the medial side of the elbow, in the depression between the ulna olecranon and the medial epicondyle of humerus. Indications: Headache, swelling of the cheeks, pain in the nape, back, shoulders, arms and elbows, epilepsy, etc. Method: Puncture perpendicularly 0.3-0.5 cun. Moxibustion is applicable.

小吉 Xiaoji

少泽穴别名。

The other name of Shaoze (SI1).

小眉刀 small eyebrow-shaped knife

针具名。刀口倾斜似眉,用于割治、泻血等。

Name of an acupuncture instrument which

is made with a small eyebrow-shaped blade to perform incision therapy, letting out blood, etc.

小溪 intermuscular septum

部位名。指全身筋肉骨节间的小间隙,多为腧穴所在部位。

Name of the body parts which are the tiny spaces among the tendons, muscles, bones or joints and where exist mostly the acupoints.

小指尖 Xiaozhijian

经外奇穴名。定位:位于两手小指尖端。针或灸治黄疸、百日咳等。

Name of extra points. Location: At the two little finger tips. Indications are jaundice, whooping cough, etc., using acupuncture or moxibustion.

小趾尖 Xiaozhijian

①经外奇穴名。位于两足小趾尖端。主催生,也治头痛,眩晕。刺或灸。②指至阴穴。

①Name of extra points which are situated at the tips of the two small toes. Indications are hasten child delivery, headache, vertigo, etc. with acupuncture or moxibustion. ② Zhiyin (BL67).

哮喘 asthma

是哮证与喘证的合称。指以呼吸急促或喘鸣有声、呼吸困难为特征的一种疾病。多因外邪侵袭、痰浊内盛、肺气不得宣肃;或肺肾虚弱,气失摄纳所致。治宜宣肺、化痰、平喘。取穴:列缺、大椎、丰隆、尺泽、肺俞、定喘。

A general name of asthma with wheezing and dyspnea. It refers to the disease characterized by tachypnea, wheezing, and difficult breathing, due to failure of dispersing and descending of lung-qi resulting from the attack of exogenous pathogens and the stagnation of phlegm-dampness, or due to the disorder of inspiration resulting from asthenia of the lung and kidney. Treatment principle: Facilitate the flow of the lung-qi and disperse phlegm to relieve asthma. Point selection: Lieque(LU7), Dazhui(GV14), Fenglong(ST40), Chize(LU5), Feishu(BL13), Dingchuan(EX-B1).

哮证 asthma with wheezing

以发作性呼吸喘促、喉间有哮喘声、咽塞胸闷、咳痰不爽为特征的疾病。多因内有伏邪,外感时邪,二者结合,闭阻气道所致。气候变化,食物不当,情志不遂或过劳常为其诱发因素。治宜宣肺、化痰、平喘。取穴:列缺、风门、尺泽、肺俞。

A disease characterized by recurrent attacks of paroxysmal rapid respiration with wheezing, feeling of oppression over the chest and difficult expectoration; caused by the accumulation of phlegm and exposure to the seasonal evils resulting in the obstruction of airway; usually induced by the change of weather, improper diet, emotional upset, or overstrain. Treatment principle: Facilitate lung-qi and disperse phlegm to relieve asthma. Point selection: Lieque(LU7), Fengmen(BL12), Chize(LU5), Feishu(BL13).

斜刺 oblique acupuncture

指针体与皮肤面成 30°～60°角刺入,以免伤及内脏,或利于获取针感。

A kind of acupuncture with an 30°-60°angle between the needle and the skin surface to avoid the visceral injuries or to get a certain sensation.

胁堂 Xietang

经外奇穴名。定位:位于腋窝下 2 寸。斜刺或灸治胸胁支满、喘逆、腹胀、目黄、肋间神经痛等。

Name of an extra point. Location: 2 cun below the axillary fossa. Oblique acupuncture or moxibustion is used to treat chest and hypochondrium fullness, asthma, abdominal distention, yellowish sclera, intercostals neuralgia, etc.

胁痛 hypochondrium pain

指胁肋一侧或两侧疼痛。多因肝胆湿热、肝气郁结、痰瘀停着,致肝胆经络气血运行不畅,或肝阴不足、肝经失养引起。治宜疏肝利胆、通络止痛。取穴:期门、支沟、阳陵泉、太冲、膈俞。

A symptom due to sluggishness of qi and blood flow in the Liver and Gallbladder Meridians resulting from the accumulation of damp-heat in the liver and gallbladder, the stagnation of liver-qi, and the retention of phlegm and blood stasis, or due to insufficiency of liver-yin resulting to the failure of nourishing the Liver Meridian. Treatment principle: Disperse stagnated liver-qi for promoting bile flow, remove obstruction in the meridians and collaterals to relieve pain. Point selection: Qimen (LR14), Zhigou (TE6), Yanglingquan (GB34), Taichong (LR3), Geshu(BL17).

泻方补圆 reducing the square and reinforcing the round

刺法补泻用语。方指气血正盛之时,宜泻;圆为正气不足之时,宜补。

A term used in reducing and reinforcing acupuncture, the square means the flourishing time of qi and blood when the reducing acupuncture is complicable, while the round means the deficiency time of qi when the reinforcing acupuncture is complicable.

泻南补北法 reducing the south and reinforcing the north

配穴法之一。南方指心,北方指肾。根据五行相互生克关系,对肝实肺虚而脾土无恙的病症,要用泻心火、补肾水的方法来治疗。

A kind of point-selecting method. The south refers to the heart and the north to the kidney. According to the theory of the inter-promoting and inter-inhibiting relationship of the five phases, the diseases of the liver excess and lung deficiency with the normal spleen function should be treated by discharging the heart-fire and tonifying the kidney-water.

泻圆补方 reducing by turning and reinforcing by remaining

为针刺补泻法的要领。意指泻法有如圆规,多旋转有利于祛邪;补法有如角尺,少转动有利于扶正。

A principle of reinforcing and reducing methods which implies that the reducing method consists in much rotating as the compasses do to expel the pathogens while the reinforcing method consists in remaining still without much rotating as an angle ruler does.

心 heart; Xin

①五脏之一,是最重要的一个脏器,主要功能是保证机体进行正常的血液循环。中医认为,高级神经系统的功能活动也和心有密切的关系。心的病变主要反映于血液循环和高级神经活动障碍,尤其是精神和意识活动障碍。此外,心与汗液的分泌、舌体的变化也有密切的关系。②耳穴名。在耳甲腔中央。主治:癔病,心悸,心律失常,失眠,盗汗,神经衰弱,无脉症,口舌生疮等。

① One of the five zang-organs and the most important organ in the body. Its main function is to maintain the normal blood circulation. In TCM, the heart is considered to be closely related to the functional activities of the high nervous. The pathological changes of the heart are reflected in the disturbance of the blood circulation and the activities of the high nervous, especially in that of the mental and emotional activities. Moreover, the secretion of the sweat glands and the changes of the tongue are also related to the heart. ②Name of an ear point. It is in the center of the cavum conchae. Indications: Hysteria, palpitation, arrhythmia, insomnia, night sweating, neurasthenia, pulseless disease, mouth sores, etc.

心包络 pericardium

脏腑之一。位于心的外围,具有保护心脏的功能,也与中枢神经系统的一些功能有关。如热入心包,可出现神昏谵语。

One of the zang-fu organs. Located at the periphery of the heart, serving as the protector of the heart. It is considered that some functions of the central nervous system have relation to the pericardium. If heat-pathogen attacks pericardium, symptom as delirium may appear.

心烦 feeling of oppression over the chest

即心胸烦闷不安。多由内热(包括实热和虚热)引起。治宜泻心火、滋心阴。取穴：劳宫、少府、阴郄、然谷。

A symptom due to disturbance of the endogenous heat-pathogen, including excessive heat and deficiency heat. Treatment principle: Purge pathogenic fire in the heart, nourish the yin-fluid of the heart. Point selection: Laogong(PC8), Shaofu(HT8), Yinxi(HT6), Rangu(KI2).

心肺之部 heart and lung site

针刺的分部，指皮肉浅层。

A term of acupuncture depth, i. e., the shallow layer of the skin and muscles.

心合小肠 heart being connected with the small intestine

指心和小肠之间的相互关联和影响。它们通过经络的联系互为表里，在生理上互相协调，在病理上互相影响。

The paired relationship between the heart and the small intestine which are connected with each other by the meridian. They cooperate in functioning and affect each other when diseased.

心悸 palpitation

自觉心跳不安的一种症状。多由气虚、血虚、停饮或气滞血瘀所致。治宜益心安神、养血定惊。取穴：心俞、巨阙、间使、神门、膈俞、通里。

Unduly beating of the heart which can be noted by the patients, usually caused by the deficiency of qi and blood, fluid retention in the body, or qi-sluggishness and blood stasis. Treatment principle: Benefit qi and tranquilize the mind, enrich the blood and arrest convulsion. Point selection: Xinshu(BL15), Juque(CV14), Jianshi(PC5), Shenmen(HT7), Geshu(BL17), Tongli(HT5).

心脾两虚 heart and spleen deficiency

心脾两脏气血虚弱的病理。症见心悸、怔忡、失眠、多梦、健忘、食欲减退、大便稀溏、倦怠或便血、皮下出血、月经过多、舌淡、脉细弱等。治宜补气养血。取穴：脾俞、心俞、足三里、三阴交、神门。

A morbid condition with the qi blood deficiency in heart and spleen; manifested as palpitation, severe palpitation, insomnia, dreaminess, amnesia, poor appetite, loose stools, fatigue, hematochezia, subcutaneous bleeding, menorrhagia, pale tongue, thin and weak pulse, etc. Treatment principle: Tonify qi and nourish blood. Point selection: Pishu(BL20), Xinshu(BL15), Zusanli(ST36), Sanyinjiao(SP6), Shenmen(HT7).

心肾相交 intercourse between heart and kidney

在正常情况下，心和肾的生理功能是相互协调，彼此沟通，保持相对的平衡。如这一平衡被破坏，就会发生心烦、怔忡、失眠等症状。

Under normal condition, the functions of the heart and kidney are kept in balance by coordinating each other. If the balance is destroyed, it would cause the symptoms such as restlessness, severe palpitation, insomnia, etc.

心俞 Xinshu (BL15)

经穴名。属足太阳膀胱经,心的背俞穴。定位:在背部,当第五胸椎棘突下,旁开1.5寸。主治:心痛、惊悸、健忘、咳嗽、吐血、梦遗、盗汗、癫狂、痫证等。操作:直刺0.5～1寸;可灸。

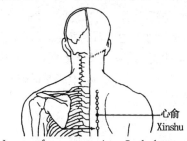
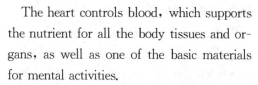

Name of an acupoint. It belongs to the Bladder Meridian of Foot-Taiyang. Back-Shu point of the heart. Location: On the back, below the spinous process of the 5th thoracic vertebra, 1.5 cun lateral to the posterior midline. Indications: Cardialgia, panic and palpitation, amnesia, coughing, spitting of blood, nocturnal emission, night sweating, mania, epilepsy, etc. Method: Puncture perpendicularly 0.5-1 cun. Moxibustion is applicable.

心痛 heart pain

①以心前区疼痛为主症的病症。②指胃脘痛。治宜活血通络、行气止痛。取穴:曲泽、少海、血海、郄门、膻中。

① Precordial pain. ② Epigastric pain. Treatment principle: Promote blood circulation to remove obstruction in the meridians and collaterals, activate qi to relieve pain. Point selection: Quze (PC3), Shaohai (HT3), Xuehai (SP10), Ximen (PC4),

Danzhong (CV17).

心系 heart vessels

指心与其他脏器相联系的脉络。

It refers to the collaterals of the heart communication with other zang-fu organs.

心血 heart-blood

即心所主的血。它是全身组织器官重要的营养物质,也是精神活动的物质基础之一。

The heart controls blood, which supports the nutrient for all the body tissues and organs, as well as one of the basic materials for mental activities.

心血虚 deficiency of heart-blood

心血不足的病理。症见头晕、面色苍白、心悸、心烦、失眠、多梦、健忘、脉细弱等。治宜补气养血。取穴:脾俞、心俞、足三里、膈俞。

A morbid condition manifested as dizziness, pallor, palpitation, restlessness, insomnia, dreaminess, amnesia, weak and thin pulse, etc. Treatment principle: Tonify qi and nourish blood. Point selection: Pishu (BL20), Xinshu (BL15), Zusanli (ST36), Geshu (BL17).

心阳虚 deficiency of heart-yang

心气虚的进一步发展。除心气虚的症状外,并见四肢厥冷,大汗出,甚至昏迷不醒、脉极微弱等症。常见于急、慢性循环衰竭。治宜温补心阳。取穴:心俞、巨阙、间使、神门。

A morbid state of further development of heart-qi deficiency, manifested as cold limbs, profuse sweating, even unconsciousness and weak pulse, in addition to the manifestations of heart qi deficiency; usually seen in acute and chronic circulatory failure. Treatment principle: Warming and tonifying heart-yang. Point selection: Xinshu(BL15), Juque (CV14), Jianshi (PC5), Shenmen (HT7).

新设 Xinshe

经外奇穴名。位于颈斜方肌外缘，后发际下1.5寸。直刺或灸治头痛、肩痛、落枕、咳嗽、气喘、咽痛等。

Name of an extra point. Located at the lateral margin of the trapezius muscle, 1.5 cun below the posterior hairline. Perpendicular acupuncture or moxibustion is used to cure headache, shoulder pain, stiff neck, cough, asthma, pharyngalgia, etc.

囟会 Xinhui (GV22)

经穴名。属督脉。定位：在头部，当前发际正中直上2寸，百会前3寸。主治：头痛，视物不清，鼻渊，小儿惊风等。操作：直刺0.3~0.8寸；可灸。

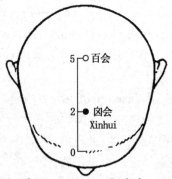

Name of an acupoint. It belongs to the Governor Vessel. Location: On the head, 2 cun directly above the midpoint of the anterior hairline and 3 cun anterior to Baihui (GV20). Indications: Headache, blurred vision, sinusitis, infantile convulsion, etc.

Method: Puncture perpendicularly 0.3-0.8 cun. Moxibustion is applicable.

囟门 fontanel

婴儿未完全骨化的颅骨所形成的空隙。

The membrane-covered space remaining in the incomplete ossified skull of an infant.

行间 Xingjian (LR2)

经穴名。属足厥阴肝经，本经荥穴。定位：在足背侧，当第一、二趾间，趾蹼缘的后方赤白肉际处。主治：胁痛，腹胀，头痛头晕，目赤肿痛，口喝，疝气，尿痛，小便不利，月经不调，癫痫，失眠等。操作：直刺0.5~1寸；可灸。

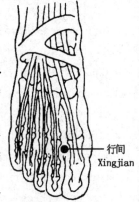

The acupoint, Xing-Spring point of the Liver Meridian of Foot-Jueyin. Location: On the instep of the foot, between the 1st and 2nd toes, at the junction of the dorso-ventral boundary proximal to the margin of the webs. Indications: Pain in the hypochondriac region, abdominal distension, headache, vertigo, redness, swelling and pain of the eyes, deviation of the mouth, hernia, odynuria, dysuria, irregular menstruation, epilepsy, insomnia, etc. Method: Puncture perpendicularly 0.5-1 cun. Moxibustion is applicable.

行气 promote qi

是疏通脏腑气机，治疗气滞证的方法。

A treatment to remove obstruction

from the circulation of qi in zang-fu organs to relieve qi stagnation.

行气法 qi-promoting method

针刺时促使针感传导的方法。

A manipulation employed in acupuncture to direct the transmission of needling sensation.

行气活血 promote qi and invigorate blood

治法名。临床上常以行气、活血、散瘀的方法或药物,治疗心、腹、胁等部位的疼痛,以及月经不调、跌打损伤、产后恶露不行等属于气滞血瘀的病证。

Name of a therapeutic method. Methods or drugs for regulating qi and invigorating blood circulation，dispersing the stagnation of blood are often used in qi stagnation with blood stasis syndrome，such as pain in the chest，abdomen and hypochondrium，menoxenia，trauma，retention of lochia，etc.

行针 performing acupuncture

①施行和运用针刺疗法。②针刺后运用手法。

① Performing and using acupuncture therapy. ②Operating manipulation techniques after acupuncture.

胸 Xiong

耳穴名。在胸椎前侧耳腔缘。主治:胸满胁痛,乳腺炎,肋间神经痛。

Name of an ear point. It is on the border of cavum conchae，anterior to Xiongzhui. Indications：Pain and stuffiness of the chest and hypochondrium，mastitis，intercostals neuralgia.

胸第二侧线 the second thoracic lateral line

经穴定位线。距胸正中线 4 寸,为足阳明胃经循行处。

Meridians and points-locating line，4 cun lateral to the thoracic midline，where passes the Stomach Meridian of Foot-Yangming.

胸第三侧线 the third thoracic lateral line

经穴定位线。距胸正中线 6 寸,为手太阴肺经和足太阴脾经循行处。

Meridians and points-locating line，6 cun lateral to the thoracic midline，where passes the Lung Meridian of Hand-Taiyin and Spleen Meridian of Foot-Taiyin.

胸第一侧线 the first thoracic lateral line

经穴定位线。距胸正中线 2 寸,为足少阴肾经循行处。

Meridians and points-locating line，2 cun lateral to the thoracic midline，where passes the Kidney Meridian of Foot-Shaoyin.

胸俞 thoracic points

指胸部第一侧线穴,左右共 12 穴。

The points situated on the first thoracic lateral line，twelve points in all on both sides.

胸通谷 Xiongtonggu

经外奇穴名。位于乳下 2 寸。灸治心胁痛、乳腺炎等。

Name of extra points. Located 2 cun below the nipple. Moxibustion is used to cure epigastric and hypochondriac pain, mastitis, etc.

胸痛　chest pain

指胸部疼痛的症状。温热犯肺,寒痰壅塞,水饮留积胸胁,心阳不足,心血瘀阻,或肝火犯上等均可引起。治宜助阳散寒、通络止痛。取穴:膻中、巨阙、心俞。

A symptom dues to attack of heat-pathogen to the lung with retention of cold-phlegm and fluid in the chest and hypochondrium, insufficiency of heart-yang, stagnation of heart-blood, or upward attack of liver-fire. Treatment principle: Strengthen yang to dispel cold and relieve pain by removing obstruction in the meridians and collaterals. Point selection: Danzhong (CV17), Juque (CV14), Xinshu(BL15).

胸乡　Xiongxiang (SP19)

经穴名。属足太阴脾经。定位:在胸外侧部,当第三肋间隙,距前正中线 6 寸。主治胸胁胀满。操作:直刺 0.5~1 寸;可灸。

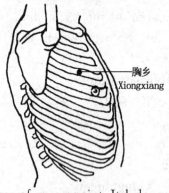

胸乡
Xiongxiang

Name of an acupoint. It belongs to the Spleen Meridian of Foot-Taiyin. Location: On the lateral side of the chest, in the 3rd intercostal space, 6 cun lateral to the anterior midline. Indication: Fullness

and pain in the chest and hypochondriac region. Method: Puncture perpendicularly 0.5-1 cun. Moxibustion is applicable.

胸正中线　the thoracic median line

经穴定位线,为任脉循行处。

Meridians and points-locating line where passes the Conception Vessel.

胸中之府　residence of the thoracic organs

指背部。

It refers to the back.

胸椎　Xiongzhui

耳穴名。在耳轮体部,将轮屏切迹至对耳轮上、下脚分叉分为 5 等份,中 2/5 为胸椎。主治:胸胁疼痛,乳腺炎。

Name of an ear point. A curved line from intertragic notch to the branching area of superior and inferior antihelix crus can be divided into 5 equal segments. The middle 2/5 is Xiongzhui. Indications: Pain in the chest and hypochondrium, mastitis.

虚寒　deficiency cold

指阳气不足,寒从内生的证候。症见面黄少华、食欲不振、怕冷、口淡不渴、精神不振、身倦乏力、小便清长、大便稀溏或泄泻清水、舌淡苔白、脉沉迟无力等。治宜温中补虚。取穴:脾俞、胃俞、章门、中脘、关元、足三里。

A morbid condition resulting from insufficiency of yang-qi with endogenous cold, manifested as sallow and lusterless complexion, poor appetite, intolerance of cold, bland taste in the mouth without thirst, languidness, fatigue, clear urine in large amounts, loose stools or watery diarrhea, pale tongue with whitish fur, deep and slow, weak pulse, etc. Treatment principle: Warm the middle jiao and tonify the deficiency. Point selection: Pishu(BL20), Weishu(BL21), Zhangmen (LR13), Zhongwan (CV12), Guanyuan(CV4), Zusanli(ST36).

虚火上炎 deficiency fire flaming upward

由于肾阴亏损,致虚火上升的病理。症见咽干、咽痛、头昏目眩、心烦不眠、手足心热、舌质嫩红、脉细数等。治宜滋阴降火。取穴:太溪、行间、照海。

A morbid condition resulting from flaring up of deficiency fire causing by the consumption of kidney-yin, manifested as dry throat, sore throat, dizziness, restlessness, insomnia, feverish sensation over the palms and soles, red and tender tongue, thin and rapid pulse, etc. Treatment principle: Nourish yin to reduce the deficiency fire. Point selecting: Taixi (KI3), Xingjian(LR2), Zhaohai(KI6).

虚里 xuli

胃之大络,位于左胸第4、5肋间,乳头下稍内侧,当心尖搏动处。

The large collateral of stomach, located at the cardiac apex between the 4th thoracic vertebra and the 5th one, inferior and medial to the left nipple, i. e. , the part of the apical impulse.

虚脉 feeble pulse

软而无力,寻按有空虚感的一种脉象。主虚证,如血虚、气虚、失水等。

A pulse condition characterized by soft and weak beats with an empty feeling while pressing, indicating deficiency syndrome, such as blood deficiency, qi deficiency, loss of fluid, etc.

虚实 deficiency and excess

八纲之一。辨别机体抵抗力强弱和病邪盛衰的两个纲领。虚,通常指机体正气不足,抵抗力弱;实,通常指邪气盛,正邪斗争剧烈。

Two principle syndromes for estimating the condition of body resistance and the evil. Deficiency usually denotes the insufficiency of vital qi and low resistance of the body, while excess denotes the hyperactivity of pathogenic evils and the violent confliction between the pathogen and the vital qi.

虚则补其母 reinforcing the mother organ when treating deficiency cases

补法之一。用药物滋补母脏以治疗子脏之虚证,如肝虚补肾。也用于针刺疗法,通过补母经、母脏、母穴以治疗有关的虚证。

One of the tonifying methods based on the theory of the five phases by administering drugs to reinforce the mother organ. For instance, to treat a deficiency syndrome of the liver, the kidney (the mother organ of the liver) should be nourished. It is also applied to acupuncture in which points pertaining to the mother organ or channel or mother points are needled with reinforcing manipulation when treating a deficiency syndrome.

虚则补之 treat deficiency by tonifi-

cation

针灸治疗原则之一。指对虚证应用补法。与"盛则泻之"相对。

One of the principles in acupuncture and moxibustion therapy, i. e., the reinforcing therapy should be adopted to cure the deficiency-natured diseases, as contrasted with the principle of "reducing the excess-natured diseases".

虚证 deficiency syndrome

由于精气不足,机体抗病能力低下,生理功能减退所产生的证候。常见于体虚久病者。表现为面色无华,精神疲惫,气短音低,心悸失眠,饮食减少,舌质胖嫩,脉虚无力等。治宜补气养血。取穴:脾俞、胃俞、足三里、三阴交、关元、气海。

A syndrome produced by the deficiency of essential qi, lowered resistance and hypofunction of the body, commonly seen in the individual with general debility and the patient suffering from a long-standing illness; manifested as lusterless complexion, fatigue, shortness of breath, weak voice, palpitation, insomnia, poor appetite, thick and tender tongue, feeble pulse, etc. Treatment principle: Invigorate qi and nourish blood. Point selection: Pishu(BL20), Weishu(BL21), Zusanli(ST36), Sanyinjiao(SP6), Guanyuan(CV4), Qihai(CV6).

徐疾补泻 slow-rapid reinforcing-reducing method

针刺补泻法之一。即徐进针而疾出针为补,疾进针徐出针为泻。

One of the reinforcing and reducing methods in acupuncture, i. e., slow insertion and rapid withdrawal of the needle mean reinforcing while rapid insertion and slow withdrawal of the needle mean reducing.

絮针 xu needle

古代针具。圆针与锋针之前身,用以调理气血。

One of the ancient acupuncture needle, the predecessor of the round and sharp needles, used to regulate qi and blood.

悬厘 Xuanli (GB6)

经穴名。属足少阳胆经。定位:在头部鬓发上,当头维与曲鬓弧形连线的上 3/4 与下 1/4 交点处。主治:偏头痛,目外眦痛,耳鸣等。操作:直刺 0.5～1 寸;可灸。

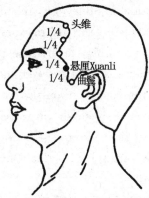

Name of an acupoint. It belongs to the Gallbladder Meridian of Foot-Shaoyang. Location: On the head, in the hair above the temple, at the junction of the upper three fourths and lower one fourth of the curved line connecting Touwei(ST8) and Qubin(GB7). Indications: Migraine, pain in the outer canthus, tinnitus, etc. Method: Puncture perpendicularly 0. 5-1 cun. Moxibustion is applicable.

悬颅 Xuanlu (GB5)

经穴名。属足少阳胆经。定位:在头部鬓发上,当头维与曲鬓弧形连线的中点处。主治:偏头痛,目外眦痛,面肿等。操作:直刺 0.5~1 寸;可灸。

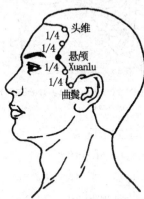

Name of an acupoint. It belongs to the Gallbladder Meridian of Foot-Shaoyang. Location:On the head,in the hair above the temple, at the midpoint of the curved line connecting Touwei (ST8) and Qubin (GB7). Indications:Migraine, pain in the outer canthus, facial swelling, etc. Method: Puncture perpendicularly 0. 5-1 cun. Moxibustion is applicable.

悬命 Xuanming

经外奇穴名。定位:位于上唇系带中点。治疗常用直刺 0.1~0.2 寸,主治神昏谵语、小儿惊痫等。

Name of an extra point. Location:At the midpoint of upper lip ligament. Perpendicular acupuncture 0. 1-0. 2 cun to cure coma and delirium, infantile convulsion, etc.

悬起灸 suspending moxibustion

艾条灸的一种。即将艾条悬于穴位上方施灸,与实按灸相对。

A kind of stick moxibustion, i. e., the stick is suspended over the point to perform moxibustion, as contrasted with the "pressing moxibustion".

悬枢 Xuanshu (GV8)

经穴名。属督脉。定位:在腰部,当后正中线上,第一腰椎棘突下凹陷中。主治:腰脊强痛,泄泻,完谷不化等。操作:直刺 0.5~1 寸;可灸。

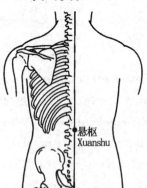

Name of an acupoint. It belongs to the Governor Vessel. Location:On the low back, on the posterior midline,in the depression below the spinous process of the 1st lumbar vertebra. Indications:Pain and stiffness of the lower back spreading to the back, diarrhea with undigested food, etc. Method: Puncture perpendicularly 0. 5-1 cun. Moxibustion is applicable.

悬阳 xuanyang

指鼻部,又称明堂。

The other name of the nose, also known as Mingtang.

悬钟 Xuanzhong (GB39)

经穴名。属足少阳胆经,八会穴之一,髓会悬钟。定位:在小腿外侧,当外踝尖上 3 寸,腓骨前缘。

主治:半身不遂,项痛,腹胀,胁痛,下肢痿痹,脚气,腿痛等。操作:直刺 1～1.5 寸;可灸。

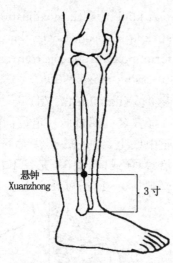

悬钟 Xuanzhong
3寸

Name of an acupoint. It belongs to the Gallbladder Meridian of Foot-Shaoyang. One of the eight influential points. Influential point of the marrow. Location: On the lateral side of the leg, 3 cun above the tip of the lateral malleolus, on the anterior border of the fibula. Indications: Hemiplegia, neck pain, abdominal distension, pain in the hypochondriac region, muscular atrophy of the lower limb, beriberi, pain of the leg, etc. Method: Puncture perpendicularly 1-1.5 cun. Moxibustion is applicable.

璇玑 Xuanji (CV21)

经穴名。属任脉。定位:在胸部,当前正中线上,天突下 1 寸。主治:咳嗽,气喘,胸痛。操作:平刺 0.3～0.5 寸;可灸。

Name of an acupoint. It belongs to the Conception Vessel. Location: On the chest and on the anterior midline, 1 cun below Tiantu (CV22). Indications: Cough, asthma, chest pain, etc. Method: Puncture horizontally 0.3-0.5 cun.

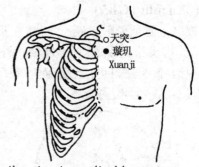

天突
璇玑
Xuanji

Moxibustion is applicable.

选穴法 point-selecting method

以经络学说为指导,根据辨证论治的原则,选取一定穴位配方进行针灸治疗。

Choosing of effective points based on TCM syndrome differentiation and the theory of the meridians and collaterals as the guide.

眩晕 vertigo

眩,即视物昏暗不明。晕,即感觉自身及周围景物旋转。其发生多与风、火、痰、虚有关。治宜平肝潜阳、调畅气血。取穴:翳风、印堂、行间、水泉、百会。

Xuan refers to blurred vision. Yun refers to the feeling of twirling of the surrounding scenery. The causes are related to wind-pathogen, fire-pathogen, phlegm, or qi and blood deficiency. Treatment principle: Suppress hyperactive liver and subside yang, regulate the movement of qi and blood. Point selection: Yifeng (TE1), Yintang(GV29), Xingjian(LR2), Shuiquan(KI5), Baihui(GV20).

眩晕听觉区 vertigo auditory area

在耳尖直上 1.5cm 处,分别向前、后各 2cm 处作一水平直线即为本区。主治:同侧头晕,耳鸣,内耳性眩晕,听力下降。

The area is defined by drawing a horizontal line 1. 5 cm above the ear apex and 2 cm forward and backward respectively. Indications：Dizziness，tinnitus，vertigo caused by the inner ear disease，and hearing loss on the same side.

穴名 name of acupoints

即穴位的名称。每穴的定名在汉语中皆有一定的意义。

The Chinese name of the acupoints. Each name has certain significance.

穴名代码 code of acupoints

指用缩写和序号方法表示经络腧穴的名称。一般以缩写的经名加上穴位的序号来表示。

The point names are usually expressed with the abbreviated meridian names and the ordinal number of the points.

穴位 acupuncture points

针灸学术语。指人体脏腑经络气血输注的部位，也是一些病痛的反应点。

A terminology of acupuncture and moxibustion. Referring to the points where the blood and qi are transmitting in and out of the organs，also the points of pain.

穴位超声刺激法 point ultrasonic stimulating therapy

使一定强度的高频声能透入穴位进行刺激的疗法。

A kind of therapy by making a certain amount of high frequency sound energy penetrate into points to give stimulation.

穴位磁疗法 point magnetic therapy

以磁性物体作用于穴位的疗法。

A kind of therapy using magnetic objects to act on the points.

穴位刺激结扎疗法 point stimulating and suture therapy

现代治疗方法之一。指在患者身体的一定部位，用手术刀切开皮肤及肌肉进行机械性刺激，并用羊肠线结扎穴位的治疗方法。

One of the newly developed acupuncture techniques. It means to apply mechanical stimulation to the patient by cutting the skin and muscle with a scalpel，and then，to suture the acupuncture point with catgut.

穴位电测定 electrical measurement of acupoints

近代有人从皮肤电现象方面来研究穴位的特性。一种方法是在有外加电流的情况下测定皮肤的电阻变化；另一种方法是在没有外加电流的情况下从皮肤导出电流，测定电位变化。

In modern times，the properties of acupoints have been studied in terms of cutaneous electrical phenomenon，one method is to measure the cutaneous resistance changes with external current；the other is to induce the cutaneous current and measure the potential changes without applying the external current.

穴位埋线法 point catgut-embedding therapy

将羊肠线埋入穴位皮下或深层，利用羊肠线对穴位的持久刺激作用治疗疾病的一种方法。

A kind of therapy of embedding a piece of

catgut into the points subcutaneously or deeply, which can provide contant stimulation to the points and cure dieases.

穴位吸引器 acupoint cupper

抽气拔罐的一种用具。用某种机械装置抽取罐内部分空气造成负压,进行拔罐治疗。

A kind of air-evacuating device for cupping, some kind of mechanical device is used to evacuate the air partly from the jar to get a negative pressure for cupping therapy.

穴位照射法 point irradiating therapy

利用光辐射作用于穴位的疗法。近代多使用红外线、紫外线及激光等。

A kind of therapy by irradiating the points. In modern times, infrared, ultraviolet and laser are mostly used.

穴位注射 point injection

将药液注入一定的穴位以治疗疾病的方法。

A method to treat diseases by injecting certain medicines into relevant acupoints.

血 blood

循行于脉管中的富有营养的红色液体,是构成人体和维持人体生命活动的基本物质之一。由水谷精微和肾精所化生。又称营血,具有营养和滋润作用,是机能活动的物质基础。

Red fluid with nutrition circulating inside vessels, one of the essential substances constructing human body and maintaining its vital activities. It transforms from food essence and kidney essence, which acts to nourish and moisten the body, thereby it is also called nutrient blood.

血崩 metrorrhagia

指不在经期内突然阴道大量流血。多发于青春期及更年期妇女。常因血热、血虚、肝肾阴虚、血瘀等致冲任不固所引起。治宜:清热凉血、理气止血。取穴:三阴交、隐白、大敦、气海。

Sudden onset of profuse uterine bleeding beyond the menstrual period, mostly seen in the women during puberty and menspause; usually due to debility of the Thoroughfare Vessel and Conception Vessel resulting from blood-heat, qi deficiency, deficiency of liver-yin and kidney-yin, blood stasis, etc. Treatment principle: Eliminate pathogenic heat from the blood, stop bleeding by regulate qi. Point selection: Sanyinjiao (SP6), Yinbai (SP1), Dadun(LR1), Qihai(CV6).

血愁 Xuechou

经外奇穴竹杖的别名。

The other name of the extra point Zhuzhang.

血管运动区 vasomotor zone

在舞蹈震颤控制区向后 1.5cm 处。主治高血压。

It is parallel to and 1.5 cm in front of the chorea and tremor controlling zone. It is used for treating hypertension.

血海 Xuehai; blood sea

①经穴名。属足太阴脾经。定位:屈膝,在大腿内侧,髌底内侧端上 2 寸,当股四头肌内侧头的隆起处。主治:月经不

调,痛经,经闭,尿血,丹毒,湿疹,瘾疹,腿内侧痛等。操作:直刺 1~1.5 寸;可灸。②血的会聚之处,一指肝脏,一指冲脉。

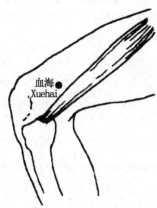

①Name of an acupoint. It belongs to the Spleen Meridian of Foot-Taiyin. Location: With the knee flexed, on the medial side of the thigh, 2 cun above the medial corner of the basis patellae, on the prominence of the medial head of the quadriceps femoris. Indications: Irregular menstruation, dysmenorrhea, amenorrhea, hematuria, erysipelas, eczema, urticaria, pain in the medial aspect of the thigh, etc. Method: Puncture perpendicularly 1-1.5 cun. Moxibustion is applicable. ②The reservoir of the blood, referring to the liver or the Thoroughfare Vessel.

血会 influential point of blood

八会穴之一。即膈俞,主治咯血、吐血及血虚等证。

One of the eight influential points, i. e., Geshu (BL17). Main indications are hemoptysis, hematemesis, blood deficiency, etc.

血络 tiny blood vessels

指细小静脉和动脉,临床上用以针刺放血。

Tiny veins and arteries, clinically used to let out blood by puncturing.

血门 Xuemen

经外奇穴名。定位:位于中脘穴旁 3 寸。主治:妇人腹中血块,胃痛,消化不良等。治疗常用直刺或灸治。

Name of an extra point. Location: 3 cun lateral to Zhongwan (CV12). Main indications are women's abdominal blood clot, gastralgia, indigestion, etc., by perpendicular acupuncture or moxibustion.

血尿 hematuria

血样尿或尿中有凝血块,但无尿痛。多因肾阴不足,心经火旺,下移小肠;或脾肾两亏、血失统摄所致。治宜养阴清热、降火止血。取穴:关元、阴谷、太溪、大敦。

Painless urination with blood or blood clot in the urine, caused by the insufficiency of kidney-yin leading to hyperactivity of fire in the Heart Meridian which attacks the small intestine, or by both the spleen and kidney deficiency leading to extravasation of blood. Treatment principle: Nourish yin, remove heat and reduce pathogenic fire to stop bleeding. Point selection: Guanyuan(CV4), Yingu(KI10), Taixi(KI3), Dadun(LR1).

血虚 blood deficiency

指血分亏损而出现虚弱症状的病理。常由于失血过多、脏腑虚损、产生精血的功能障碍等原因所致。一般可见面白、唇色淡白、头晕眼花、心悸、失眠、手足发麻、脉细无力等症状。治宜补气养血。取穴:脾俞、胃俞、足三里、三阴交、关元、气海。

A morbid condition of general debility

caused by profuse bleeding and deficiency of the viscera, leading to dysfunction of blood and essence production; manifested as pallor, dizziness, palpitation, insomnia, numbness of extremities, thin and weak pulse, etc. Treatment principle: Tonify qi and nourish blood. Point selection: Pishu(BL20), Weishu(BL21), Zusanli (ST36), Sanyinjiao(SP6), Guanyuan(CV4), Qihai(CV6).

血瘀 blood stasis

血流瘀滞或离经之血凝结不化的病证。多因气滞、气虚、血虚、血寒、血热或跌打损伤所致。治宜活血化瘀。取穴：膈俞、地机、气海、归来、血海。

A morbid condition with stagnation of blood circulation or coagulation of the extravasated blood; mostly caused by stagnation of qi, deficiency of qi and blood, blood-heat or trauma. Treatment principle: Promote blood circulation to remove blood stasis. Point selection: Geshu(BL17), Diji(SP8), Qihai(CV6), Guilai(ST29), Xuehai(SP10).

熏脐法 navel moxibustion

根据病情选用不同药物放入脐中，在药物上施灸，为间接灸的一种。主治各种虚证，也可延年益寿。

A kind of indirect moxibustion, i. e., according to the diseases, different drugs are put into the navel and moxibustion is performed on these drugs to cure all the deficiency-natured diseases or to prolong life.

熏蒸法 fumigation and steaming methods

又称熏灸。指利用药物燃烧时产生的烟雾或药物煮沸后产生的蒸气来熏蒸患部或全身的一种疗法。

Also named fuming or steaming moxibustion. A kind of therapy of using the smoke of burning drug or steam of hot decoction to heat the affected part or the whole body.

循法 meridian-massaging method

留针时，用手指循着经脉轻轻按压的辅助方法。

A procedure for promoting the effect of needling by pressing with fingers gently along the related meridian.

循经取穴 selecting acupoints of the corresponding meridian

取穴方法之一，指本经患病即在本经的循行路线上选取穴位的方法。

One of the point-selecting methods. It means to select the points along the affected meridian.

循针 guiding the needle

针刺手法之一。即针刺前用手指或指甲按压要针刺的穴位及其所属经脉的准备动作。

One of the acupuncture techniques. Before inserting the needle, press the designated point and the related meridian with finger or fingernail as a preparatory procedure.

Y

压痛点 tenderness point

按压或捏拿体表时所发现的敏感和疼痛之处。即阿是穴。

The sensitive or painful point found by pressing or kneading the body surface, also known as Ashi point.

压诊 pressure diagnosis

是以按、压、推、捏等手法寻找经络穴位上的异常变化的一种辅助诊断法。

A supplementary diagnostic method by pressing, pushing and kneading manipulations to find the pathological changes in the meridians and acupoints.

押手 pressing hand

辅助进针的手,一般为左手,与"刺手"相对。

The hand preparing for acupuncture, usually the left hand, as contrasted with "puncturing hand" (usually the right hand).

牙痛 toothache

多因龋齿所致,也可因风火、风寒、虚火所致。治宜清热止痛。取穴:合谷、下关、颊车、外关。

A symptom usually caused by dental caries, and also by pathogenic wind-fire, wind-cold and deficiency fire. Treatment principle:Clear the heat to alleviate pain. Point selection: Hegu (LI4), Xiaguan (ST7),Jiache(ST6),Waiguan(TE5).

哑门 Yamen (GV15)

经穴名。属督脉。定位:在项部,当后发际正中直上 0.5 寸,第一颈椎下。主治:癫狂,痫症,聋哑,暴喑,中风,舌强失语,后头痛,项强等。操作:直刺 0.5～1 寸;禁灸。

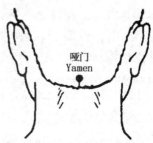

Name of an acupoint. It belongs to the Governor Vessel. Location:On the nape, 0.5 cun directly above the midpoint of the posterior hairline,below the 1st cervical vertebra. Indications:Mental disorders, epilepsy, deaf-mutism, sudden aphonia, apoplexy, stiffness of the tongue and aphasia, occipital headache, neck stiffness, etc. Method:Puncture perpendicularly 0.5-1 cun. Moxibustion is prohibited.

咽喉 Yanhou

耳穴名。在耳屏内侧上 1/2 处,主治:急慢性咽炎,扁桃体炎等。

Name of an ear point. Location:Upper half of the medial aspect of tragus. Indications:Acute and chronic pharyngitis, tonsillitis, etc.

沿皮刺 subcutaneous acupuncture

指针体与皮肤表面成 10°～20°角沿皮下刺入,又称横刺。

A kind of acupuncture with a 10°-20° angle between the needle and the skin surface, also known as horizontal acupuncture.

眼 eye; Yan

①五官之一,是视觉器官。眼的功能与机体脏腑经络的功能有关。眼为肝之窍,肝的病变可以反映在眼上,眼的疾病常从肝论治。②耳穴名。在耳垂 5 区。主治:急性结膜炎,电光性眼炎,睑腺炎(麦粒肿),假性近视等。

①One of the five sense organs, i. e., the organ of vision. The normal function of the eyes bear a close relationship to the physiological activities of the viscera and meridians. It is considered as the orifice to the liver, hence, the disorder of the liver may be reflected on the eyes and the eye diseases may be cured by treating the liver. ②Name of an ear point. It is in the section 5 of ear lobes. Indications: Acute conjunctivitis, electric ophthalmia, hordeolum, pseudo myopia, etc.

眼偷针 hordeolum

即针眼。症见胞睑边缘长出小疖,初起形如麦粒,有轻微痛痒,继而出现红肿,多由风热或脾胃热毒所致。相当于麦粒肿。治宜疏风清热。取穴:睛明、攒竹、行间、太阳。

Also named stye. A purulent infection of one or more sebaceous glands of the eyelid, marked by localized swelling like grains of wheat, mild itching and pain, and redness and swelling; caused by the attack of exogenous wind-heat pathogens or the accumulation of heat-evil in the spleen and stomach. Treatment principle: Dispel wind and remove heat. Point selection: Jingming (BL1), Cuanzhu (BL2), Xingjian (LR2), Taiyang (EX-HN5).

燕口 Yankou

经外奇穴名。定位:位于两口角赤白肉际处。沿皮刺主治癫狂、口眼歪斜、小儿痉挛、便秘、尿闭、三叉神经痛等。

Name of extra points. Location: At the junction of the dorso-ventral boundary of the two mouth corners. Subcutaneous acupuncture is used to treat mania, deviation of mouth and eyes, infantile convulsion, constipation, anuria, trigeminal neuralgia, etc.

扬刺 centro-square puncture

十二刺法之一。用于治疗范围较大、病位较浅的寒痹(寒邪阻滞)。刺法是在患处局部中央刺 1 针,四围再浅刺 4 针。

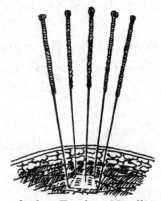

One of the Twelve Needling Techniques for treating a relatively large and shallow area caused by cold bi. It is to puncture the center of the affected area with one needle and four superficially around it.

羊矢 yangshi

①部位名。指腹股沟内的淋巴结。

②经外奇穴名。位于腹股沟淋巴结上。治疗常用斜刺或艾灸,治疗瘿瘤、小腹胀痛、疝气等。

①Name of the body part, i. e., the inguinal lymph nodes. ②Name of the extra points located on the inguinal lymph nodes. Slanting acupuncture or moxibustion is used to treat goiter tumor, lower abdominal fullness and pain, hernia, etc.

仰卧位 supine position

针灸体位名。患者身体平卧于床,头面胸腹朝上的体位。适用于取头、面、颈、胸、腹及上、下肢的部分腧穴。

Posture for acupuncture or moxibustion, with the patient lying on a bed, his/her face, chest and abdomen facing upwards for the convinence of selecting acupoints on the head, face, neck, chest, abdomen, upper and lower limbs.

阳 yang

中医学中的阴阳学说所指的与"阴"相对的一类事物或性质。凡是活动的、外在的、上升的、温热的、明亮的、功能的、兴奋的、亢进的,都属于"阳"。中医学广泛应用这一术语解释人体的生理、病理现象和指导疾病的诊断、治疗。例如把疾病的表证、热证、实证归属于"阳"。

A philosophical term in ancient China, referring to the things or characters opposite to "yin". The condition which appears as active, external, upward, hot, bright, functional, exciting and hyperactive are attributive to "yang". In TCM, it is widely used for explaining the physiological and pathological phenomena of the human body, and for directing the diagnosis and treatment of the diseases. For example, superficies syndrome, heat syndrome, excess syndrome are ascribed to "yang".

阳白 Yangbai (GB14)

经穴名。属足少阳胆经。定位:在前额部,当瞳孔直上,眉上 1 寸。主治:前额痛,目眶痛,眩晕,眼痛,眼睑眴动,眼睑下垂等。操作:平刺 0.5～1 寸;可灸。

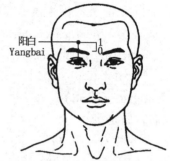

阳白 Yangbai

Name of an acupoint. It belongs to the Gallbladder Meridian of Foot-Shaoyang. Location: On the forehead, directly above the pupil, 1 cun above the eyebrow. Indications: Forehead pain, pain of the orbital ridge, vertigo, eye pain, twitching of the eyelids, ptosis of the eyelids, etc. Method: Puncture horizontally 0. 5-1 cun. Moxibustion is applicable.

阳池 Yangchi (TE4)

经穴名。属手少阳三焦经,本经原穴。定位:在腕背横纹中,当指伸肌腱的尺侧缘凹陷处。主治:肩臂腕痛,疟疾,耳聋,口渴等。操作:直刺 0.3～0.5 寸;可灸。

The acupoint, Yuan-Primary point of the Sanjiao Meridian of Hand-Shaoyang. Location: At the midpoint of the dorsal crease of the wrist, in the depression on

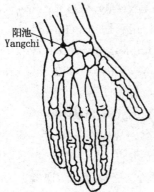

阳池
Yangchi

the ulnar side of the extensor tendon. Indications: Pain in the shoulder, arm and wrist, malaria, deafness, thirst, etc. Method: Puncture perpendicularly 0.3-0.5 cun. Moxibustion is applicable.

阳辅 Yangfu（GB38）

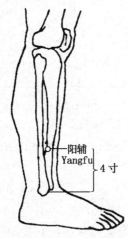

阳辅
Yangfu
4寸

经穴名。属足少阳胆经,本经经穴。定位:在小腿外侧,当外踝尖上4寸,腓骨前缘稍前方。主治:偏头痛,目外眦痛,腋痛,瘰疬,腰痛,下肢外侧痛,疟疾等。操作:直刺1～1.5寸;可灸。

The acupoint, Jing-River point, belongs to Gallbladder Meridian of Foot-Shaoyang. Location: On the lateral side of the leg, 4 cun above the tip of the external malleolus, slightly anterior to the anterior border of the fibula. Indications: Migraine, pain of the outer canthus, pain in the axillary region, scrofula, lumbago, pain in the lateral aspect of the lower extremities, ma-

laria, etc. Method: Puncture perpendicularly 1-1.5 cun. Moxibustion is applicable.

阳刚 Yanggang

①阳纲穴别名。②经外奇穴名。位于命门旁开1寸。主治:消渴,黄疸,腰痛,痔疮,遗尿,遗精等。治疗常直刺0.5～1寸或灸。

①The other name of Yanggang (BL48). ②Name of an extra point. Located 1 cun lateral to Mingmen (GV4). Indications: Consumptive thirst, jaundice, lumbago, hemorrhoids, enuresis, nocturnal emission, etc. Perpendicular acupuncture 0.5-1 cun or moxibustion is often used for treating.

阳纲 Yanggang（BL48）

经穴名。属足太阳膀胱经。定位:在背部,当第十胸椎棘突下,旁开3寸。主治:肠鸣,腹痛,腹泻,黄疸,胁痛等。操作:直刺0.5～1寸;可灸。

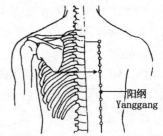

阳纲
Yanggang

Name of an acupoint. It belongs to the Bladder Meridian of Foot-Taiyang. Location: On the back, below the spinous process of the 10th thoracic vertibra, 3 cun lateral to the posterior midline. Indications: Borborygmus, abdominal pain, diarrhea, jaundice, pain in the hypochondriac region, etc. Method: Puncture perpendicularly 0. 5-1 cun. Moxibustion is applicable.

阳谷 Yanggu (SI5)

经穴名。属手太阳小肠经,本经经穴。定位:在手腕背横纹尺侧端,当尺骨茎突与三角骨之间的凹陷处。主治:颈痛,颌肿痛,手腕痛,热病等。操作:直刺 0.3～0.5寸;可灸。

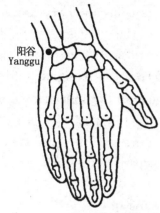

Name of an acupoint, Jing-River point, belongs to the Small Intestine Meridian of Hand-Taiyang. Location: At the ulnar end of the transverse crease of the dorsal aspect of the wrist, in the depression between styloid process of ulna and trianguar bone. Indications: Neck pain, pain and swelling of the submandibular region, pain of the wrist, febrile diseases, etc. Method: Puncture perpendicularly 0. 3-0. 5 cun. Moxibustion is applicable.

阳交 Yangjiao (GB35)

经穴名。属足少阳胆经,阳维脉郄穴。定位:在小腿外侧,当外踝尖上7寸,腓骨后缘。主治:胸胁胀满,下肢痿痹等。操作:直刺 1～1.5寸;可灸。

Name of an acupoint. It belongs to the

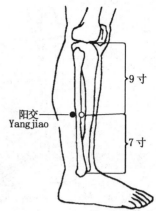

Gallbladder Meridian of Foot-Shaoyang. Xi-Cleft point of Yang Link Vessel. Location: On the lateral side of the leg, 7 cun above the tip of the external malleolus, on the posterior border of the fibula. Indications: Fullness of the chest and hypochondriac region, muscular atrophy and paralysis of the lower limbs, etc. Method: Puncture perpendicularly 1-1. 5 cun. Moxibustion is applicable.

阳经 yang meridians

又称阳脉。属阳的经脉,包括阳明经、太阳经、少阳经、督脉、阳维脉、阳跷脉。

The meridians ascribed to yang, including Yangming Meridian, Taiyang Meridian, Shaoyang Meridian, Governor Vessel, Yang Link Vessel, Yang Heel Vessel.

阳陵泉 Yanglingquan (GB34)

经穴名。属足少阳胆经,本经合穴,八会穴之一,筋会阳陵泉。定位:在小腿外侧,当腓骨小头前下方凹陷处。主治:偏瘫,下肢痿痹无力,膝肿痛,脚气,胁痛,口苦,呕吐,小儿惊风。操作:直刺 1～1.5寸;可灸。

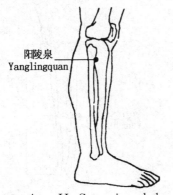

阳陵泉
Yanglingquan

The acupoint, He-Sea point, belongs to the Gallbladder Meridian of Foot-Shaoyang. One of the eight influential points. Influential point of tendons. Location: On the lateral side of the leg, in the depression anterior and inferior to the head of the fibula. Indications: Hemiplegia, weakness and atrophy of the lower extremities, swelling and pain of the knees, beriberi, hypochondriac pain, bitter taste in the mouth, vomiting, infantile convulsion, Method: Puncture perpendicularly 1-1.5 cun. Moxibustion is applicable.

阳络 yangluo

①阳经分出来的络脉。②位置较浅的络脉。

① The collaterals branched from the yang meridians. ② The collaterals that located superficially on the skin.

阳脉之海 the convergency of yang meridians

指督脉。因督脉对阳经气血有调节作用,故名。

It refers to the Governor Vessel. It is named after its function of regulating qi and blood in the yang meridians.

阳明 yangming

经脉名称之一,是阳气发展的最后阶段。

A collective name for a group of meridians. It means that the yang-qi is at the final stage of its development.

阳明经 Yangming Meridians

手阳明大肠经与足阳明胃经的合称。

A collective name for a group of meridians, including the Large Intestine Meridian of Hand-Yangming and the Stomach Meridian of Foot-Yangming.

阳明为阖 the Yangming Meridians analogous to the inner closed door

指阳明经位于身体三阳经的最里部位。

The Yangming Meridians are in the innermost part of the three Yang Meridians.

阳气 yang-qi

与阴气相对。就功能与形态来说,阳气指功能;就人体生理活动与病理变化来说,凡属外表的、向上的、亢盛的、增强的、轻清的均为阳气。

It is opposite to yin-qi as for the function and form, yang-qi stands for function. As for the physiological and pathological changes, yang-qi stands for those which are external, upward, hyper-functioning, reinforcing, light, etc.

阳跷脉 Yang Heel Vessel

奇经八脉之一。起于足跟外侧,沿外踝向上,经下肢外侧、侧胸腹部、肩部、面颊,止于后颈部。本经有病时,主要有肢体内侧肌肉弛缓而外侧肌肉拘急、癫狂、失眠等病症。

One of the eight extra meridians. It

starts from the lateral aspect of the heel, travels up along the lateral malleolus, via the lateral aspect of the lower limb, the lateral aspect of the abdomen and chest to the shoulder, and the cheek, terminates at the back of the neck. When it is diseased, it manifested as flaccidity of the medial group of muscles and spasm of the lateral muscles of the limbs, mania, insomnia, etc.

阳跷穴 Yangqiao point

①阳跷脉交会穴。②指申脉穴,八脉交会穴之一。

①All the crossing points of Yang Heel Vessel with the other meridians. ②Shenmai (BL62), one of the eight confluence points of the eight extra meridians.

阳燧 yangsui

古代取火用的凹面铜镜,用以点燃艾火。

Concave copper mirror which was used to get fire to light moxa in ancient China.

阳维脉 Yang Link Vessel

奇经八脉之一。起于外踝下方,与足少阳胆经并行,沿下肢外侧向上,经躯干部外侧,从胁后上肩,至头部,与督脉会合。具有维络诸阳经的功能。

One of the eight extra meridians. It starts below the lateral malleolus and travels along the Gallbladder Meridian of Foot-Shaoyang, ascends along the lateral aspect of the lower limb, passes the lateral aspect of the trunk and shoulder to the head, where it converges with the Governor Vessel. It functions to commu-

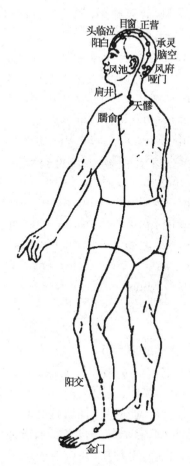

nicate all the yang meridians.

阳维穴 Yangwei point

①阳维脉的交会穴。②指外关穴,为八脉交会穴之一。

①All the crossing points of Yang Link Vessel with the other meridians. ②Waiguan (TE5), one of the eight confluence points of the eight extra meridians.

阳痿 impotence

指男性未到性功能衰退时期,出现阴茎不能勃起,或举而不坚、不久的症候。多因房劳过度,命门火衰所致;也有因肝肾虚火,心脾受损,或湿热下注所致。治宜温补肾阳，清热利湿。取穴：肾俞、命门、腰阳关、关元、阴陵泉。

Inability to have erection of the penis or lack of copulative power in the male before sexual decline; usually due to sexual excess and hypofunction of the fire of the life-gate; and also the hyperactivity of the deficiency fire of the liver and kidney, impairment of the heart and spleen, or the attack of damp-heat pathogens. Treatment principle: Warm and tonify the kidney-yang, eliminate damp and heat-pathogens. Point selection: Shenshu (BL23), Mingmen(GV4), Yaoyangguan (GV3), Guanyuan (CV4), Yinlingquan (SP9).

阳溪 Yangxi(LI5)

经穴名。属手阳明大肠经，本经经穴。定位：在腕背横纹桡侧，拇指向上跷起时，当拇短伸肌腱与拇长伸肌腱之间凹陷中。主治：头痛，目赤肿痛，齿痛，咽喉肿痛，腕痛等。操作：直刺0.3～0.5寸；可灸。

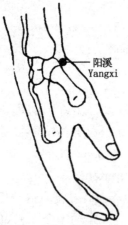

阳溪 Yangxi

The acupoint, Jing-River point, belongs to the Large Intestine Meridian of Hand-Yangming. Location: At the radial end of the transverse crease of the wrist, in the depression bewteen the extensor pollicis brevis tendon and the extensor pollicis longus tendon when the thumb is tilted upward. Indications: Headache, redness, swelling and pain of the eyes, toothache, sore throat, pain of the wrist, etc. Method: Puncture perpendicularly 0.3-0.5 cun. Moxibustion is applicable.

阳虚 yang deficiency

阳气不足，虚寒内生的证候。症见神疲乏力、少气懒言、畏寒肢冷、自汗、面色淡白、小便清长、大便稀溏、舌质淡嫩、脉虚大或沉细等。治宜温阳补虚。取穴：肾俞、命门、关元、百会、气海。

An endogenous cold syndrome resulting from the insufficiency of yang-qi; manifested as fatigue, shortness of breath, intolerance of cold extremities, spontaneous sweating, pallor, polyuria with watery urine, diarrhea, pale and tender tongue, feeble and large or deep and thin pulse, etc. Treatment principle: Warm the yang and supplement the deficiency. Point selection: Shenshu(BL23), Mingmen (GV4), Guanyuan (CV4), Baihui(GV20), Qihai(CV6).

阳中隐阴 yin hidden in yang

针刺手法名。为先补后泻法，与"阴中隐阳"相对。

Name of the acupuncture technique, i.e., the technique of reinforcing first and reducing after, as contrasted with "yang hidden in yin".

杨继洲 Yang Jizhou

明代著名针灸学家。编有《针灸大成》一书。

A noted expert in acupuncture and moxibustion in the Ming Dynasty, the compiler of *Compendium of Acupuncture and Moxibustion*.

养老 Yanglao (SI6)

经穴名。属手太阳小肠经,本经郄穴。定位:在前臂背面尺侧,当尺骨小头近端桡侧凹陷中。主治:目视不明,肩肘臂痛等。操作:直刺或斜刺 0.3～0.5 寸;可灸。

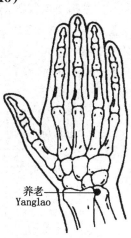

养老
Yanglao

The acupoint, Xi-Cleft point, belongs to the Small Intestine Meridian of Hand-Taiyang. Location: On the ulnar side of the posterior side of the forearm, in the depression proximal to and on the radial side of the capitulum of ulna. Indications: Blurred vision, pain in the shoulder, elbow and arm, etc. Method: Puncture perpendicularly or obliquely 0.3-0.5 cun. Moxibustion is applicable.

养心安神 tranquilizing of mind by nourishing the heart

治疗阴虚心神不安的方法。常用于心血不足,症见心悸易惊、健忘失眠、精神恍惚、多梦遗精、大便干燥或秘结、口舌生疮、舌红少苔、脉细数等。

A treatment for restlessness due to yin deficiency, applicable to the case with insufficiency of heart-blood, manifested as palpitation, timidness, amnesia, insomnia, dreaminess, nocturnal emission, dry stools or constipation, aphthae, red tougue with less fur, thin and rapid pulse, etc.

腰背痛 pain over the back and loins

指腰及背部疼痛。肾气虚弱、风湿之邪乘袭经络等均可引起。治宜祛寒利湿、温通经络。取穴:肾俞、委中、腰阳关、风池、膈俞、阴陵泉。

A disorder due to deficiency of kidney-qi or attack of wind-damp pathogens to the meridians. Treatment principle: Dispel cold and dampness, promote the flow of qi by warming the meridians and dredging the collaterals. Point selection: Shenshu (BL23), Weizhong (BL40), Yaoyangguan (GV3), Fengchi (GB20), Geshu (BL17), Yinlingquan (SP9).

腰骶椎 Yaodizhui

耳穴名。在对耳轮体部,将轮屏切迹至对耳轮上、下脚分叉处分为 5 等份,上 2/5 为腰骶椎。主治脊椎相应部位的疼痛。

Name of an ear point. A curve line from intertragic notch to the branching area of superior and inferior antihelix crus can be divided into 5 equal segments. The upper 2/5 is Yaodizhui. It is used for treating pain at corresponding part of the spine.

腰脊痛 pain along the spinal column

指腰椎及其周围疼痛。腰部外伤,瘀血

停滞,或肾虚内热均可引起。治宜祛寒利湿、温经通络。取穴:肾俞、委中、腰阳关、秩边、阴陵泉。

A symptom caused by formation of blood stasis following injury, or by kidney deficiency with heat accumulation internally. Treatment principle: Dispel cold and dampness, promote the flow of qi by warming the meridians and dredging the collaterals. Point selection: Shenshu (BL23), Weizhong (BL40), Yaoyangguan (GV3), Zhibian (BL54), Yinlingquan (SP9).

腰尻痛 lumbosacral pain

指腰骶部疼痛。腰尻痛多由肾脏虚亏所致。治宜益肾填精、通络止痛。取穴:命门、志室、太溪、肾俞、委中。

A symptom usually due to deficiency of the kidney. Treatment principle: Tonify the kidney and replenish essence, activate collaterals to relieve pain. Point selection: Mingmen (GV4), Zhishi (BL52), Taixi (KI3), Shenshu (BL23), Weizhong (BL40).

腰孔 Yaokong

十七椎穴(经外奇穴)别名。

The other name of the extra point Shiqizhui (EX-B8).

腰奇 Yaoqi (EX-B9)

经外奇穴名。定位:位于尾骨尖直上 2 寸处。向上沿皮刺主治癫痫、头痛、失眠等。

Name of an extra point. Location: 2 cun directly above the coccygeal tip. Upward subcutaneous acupuncture can be adopted to cure epilepsy, headache, in-

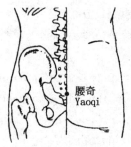

somnia, etc.

腰俞 Yaoshu (GV2)

经穴名。属督脉。定位:在骶部,适对骶管裂孔处。主治:月经不调,腰脊强痛,痔疾,下肢痿痹,癫痫等。操作:向上斜刺0.5～1寸;可灸。

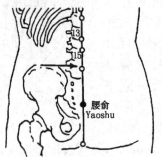

Name of an acupoint. It belongs to the Governor Vessel. Location: On the lower back, just opposite to the hiatus of the sacrum. Indications: Irregular menstruation, pain and stiffness of the lower back, hemorrhoids, muscular atrophy of the lower extremities, epilepsy, etc. Method: Puncture obliquely upward 0.5-1 cun. Moxibustion is applicable.

腰痛 lumbago

指腰部一侧或两侧疼痛或痛连脊椎的证候。凡因劳累过度,肾气亏损,或因感受外邪、外伤等致腰部经络受阻,气血运行不畅,均可发生腰痛。治宜祛寒利湿、通络止痛。取穴:肾俞、委中、命门、志室、太溪。

Pain over the lumbar region due to deficiency of kidney-qi resulting from overstrain, or obstruction of qi and blood circulation in the meridians resulting from the attack of exogenous pathogens or injury, etc. Treatment principle: Dispel cold and dampness, promote the flow of qi by warming the meridians and dredging the collaterals. Point selection: Shenshu (BL23), Weizhong (BL40), Mingmen (GV4), Zhishi(BL52), Taixi(KI3).

腰眼　Yaoyan(EX-B7)

经外奇穴名。定位：在第四腰椎棘突下,旁开约 3.5 寸凹陷中。主治：腰痛,尿频,月经不调等。

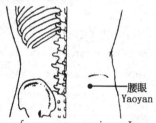

腰眼
Yaoyan

Name of an extra point. Location: About 3.5 cun lateral to the lower border of the spinous process of the 4th lumbar vertebra. Indication: Lumbago, frequent urination, irregular menstruation, etc.

腰阳关　Yaoyangguan(GV3)

经穴名。属督脉。定位：在第四腰椎棘突下。主治：月经不调,遗精阳痿,腰骶痛,下肢痿痹等。操作：向上斜刺 0.5～1 寸;可灸。

Name of an acupoint. It belongs to the Governor Vessel. Location: Below the spinous of the 4th lumbar vertebra. Indication: Irregular menstruation, nocturnal emission, impotence, pain in the lumbo-

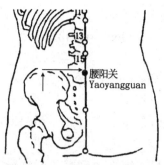

腰阳关
Yaoyangguan

sacral region, numbness and pain of the lower limbs, etc. Method: Puncture obliquely upward 0.5-1 cun. Moxibustion is applicable.

摇针　shaking the needle

针刺手法之一。即将针刺入体内后,用手轻轻摇动的方法。

One of the acupuncture techniques to slightly shake the inserted needle.

药饼灸　medicinal cake-partitioned moxibustion

间接灸的一种。采用辛温芳香的药物制成药饼放在穴位上,在药饼上再施以艾炷灸,具温中散寒、行气活血的作用。

A kind of indirect moxibustion, i. e., the medicinal cake made of drugs of pungent, warm and aromatic nature is placed on the point and moxa cone moxibustion is performed on the cake, this kind of therapy has the functions of warming the middle jiao to dispel cold, promote qi and activate blood.

药罐　medicinal cupping

指将竹制的火罐放在中药煎剂中煮沸后取出,再进行拔罐的疗法。

A bamboo cup is boiled in a decoction of Chinese drugs, and then, used for cupping.

药条灸 medical moxibustion

用混有中药的艾条施灸的方法。

Moxibustion with the moxa-stick made of mugwort and various herbal medicine.

药物艾卷 a roll of medicated mugwort

指将粗艾绒掺加一定的药物粉末卷成的长 20 厘米、直径 1.2 厘米的圆柱体。

A roll of coarse mugwort mixed with powdered drugs, it is 20 cm in length and 1.2 cm in diameter.

药物离子透入法 method of medicinal irons infiltrating into the acupoints

选用直流电的电解作用,将药物离子透入穴位的疗法。

A kind of therapy by infiltrating the medicinal irons into the acupoints by means of the electrolytic ionization of the direct current.

药线 medicated thread

又称药捻。用桑白纸搓成线状,沾上药物或内裹药物,用于治疗瘘管或排脓。

A mulberry paper thread or roll with medicine in or on it to be inserted into a fistula for treating purpose or for draining pus.

噎膈 dysphagia

以吞咽困难为主症的疾病。多因忧思气结生痰,痰气交阻于胸膈,或肾阴亏损,阴虚火旺,瘀热交阻所致。治宜调理脾胃、滋阴降逆。取穴:天突、膻中、足三里、内关、上脘、胃俞、脾俞、膈俞。

A symptom caused by the stagnation of phlegm and qi in the chest resulting from anxiety, or by the accumulation of blood stasis and heat-pathogen resulting from the consumption of kidney-yin and hyperactivity of fire due to yin deficiency. Treatment principle: Regulate the spleen and stomach, nourish yin and lower the adverse flow of qi. Point selection: Tiantu (CV22), Danzhong (CV17), Zusanli (ST36), Neiguan (PC6), Shangwan (CV13), Weishu(BL21), Pishu(BL20), Geshu(BL17).

掖门 Yemen

①即液门穴。②经外奇穴名。在腋窝直下 1 寸处。灸治诸风惊妄、呃逆、瘰疬等。

①The acupoint Yemen (TE2). ②Name of the extra point located 1 cun directly below the armpit. Moxibustion is used to cure convulsions due to various wind, hiccup, scrofula, etc.

液门 Yemen (TE2)

经穴名。属手少阳三焦经,本经荥穴。定位:在手背部,当第四、五指间,指蹼缘后方赤白肉际处。主治:头痛,目赤,暴聋,咽喉肿痛,疟疾,臂痛等。操作:直刺 0.3~

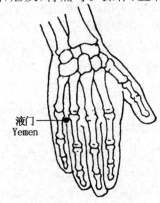

液门
Yemen

0.5寸;可灸。

The acupoint, Xing-Spring point, belongs to the Sanjiao Meridian of Hand-Shaoyang. Location: On the dorsum of the hand, between the 4th and 5th fingers, at the junction of the dorso-ventral boundary, proximal to the margin of the web. Indications: Headache, redness of the eye, sudden deafness, sore throat, malaria, pain in the arm, etc. Method: Puncture perpendicularly 0.3-0.5 cun. Moxibustion is applicable.

腋门 Yemen

①即液门。②大巨穴别名。

①Yemen (TE2). ②The other name of Daju (ST27).

腋下 Yexia

经外奇穴名。位于腋窝直下 1.5 寸处。治疗常用斜刺或灸治肋间神经痛、狐臭等。

Name of an extra point. Located 1.5 cun directly below the axillary fossa. Oblique acupuncture or moxibustion is used to cure intercostals neuralgia, bromhidrosis, etc.

一夫法 yifu method

同身寸的一种。即以第 2～5 指并合,当中节上横度,其两侧间距离为一夫,相当于 3 寸。

One of the proportional measurements. The breadth of the four fingers (index, middle, ring and little fingers) close together at the level of the skin crease of the proximal interphalangeal joint at the dorsum of the middle finger is

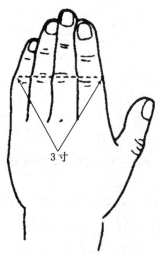

3寸

taken as yifu, equal to 3 cun.

一进三退 direct insertion with 3-stepped lifting

刺法用语。一直进针至深层,分三层退针,可反复进行。为泻法,透天凉刺法中常用此。

A term of needle manipulation. The skill is to insert the needle directly into the deep site of the point and draw it outward in three steps and this can be done repeatedly. This is a kind of manipulation for reducing and often used in the acupuncture skill called "heaven-penetrating cooling method".

一阳 One yang

经络名,指少阳。

The other name of the Shaoyang Meridian.

一阴 One yin

经络名,指厥阴。

The other name of the Jueyin Meridian.

医学纲目 *Compendium of Medicine*

明代楼英撰。论述临床各科证治。

A medical work written by Lou Ying in the Ming Dynasty, in which the diagnosis and treatment of various branches of clinical medicine were discussed.

医学入门 *Introduction to Medicine*

明代李梴撰。正文为歌赋,附注说明。

A medical work of the Ming Dynasty, written in a style of verse with annotations by Li Chan.

医学源流论 *Treatise on Origin and Development of Medicine*

书名。清代徐大椿撰。包括短论多篇,内容广泛。

A medical work written by Xu Dachun in the Qing Dynasty , with short discourses on miscellaneous medical problems.

医宗金鉴 *Golden Mirror of Medicine*

清政府组织编写的大型医学全书。吴谦等主编。本书涉及医学各科,内容系统扼要,选方实用。

A voluminous medical work compiled by the medical officers of the Qing government, headed by Wu Qian, et al. The series systematically and concisely covers various branches of medicine and records selected prescription of practical nature.

胰胆 Yidan

耳穴名。在肝、肾两穴之间。主治:胆囊炎,胆石症,偏头痛,带状疱疹,胰腺炎,耳鸣等。

Name of an ear point between Gan and Shen. Indications: Cholecystitis, cholelithiasis, migraine, herpes zoster, pancreatitis, tinnitus, etc.

遗精 nocturnal emission

指精液不因性交而外泄的一种疾病。心肾不交、肾气不固、相火炽盛或湿热下注等均可引起本病。治宜清心降火、滋阴涩精。取穴:心俞、肾俞、关元、神门、中封。

Involuntary discharge of semen due to imbalance between heart-yang and kidney-yin, deficiency of kidney-qi, overabundance of minitsterial fire, or damp-heat diffusing downward. Treatment principle: Clear heart-fire, nourish yin and astringe essence. Point selection: Xinshu (BL15), Shenshu(BL23), Guanyuan(CV4), Shenmen(HT7), Zhongfeng(LR4).

遗尿 enuresis

指小便不能控制而自遗或睡眠中小便遗出。治宜补益脾肺。取穴:气海、太渊、足三里、三阴交、百会、脾俞、肺俞。

It refers to the uncontrollable urnation or urination during sleep. Treatment principle: Tonify the spleen and lung. Point selection: Qihai (CV6), Taiyuan (LU9), Zusanli (ST36), Sanyinjiao (SP6), Baihui (GV20), Pishu (BL20), Feishu(BL13).

颐 yi

部位名。指面颊。

Name of a body part. It refers to the cheeks.

以痛为腧 tender-point needling

以压痛点为穴位。

Select the tender point as the acupuncture point.

以右治左 puncturing the right to

treat the left

是针灸取穴治疗的一种方法。针灸身体右侧的穴位可以治疗身体左侧的病患。

The method to select the acupuncture points for therapy, i. e. , a disease on the left side of the body may be treated by puncturing the points on the right side.

以左治右 puncturing the left to treat the right

是针灸取穴治疗的一种方法。针灸身体左侧的穴位可以治疗身体右侧的病患。

The method to select the acupuncture points for therapy, i. e. , a disease on the right side of the body may be treated by puncturing the points located on the left side.

异病同治 same treatment for different diseases

不同的疾病,若病机相同,可用同一种方法治疗。如脱肛、泄泻、子宫脱垂,其病机均属脾虚中气下陷者,都可用补中益气的方法治疗。

A principle for treatment in which the same therapy is applied to treat the different diseases with the same pathogenesis. For instance, prolapse of rectum, diarrhea, and uterine prolapse can be treated by the therapy of nourishing the middle jiao and tonify qi if the pathogenesis of these diseases are deficiency of spleen and collapse of the middle qi.

异经取穴 selecting points on the other meridians

取穴法的一种。与本经取穴相对,在表里、同名经上取穴。

One of the point-selecting methods, i. e. , selecting points on the other related meridians such as the interior-exterior correlated meridians or the identically named meridians, by contrast with "selecting points on the diseased meridian".

益气健脾 benefiting qi and strengthen spleen

用具有补脾益气作用的方法或药物治疗脾胃虚弱的病症。适用于脾胃虚弱所致的食欲不振、泄泻、呕吐等。

A treatment for the hypofunction of the spleen and stomach by the application of certain methods or drugs with the action of tonifying the spleen and qi, applicable to the disorders such as anorexia, diarrhea, vomiting, etc. , which are resulting from the hypofunction of the spleen and stomach.

益气养血 benefit qi and nourish blood

补气和补血药并用的治法。适用于气血俱虚。症见面色苍白或萎黄、心悸怔忡、食欲不振、气短懒言、四肢倦怠、头晕目眩、舌质淡苔白、脉细弱或虚大无力等。

A treatment for deficiency of both qi and blood with qi and blood tonification herbs, applicable to the cases manifested as pale or sallow complexion, palpitation, poor appetite, shortness of breath, fatigue, dizziness, pale tongue with whitish fur, thin and weak pulse or feeble, large and weak pulse, etc.

意舍 Yishe (BL49)

经穴名。属足太阳膀胱经。定位:在背

部,当第十一胸椎棘突下,旁开 3 寸。主治:腹胀,肠鸣,呕吐,泄泻,饮食不下等。操作:斜刺 0.5～0.8 寸;可灸。

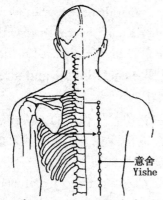

意舍
Yishe

Name of an acupoint. It belongs to the Bladder Meridian of Foot-Taiyang. Location: On the back, below the spinous process of the 11th thoracic vertebra, 3 cun lateral to the posterior midline. Indications: Abdominal distension, borborygmus, vomiting, diarrhea, difficulty in swallowing, etc. Method: Puncture obliquely 0. 5-0. 8 cun. Moxibustion is applicable.

谚谚 Yixi (BL45)

经穴名。属足太阳膀胱经。定位:在背部,当第六胸椎棘突下,旁开 3 寸。主治:气喘,咳嗽,肩背痛等。操作:斜刺 0.5～0.8 寸;可灸。

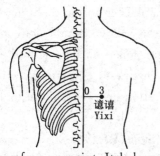

0 3

谚谚
Yixi

Name of an acupoint. It belongs to the Bladder Meridian of Foot-Taiyang. Location: On the back, below the spinous process of the 6th thoracic vertebra, 3 cun lateral to the posterior midline. Indications: Asthma, cough, pain in the shoulder and back, etc. Method: Puncture obliquely 0. 5-0. 8 cun. Moxibustion is applicable.

翳风 Yifeng (TE17)

经穴名。属手少阳三焦经。定位:在耳垂后方,当乳突与下颌角之间的凹陷处。主治:耳鸣耳聋,面瘫,牙痛颊肿,瘰疬,牙关紧闭等。操作:直刺 0.5～1 寸;可灸。

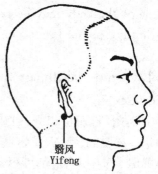

翳风
Yifeng

Name of an acupoint. It belongs to the Sanjiao Meridian of Hand-Shaoyang. Location: Posterior to the ear lobe, in the depression between the mastoid process and mandibular angle. Indications: Tinnitus, deafness, facial paralysis, toothache, swelling of the check, scrofula, trismus, etc. Method: Puncture perpendicularly 0. 5-1 cun. Moxibustion is applicable.

翳明 Yiming (EX-HN14)

经外奇穴名。定位:在翳风穴后 1 寸。主治:目疾,耳鸣,失眠等。

Name of an extra point. Location: 1 cun posterior to Yifeng(TE17). Indica-

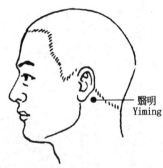

翳明
Yiming

tions: Eye diseases, tinnitus, insomnia, etc.

因地制宜 treatment in accordence with local conditions

由于地区气候环境等因素的不同,对人体产生的影响也不同,治疗时应注意根据地区的特点制定适宜的治疗方法。如南方炎热多雨地区,往往多湿热证候,治疗时要注意清热化湿。

A therapeutical principle that the treatment should be chosen according to the environment, since the human body may be influenced by the environmental variations. For example, the method of clearing heat and resolving dampness are usually applied in the southern areas because of its hot and rainy weather.

因人制宜 treatment in accordence with individual

在治疗上要根据患者的具体情况,如患者的生理、病理特点和患者的体质,以及患者所处的环境等来考虑治疗方法,使其能切合病情变化。

A therapeutical principle that the treatment should be chosen according to the physiological and pathological characteristics of the patient and also his constitu-

tion and environment.

因时制宜 treatment in accordence with seasonal conditions

因人生活在自然界中,四季的气候变化对人体产生一定的影响,故治疗时应考虑气候变化的特点。

A therapeutical principle that the treatment should be chosen according to the climate, since the human body may be influenced by the climatic variations of the four seasons.

阴 yin

中医学中的阴阳学说所指的与阳相对的一类事物或性质。凡是沉静的、内在的、下降的、寒冷的、晦暗的、物质的、抑制的、衰减的,都属于阴。中医学广泛应用这一术语解释人体的生理、病理现象和指导疾病的诊断、治疗。例如把疾病的里证、寒证、虚证归属于阴。

A philosophical term in ancient China, referring to the things or characters opposite to yang. The condition which appears as inert, internal, downward, cold, dim, material, inhibitory and declining is attributed to yin. In TCM, it is widely used for explaining the physiological and pathological phenomena of the human body, and for directing the diagnosis and treatment of the diseases. For example, interior syndrome, cold syndrome, deficiency syndrome are ascribed to "yin".

阴包 Yinbao (LR9)

经穴名。属足厥阴肝经。定位:在大腿内侧,当股骨内上髁上 4 寸,股内肌与缝匠肌之间。主治:腰骶痛,少腹痛,遗尿,小便不利,月经不调等。操作:直刺1~2寸;可灸。

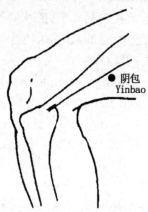

Name of an acuppoint. It belongs to the Liver Meridian of Foot-Jueyin. Location:On the medial side of the thigh,4 cun above the medial epicondyle of the femur, between the medial vastus muscle and sartorius muscle. Indications:Pain in the lumbosacral region, lower abdominal pain, enuresis, dysuria, irregular menstruation, etc. Method:Puncture perpendicularly 1-2 cun. Moxibustion is applicable.

阴刺 yin needling

十二刺法之一。用于治疗寒厥。刺法是针刺两侧足内踝后足少阴肾经的太溪穴。

One of the twelve needling techniques for treating the cold syncope. It is to puncture Taixi(KI3) behind the medial malleolus on both sides.

阴都 Yindu (KI19)

经穴名。属足少阴肾经。定位:在上腹部,当脐中上4寸,前正中线旁开0.5寸。主治:肠鸣,腹痛,胃脘痛,便秘,呕吐等。

操作:直刺1~1.5寸;可灸。

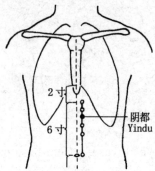

Name of an acupoint. It belongs to the Kidney Meridian of Foot-Shaoyin. Location:On the upper abdomen,4 cun above the center of the umbilicus and 0.5 cun lateral to the anterior midline. Indications:Borborygmus, abdominal pain, epigastric pain, constipation, vomiting, etc. Method:Puncture perpendicularly 1-1.5 cun. Moxibustion is applicable.

阴独八穴 eight Yindu points

经外奇穴名,即八风或八冲穴,治妇人月经不调。

Name of extra points, i. e., Bafeng (EX-LE10) or Bachong, with the indication of irregular menstruation.

阴谷 Yingu (KI10)

经穴名。属足少阴肾经,本经合穴。定位:在胭窝内侧,屈膝时,当半腱肌肌腱与半膜肌肌腱之间。主治:阳痿,疝气,尿少,崩漏,膝胭酸痛等。操作:直刺1~1.5寸;可灸。

The acupoint, He-Sea point of the Kidney Meridian of Foot-Shaoyin. Location:On the medial side of the poploteal fossa, between the tendons of the semitendinosus and semimembranosus when the knee

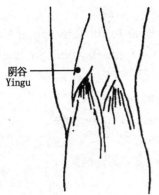

is flexed. Indications:Impotence, hernia, dysuria, metrorrhagia and metrostaxis, pain in the knee and popliteal fossa. Method:Puncture perpendicularly 1-1. 5 cun. Moxibustion is applicable.

阴交 Yinjiao (CV7)

经穴名。属任脉。定位:在下腹部,前正中线上,当脐中下1寸。主治:腹胀,水肿,疝气,月经不调,崩漏,带下,阴痒,产后出血,脐周痛等。操作:直刺0.5～1寸;可灸。孕妇慎灸。

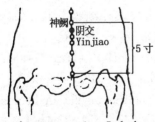

Name of an acupoint. It belongs to the Conception Vessel. Location:On the lower abdomen and on the anterior midline,1 cun below the center of the umbilicus. Indications: Abdominal distension, edema, hernia, irregular menstruation, uterine bleeding, leukorrhea, pruritus vulvae, postpartum hemorrhage, pain around the umbilicus, etc. Method:Puncture perpendicularly 0. 5-1 cun. Moxibus-

tion is applicable. Be cautious to apply moxibustion in pregnant women.

阴经 yin meridians

又称阴脉。为属阴的经脉,包括太阴经、少阴经、厥阴经、任脉、冲脉、阴维脉、阴跷脉等。

The meridians that pertain to yin, include Taiyin Meridians, Shaoyin Meridians, Jueyin Meridians, Conception Vessel, Thoroughfare Vessel, Yin Link Vessel, Yin Heel Vessel, etc.

阴廉 Yinlian (LR11)

经穴名。属足厥阴肝经。定位:在大腿内侧,当气冲直下2寸,大腿根部耻骨结节的下方,长收肌的外缘。主治:月经不调,带下,小腹痛,腿痛等。操作:直刺1～1.5寸;可灸。

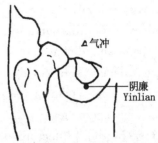

Name of an acupoint. It belongs to the Liver Meridian of Foot-Jueyin. Location: On the medial side of the thigh,2 cun directly below Qichong(ST30), at the proximal end of the thigh, below the pubic tubercle and on the lateral border of the adductor longus of the thigh. Indications:Irregular menstruation, leukorrhea, lower abdominal pain, pain in the lower limbs, etc. Method:Puncture perpendicularly 1-1. 5 cun. Moxibustion is applicable.

阴陵泉 Yinlingquan(SP9)

经穴名。属足太阴脾经,本经合穴。定位:在小腿内侧,当胫骨内侧髁后下方凹陷处。主治:腹痛腹胀,泄泻,痢疾,水肿,黄疸,小便不利或失禁,外阴痛,痛经,膝痛等。操作:直刺1~2寸;可灸。

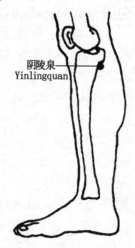

阴陵泉
Yinlingquan

The acupoint, He-Sea point, belongs to the Spleen Meridian of Foot-Taiyin. Location:On the medial side of the leg,in the depression posterior and inferior to the medial condyle of the tibia. Indications:Abdominal pain and distension, diarrhea, dysentery, edema, jaundice, dysuria, incontinence of urine, pain in the external genitalia, dysmenorrhea, pain in the knees, etc. Method:Puncture perpendicularly 1-2 cun. Moxibustion is applicable.

阴络 yinluo

①阴经分支出来的络脉。②位置较深的络脉。

① The collaterals branched from the yin meridians. ②The deeper located collaterals.

阴脉之海 the convergency of yin meridians

指任脉。任脉与全身阴经相连,总任一身阴经之气,故称。

It refers to the Conception Vessel, because it connects with yin meridians of the whole body and governs the qi of all yin meridians.

阴囊缝 Yinnangfeng

经外奇穴名。又名囊下缝。位于阴囊下正中线。灸治癫狂。

Name of an extra point, also known as Nangxiafeng. Located on the inferior medial line of scrotum. Moxibustion is used to cure epilepsy and mania.

阴器 yin organs

指外生殖器,又称前阴。

It implies the external genital organs, also known as anterior yin organs.

阴跷脉 Yin Heel Vessel

奇经八脉之一。起于足跟内侧,沿内踝向上,经下肢内侧、前阴部、腹部、胸部、颈部、鼻的两侧,止于眼部。本经有病时,主要表现为肢体外侧肌肉弛缓而内侧肌肉拘急、喉痛、嗜睡等症状。

One of the eight extra meridians. It arises from the medial side of the heel and travels via the medial malleolus, along the medial side of the lower limbs, pubic area, abdomen, chest, neck, both sides of the nose and ends at the eye. When it is diseased, it manifests as flaccidity of muscles on the lateral aspect of the limb but spasm of those on the medial aspect, sore throat, and somnolence, etc.

阴跷穴 Yinqiao point

①阴跷脉的交会穴。②指照海穴。为八脉八穴之一。

①All the crossing points of Yin Heel Vessel with the other meridians. ②Zhaohai（KI6）, one of the eight crossing points of the eight extra meridians.

阴市 Yinshi (ST33)

经穴名。属足阳明胃经。定位：在大腿前面，当髂前上棘与髌底外侧端的连线上，髌底上 3 寸。主治：腿膝麻痹、酸痛，下肢不遂等。操作：直刺 1～1.5 寸；可灸。

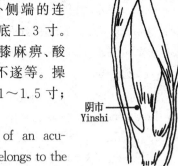

阴市
Yinshi

Name of an acupoint. It belongs to the Stomach Meridian of Foot-Yangming. Location：On the anterior side of the thigh and on the line connecting the anterior superior iliac spine and the lateral corner of the patella base,3 cun above this corner. Indications：Numbness, soreness, and motor impairment of the legs and knees, motor impairment of the lower extremities. Method：Puncture perpendicularly 1-1.5 cun. Moxibustion is applicable.

阴挺 uterine prolapse

相当于子宫脱垂、阴道壁膨出等病，多因气虚下陷或肾气不足所致。治宜益气升阳、固摄胞宫。取穴：百会、气海、维道、足三里、三阴交。

A disorder caused by the deficiency of middle qi or insufficiency of kidney-qi, e-quivalent to hysteroptosis, vaginal wall pro-lapse, etc. Treatment principle：Tonify qi , elevate yang and consolidate the uterus. Point selection：Baihui（GV20）, Qihai（CV6）, Weidao（GB28）, Zusanli（ST36）, Sanyinjiao（SP6）.

阴维脉 Yin Link Vessel

奇经八脉之一。起于内踝上方，经下肢内侧腹部、胸部、咽喉，止于后颈部。本经有病时，主要表现为心痛、胃脘痛等症状。

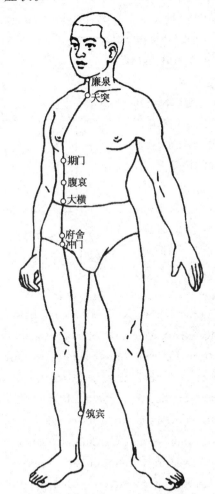

廉泉
天突
期门
腹哀
大横
府舍
冲门
筑宾

One of the eight extra meridians. It a-rises above the medial malleolus and tra-vels along the medial aspect of the lower limbs, abdomen, chest, throat, and terminates in the nape. When this meridian is diseased, it manifests as cardiac pain, pain in the epigastric region, etc.

阴维穴 Yinwei point

①阴维脉交会穴。②指内关穴,八脉八穴之一。

①All the crossing points of Yin Link Vessel with the other meridians. ② Neiguan (PC6), one of the eight crossing points of the eight extra meridians.

阴郄 Yinxi (HT6)

经穴名。属手少阴心经,本经郄穴。定位:在前臂掌侧,当尺侧腕屈肌腱的桡侧缘,腕横纹上 0.5 寸。主治:心痛,癔病,盗汗,咯血,衄血,暴暗等。操作:直刺 0.3~0.5 寸;可灸。

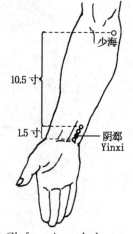

The acupoint, Xi-Cleft point, belongs to the Heart Meridian of Hand-Shaoyin. Location: On the palmar side of the forearm and on the radial side of the ulnar tendon of flexor muscle of the wrist, 0.5cun proximal to the crease of the wrist. Indications: Cardialgia, hysteria, night sweating, hemoptysis, epistaxis, sudden loss of voice, etc. Method: Puncture perpendicularly 0.3-0.5 cun. Moxibustion is applicable.

阴虚 yin deficiency

指阴液不足,津血亏损。常见低热、手足心热、午后潮热、消瘦盗汗、唇红口干、小便短黄、便秘、舌红少苔、脉细数无力等症状。治宜滋阴降火。取穴:太溪、阴谷、三阴交、照海。

A morbid state of yin-fluid insufficiency and consumption of fluid and blood; manifested as low fever, feverish of palms and soles, tidal fever in the afternoon, emaciation, night sweating, red lips, dry mouth, oliguria with yellowish urine, constipation, red tongue with less tongue fur, thin, rapid and weak pulse, etc. Treatment principle: Nourish yin to remove heat. Point selection: Taixi (KI3), Yingu(KI10), San-yinjiao(SP6), Zhaohai(KI6).

阴阳 yinyang

即阴阳学说中的内容。阴阳源于中国古代的哲学思想。古代哲学家认为,阴阳是存在于任何一事物中的两个对立面,它的对立统一是一切事物发展、变化的根源。就事物的属性来说,在外的、向上的、功能的、兴奋的、旺盛的、强壮的等属于阳;相反,在内的、向下的、物质的、抑制的、虚弱的等属于阴。中医学运用这一理论阐明人体生理现象和病理变化规律,同时指导疾病的诊断和治疗。

A concept originating from ancient Chinese philosophy, in which "yin" and "yang" represent two contradictories in everything. The unity and opposites of "yin" and "yang" are the fundamental cause which brings about development and changes of everything. Matters which are hot, external, upward, functional, exciting, vigorous, etc., belong to "yang", while those which are internal, downward, material, inhibitive, weak, etc., belong to "yin". In TCM, the theory of "yin" and "yang" is used to explain physiological and pathological phenomena of the body. It is also a principle of diagnosing and treating diseases.

阴阳配穴法 point-combining method of yin meridian and yang meridian

指阴经穴与阳经穴相配伍应用的配穴法。在阴阳两经相表里的情况下,则称表里配穴法。

A kind of point-combining method by using the yin meridian points and yang meridian points together. In case of the exterior and interior correlation between the two meridians, it can be named as point-combining method of exterior and interior correlated meridians.

阴痒 pruritus vulae

指外阴瘙痒。多因外阴不洁、感染,或湿热蕴结,流注于下而致;也有因阴虚血燥而致。治宜清热利湿,佐以疏肝。取穴:中极、下髎、血海、三阴交、蠡沟、曲骨、大敦、间使。

Intense itching of the external genitals of the female, caused by local infection or accumulation of damp-heat pathogens, or yin and blood deficiency lead to dryness. Treatment principle: Clear heat and promote diuresis with dispersing the stagnated liver-qi. Point selection: Zhongji (CV3), Xialiao(BL34), Xuehai(SP10),

Sanyinjiao (SP6), Ligou (LR5), Qugu (CV2), Dadun(LR1), Jianshi(PC5).

阴中隐阳 yang hidden in yin

针刺手法名。为先泻后补法,与阳中隐阴相对。

Name of the acupuncture technique, i. e., the technique of reducing first and reinforcing after, contrary to "yin hidden in yang".

殷门 Yinmen (BL37)

经穴名。属足太阳膀胱经。定位:在大腿后面,当承扶与委中的连线上,承扶下6寸。主治:腰腿疼痛,下肢痿痹等。操作:直刺1~1.5寸;可灸。

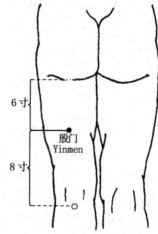

Name of an acupoint. It belongs to the Bladder Meridian of Foot-Taiyang. Location: On the posterior side of the thigh and on the line connecting Chengfu (BL36) and Weizhong(BL40), 6 cun below Chengfu (BL36). Indications: Pain in lower back and thigh, pain, numbness and motor impairment of the lower extremities, etc. Method: Puncture perpendicularly 1-1. 5 cun. Moxibustion is applicable.

银针 silver needle

以银为主要材料制成的针具,其传热及导电性能良好,多用于温针。

A kind of needle mainly made by silver and used in warm acupuncture because of its good conductivity of heat and electricity.

龈交 Yinjiao (GV28)

经穴名。属督脉。定位:在上唇内,唇系带与上齿龈的相接处。主治:癫狂,齿龈肿痛,鼻渊等。操作:向上斜刺 0.2～0.3 寸;禁灸。

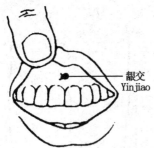

Name of an acupoint. It belongs to the Governor Vessel. Location: Inside the upper lip, at the junction of labial frenum and upper gum. Indications: Mental disorders, pain and swelling of the gums, sinusitis, etc. Method: Puncture obliquely upward 0.2-0.3 cun. Moxibustion is prohibited.

饮郄 Yinxi

经外奇穴名。位于胸骨中线外 6 寸第六肋间隙中。斜刺或灸治腹痛、肠鸣、肺炎、胸膜炎等。

Name of an extra point. Located at the 6th intercostal space, 6 cun lateral to the midsternal line. Oblique acupuncture or moxibustion is used to cure abdominal pain, borborygmus, pneumonia, pleuritis, etc.

隐白 Yinbai (SP1)

经穴名。属足太阴脾经,本经井穴。定位:在足大趾末节内侧,距趾甲角 0.1 寸。主治:腹胀,便血,尿血,多梦,惊风,痛经等。操作:直刺 0.1 寸,或斜刺 0.2～0.3 寸;可灸。

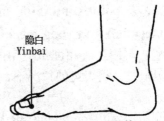

The acupoint, Jing-Well point, belongs to the Spleen Meridian of Foot-Taiyin. Location: On the medial side of the distal segment of the great toe, 0.1 cun from the corner of the toenail. Indications: Abdominal distension, hematochezia, hematuria, dreaminess, convulsion, dysmenorrhea, etc. Method: Puncture perpendicularly 0.1 cun or obliquely 0.2-0.3 cun. Moxibustion is applicable.

瘾疹 urticaria

因湿热内蕴,复感风寒,郁于皮腠而发;或对某些物质过敏所致。皮肤出现大小不等的风团,甚则成块成片,剧痒,时隐时现,即荨麻疹。治宜疏风和营。取穴:风池、大椎、肩髃、曲池、外关、足三里、三阴交。

A condition due to accumulation of damp-heat pathogens and attack of wind-cold pathogens to the skin as well, or due to hypersensitivity to certain substances;

marked by the intermittent occurrence of various sizes of elevated patches which are attended by intense itching. Treatment principle: Dispel wind and regulate the nutrient qi. Point selection: Fengchi (GB20), Dazhui(GV14), Jianyu(LI15), Quchi(LI11), Waiguan(TE5), Zusanli (ST36), Sanyinjiao(SP6).

印堂 Yintang (GV29)

经穴名。属督脉。定位：在两眉头连线的中点。主治：头痛头重，衄血，小儿惊风，前头痛，失眠等。操作：平刺 0.3～0.5 寸；可灸。

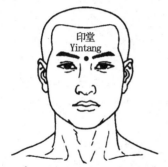

Name of an acupoint. It belongs to the Governor Vessel. Location: At the midpoint of the medial ends of the two eyebrows. Indications: Headache, head heaviness, epistaxis, rhinorrhea, infantile convulsion, frontal headache, insomnia, etc. Method: Puncture horizontally 0.3-0.5 cun. Moxibustion is applicable.

膺窗 Yingchuang (ST16)

经穴名。属足阳明胃经。定位：在胸部，当第三肋间隙，距前正中线 4 寸。主治：胸胁满痛，咳嗽，气喘，乳痈等。操作：直刺 0.2～0.4 寸；可灸。

Name of an acupoint. It belongs to the

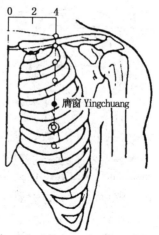

膺窗 Yingchuang

Stomach Meridian of Foot-Yangming. Location: On the chest, in the 3rd intercostal space, 4 cun lateral to the anterior midline. Indications: Fullness and pain in the chest and hypochondrium, cough, asthma, acute mastitis, etc. Method: Puncture perpendicularly 0.2-0.4 cun. Moxibustion is applicable.

膺俞 yingshu

①指胸部第三侧线上各穴。②泛指胸部各经穴。③指中府穴。

① All the acupoints on the third thoracic lateral line. ② All the acupoints on the thorax in the general meaning. ③Zhongfu (LU1).

迎香 Yingxiang (LI20)

经穴名。属手阳明大肠经。定位：在鼻翼外缘中点旁，当鼻唇沟中。主治：鼻塞不闻香臭，鼻衄，鼻渊，口㖞，面痒面肿等。操作：直刺 0.1～0.2 寸；不宜灸。

Name of an acupoint. It belongs to the Large Intestine Meridian of Hand-Yangming. Location: In the nasolabial groove, beside the midpoint of the lateral border

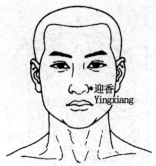

迎香
Yingxiang

of the nasal ala. Indications: Nasal obstruction, hyposmia, epistaxis, sinusitis, deviation of the mouth, itching and swelling of the face, etc. Method: Puncture perpendicularly 0.1-0.2 cun. Moxibustion is forbidden.

迎而夺之 inverse acupuncture to reduce

针刺用语。指针刺泻法要迎着经气,与"随而济之"相对。

A term of acupuncture implying that the reducing acupuncture must be performed against the moving direction of the meridian qi, as contrasted with "following the moving direction of the meridian qi to reinforce".

迎随补泻 directional supplementation and draining

针刺时使针尖顺着经脉循行方向进针和操作的属"补"法,针刺时使针尖逆着经脉循行方向进针和操作的属"泻"法。

When the needle is inserted and manipulated along the travel direction of the meridian, it is "supplementation". When it is inserted and manipulated against the travel direction of the meridian, it is "draining".

荥输治外经 Xing-Spring points and Shu-Stream points can be used to cure the diseases of the exterior meridians

取穴法之一,意指各经的荥穴和输穴可主治外行经脉所过处的疾病。

One of the point-selecting methods, i.e., the Xing-Spring points and the Shu-Stream points can be used as the main points to cure the diseases of the parts where the exterior meridians pass.

荥穴 Xing-Spring point

位于手足部远端掌指或跖趾关节附近,十二经各1个。如水之上游流出的细小水流,故名。为五输穴之一。

One of the five Shu points near the metacarpophalangeal joints of the fingers and the metatarsophalangeal joints of the feet, analogous to the springs at the upper part of a river.

营池 Yingchi

经外奇穴名。定位:位于足内踝下缘前、后方凹陷处,左、右足共4穴。直刺或灸治月经过多、赤白带下。

Name of extra points. Location: In the depressions of the inferior margin of the medial ankle, four points in all on both feet. Perpendicular acupuncture or moxibustion is used to cure red and white vaginal discharge, etc.

营气 nutrient-qi

运行于脉中的精华物质。具有化生血液和营养全身的功能。

Essential substance circulating in the vessels, responsible for the production of blood and the nourishment of body tissues.

营卫 nutrient-qi and defensive-qi

营气和卫气的合称。两者皆属于水谷精微之气，对内起营养作用者为营，对外起捍卫作用者为卫。

The collective name of nutrient-qi and defensive-qi which are both formed by the essence of water and food, as the nutrient-qi acts to nourish the body while the defensive-qi acts to defend and resist to the exogenous pathogens.

瘿 goiter

指颈前生长的肿物，红而高凸，或蒂小而下垂，如"缨络"形状。发病与水土有关；或忧思郁怒，肝郁不舒，脾失健运，致气滞痰凝而成。相当于甲状腺肿大一类的疾患。治宜滋阴降火。取穴：合谷、天鼎、天突、关元、照海。

A mass over the neck, esp. , referring to the enlargement of the thyroid gland. The pathogenic factor is normally related with acclimatization; or emotions such as anxiety, thought, depressed and anger, causing the qi stagnation with phlegm accumulation due to the liver-qi constrained and spleen failing in transportation. Treatment principle: Nourish yin to reduce pathogenic fire. Point selection: Hegu (LI4), Tianding (LI17), Tiantu (CV22), Guanyuan (CV4), Zhaohai (KI6).

涌泉 Yongquan (KI1)

经穴名。属足少阴肾经，本经井穴。定位：在足底部，卷足时足前部凹陷处，约当足第二、三趾趾缝纹头端与足跟连线的前1/3与后2/3交点上。主治：头痛咽痛，目眩头晕，舌干，失音，小便不利，小儿惊风，足心热，昏厥等。操作：直刺0.5～1寸；可灸。

The acupoint, Jing-Well point, belongs to the Kidney Meridian of Foot-Shaoyin. Location: On the sole, in the depression appearing on the anterior part of the sole when the foot is in the plantar flexion, approximately at the junction of the anterior 1/3 and

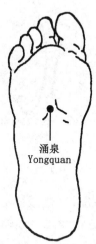

涌泉
Yongquan

posterior 2/3 of the line connecting the base of the 2nd and 3rd toes with the heel. Indications: Headache, sore throat, blurred vision, dizziness, dryness of the tongue, loss of voice, dysuria, infantile convulsion, feverish sensation in the sole, syncope, etc. Method: Puncture perpendicularly 0. 5-1 cun. Moxibustion is applicable.

幽门 Youmen(KI21); pylorus

①经穴名。属足少阴肾经。定位：在上腹部，当脐中上6寸，前正中线旁开0.5寸。主治：腹痛，腹胀，消化不良，呕吐，泄泻，恶心，孕妇晨吐等。操作：直刺0.5～1寸；可灸。②七冲门之一。即胃的下口，连接胃与十二指肠。

①Name of an acupoint. It belongs to the Kidney Meridian of Foot-Shaoyin. Location: On the upper abdomen, 6 cun

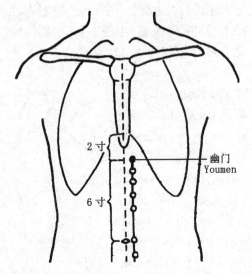

above the centre of the umbilicus and 0.5 cun lateral to the anterior midline. Indications: Abdominal pain and distension, indigestion, vomiting, diarrhea, nausea, morning sickness, etc. Method: Puncture perpendicularly 0.5-1 cun. Moxibustion is applicable. ②One of the seven important openings, the lower opening of the stomach, connecting with duodenum.

油捻灸 lampwick moxibustion

灸法的一种。以纸捻蘸植物油点燃后在穴位处进行熏灸的方法。

A kind of moxibustion, i. e., using lampwick absorbed with plant oil and lighted to perform fuming moxibustion on the points.

瘀血 blood stasis

血瘀滞于体内，包括溢出经脉或积存于组织间隙，或因血液运行受阻而滞留于经脉内或器官内，引起气机阻滞，经脉阻塞，出现局部固定性刺痛、拒按，紫斑，血肿等。多因跌打损伤所致。

A condition with stagnation of qi and obstruction of meridians, usually caused by the accumulation of extravasated blood in the tissue space or stagnation of blood in the meridians or viscera resulting from trauma; manifested as localized stabbing pain and tenderness, bruise, hematoma, etc.

瘀血阻络 obstruction of collaterals by blood stasis

因外伤或久痛不愈所致的一种病理。由于瘀血阻滞脉络，气血运行受阻，常引起以局部固定性刺痛为特点的各种痛症。如瘀血头痛、瘀血胃脘痛等。此外，某些出血性疾病也被认为与瘀血阻络有关。治宜活血化瘀。取穴：膈俞、地机、气海、归来、血海。

A morbid condition due to trauma or obstinate pain. Since the collaterals are obstructed by blood stasis and the circulation of qi and blood is disrupted, it causes various disorders characterized by stabbing pain in fix location such as headache due to blood stasis, stomachache due to blood stasis, etc. Furthermore, certain hemorrhagic diseases are also considered to be related to such condition. Treatment principle: Invigorate blood to resolve stasis. Point selection: Geshu (BL17), Diji(SP8), Qihai(CV6), Guilai (ST29), Xuehai(SP10).

鱼 thenar eminence

部位名。即鱼际。

Name of a body part, i. e., the thenar.

鱼腹 Yufu

承山穴别名。

The other name of Chengshan (BL57).

鱼际 Yuji; thenar

①经穴名。属手太阴肺经，本经荥穴。定位：在手拇指本节（第一掌指关节）后凹陷处，约第一掌骨中点桡侧，赤白肉际处。主治：咳嗽，咽喉肿痛，失音，发热等。操作：直刺 0.5～1 寸；可灸。②拇指后方掌面及踇指后方跖面肌肉隆起的边缘。

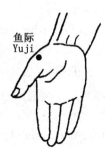

① The acupoint, Xing-Spring point, belongs to Lung Meridian of Hand-Taiyin. Location：In the depression posterior to the first metacarpophalangeal joint, on the radial aspect of the midpoint of the first metacarpal bone, and on the junction of dorso-ventral boundary. Indications：Cough, sore throat, loss of voice, fever, etc. Method：Puncture perpendicularly 0. 5-1 cun. Moxibustion is applicable. ②The edge of the prominence of the palm proximal to the thumb or that of sore proximal to the big toe.

鱼络 thenar eminence collaterals

指位于手内侧鱼际部的络脉。

The collaterals located at the thenar eminence of the hand.

鱼尾 Yuwei

①经外奇穴名。位于目外眦横纹尽处。沿皮刺治疗头痛、偏头痛、目疾、面神经麻痹等。②瞳子髎穴别名。

①Name of an extra point. Situated at the end of the lateral canthus crease. Subcutaneous acupuncture is used to cure headache, migraine, eye diseases, facial nerve paralysis, etc. ②The other name of Tongziliao (GB1).

鱼腰 Yuyao (EX-HN4)

经外奇穴名。定位：在额部，瞳孔直上，当眉毛的中点处。主治：眉棱骨痛，眼睑瞤动、下垂，目翳，目赤肿痛。

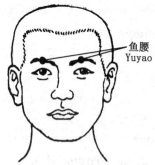

Name of an extra point. Location：At the frontal part, directly above the pupil, at the midpoint of the eyebrow. Indications：Pain in the supraorbital region, twitching of the eyelids, ptosis, cloudiness of the cornea, redness, swelling and pain of the eyes.

语言二区 speech zone Ⅱ

从顶骨结节后下 2cm 处，向后平行于后正中线延长 3cm 的直线处。主治命名性失语。

From the point 2 cm behind the parital protuberance draw a line downward, 3 cm long, parallel to the posterior midline. It is used for treating nominal aphasia.

语言三区 speech zone Ⅲ

从眩晕听觉区中点向后平移 4cm 处。主治：感觉性失语。

It is on a line, 4 cm long, behind the midpoint of the vertigo auditory zone. Indications: Sensory aphasia.

玉房 yufang

指藏精之所,即睾丸。

The place where stores sperms, i. e. , the testicle.

玉户 Yuhu

天突穴别名。

The other name of Tiantu (CV22).

玉环 yuhuan

部位名。指心、肾、肝、脾之中间与脐相对处。

Name of a body part. Located at the middle of heart, kidney, liver and spleen, just opposite to the umbilicus.

玉龙歌 *Jade Dragon Poem*

针灸歌赋名。全名《一百二十穴玉龙歌》,元代王国瑞编。

A poem about acupuncture and moxibustion with the full name *Jade Dragon Poem of 120 Acupoints*, complied by Wang Guorui in the Yuan Dynasty.

玉门头 Yumentou

经外奇穴名。定位:位于女性外生殖器,阴蒂头是穴。主治妇人阴疮、癫狂,针3分,艾条灸3~7分钟。

Name of an extra point. Location: At the end of the clitoris in the woman's vulva. Main indications are vulval ulcer, mania, with acupuncture to depth of 0. 3 cun or moxibustion with moxa stick for 3-7 minutes.

玉泉 Yuquan

①中极穴别名。②经外奇穴名。位于脐下 6.5 寸,男子阴茎根上,主治阳痿、睾丸炎等。操作:直刺 0.3~0.5 寸或灸治。③经外奇穴名。位于玉枕穴下 1 寸。主治失音不语。

①The other name of Zhongji (CV3). ②Name of the extra point located 6. 5 cun directly below the umbilicus or at the root of the penis. Main indications are impotence, testitis, etc. Method: Puncture perpendicularly 0. 3-0. 5 cun. Moxibustion is applicable. ③Name of an extra point. Located 1 cun below Yuzhen (BL9) with main indication of aphasia.

玉堂 Yutang (CV18)

经穴名。属任脉。定位:在胸部,当前正中线上,平第三肋间。主治:胸痛,咳嗽,气喘,呕吐。操作:平刺 0.3~0.5 寸;可灸。

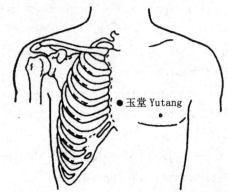

Name of an acupoint. It belongs to the Conception Vessel. Location: On the chest, at the anterior midline, level with the 3rd intercostal space. Indications: Chest pain, cough, asthma, vomiting, etc. Method: Puncture horizontally 0. 3-0. 5 cun. Moxibustion is applicable.

玉田 Yutian

经外奇穴名。定位:在第四骶椎棘突下

凹陷处。沿皮刺或灸。治难产、腰骶痛等。

Name of an extra point. Location：In the depression below the spinous process of the 4th sacral vertebra. Subcutaneous acupuncture or moxibustion is used to cure dystocia，lumbosacral pain，etc.

玉英 yuying

①玉堂穴别名。②部位名。指前阴部。

①The other name of Yutang (CV18). ②Name of a body part，i. e. ，the external genitalia.

玉枕 Yuzhen (BL9)

经穴名。属足太阳膀胱经。定位：在后头部，当后发际正中直上2.5寸，旁开1.3寸，平枕外隆凸上缘凹陷中。主治：

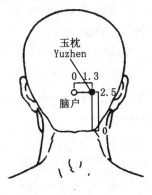

头痛，颈痛，头晕，目痛，鼻塞等。操作：平刺0.3～0.5寸；可灸。

Name of an acupoint. It belongs to the Bladder Meridian of Foot-Taiyang. Location：On the occiput, 2. 5 cun directly above the midpoint of the posterior hairline and 1. 3 cun lateral to the midline, in the depression level with the upper border of the external occipital protuberance. Indications：Headache, neck pain, dizziness，eye pain，nasal obstruction, etc. Method：Puncture horizontally 0. 3-0. 5 cun. Moxibustion is applicable.

玉柱 Yuzhu

承山穴别名。

The other name of Chengshan (BL57).

宛陈则除之 chronic diseases should be cured by letting out blood

指对气血瘀滞、邪在血分的一些病症，宜用针刺出血的办法。

Some diseases with qi and blood stagnation and with evils in the blood should be cured by acupuncture to let out blood.

郁证 depressive-syndrome

由于情志不畅、气机郁滞所引起的证候。症见心情抑郁、情绪不宁、胁肋窜痛，或易怒善哭、咽中如有物梗、咳之不出等。治宜疏肝解郁、清化痰火。取穴：太冲、内关、丰隆、天突、上星、印堂。

A syndrome due to emotions and the stagnation of qi，manifested as mental depression，hypochondriac pain，liability to be angry and crying，obstructive sensation in the throat，etc. Treatment principle：Disperse stagnated liver-qi to relieve qi stagnation， clear and resolve phlegm-fire. Point selection：Taichong (LR3)，Neiguan(PC6)，Fenglong(ST40)，Tiantu(CV22)，Shang-xing(GV23)，Yin-tang(GV29).

彧中 Yuzhong (KI26)

经穴名。属足少阴肾经。定位：在胸部，当第一肋间隙，前正中线旁开2寸。主治：咳嗽，气喘，痰壅，胸胁胀满等。操作：斜刺或平刺0.5～0.8寸；可灸。

Name of an acupoint. It belongs to the Kidney Meridian of Foot-Shaoyin. Location：On the chest，in the 1st intercostal

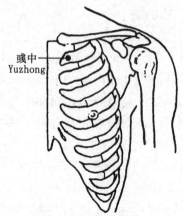

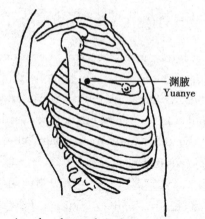

space, 2 cun lateral to the anterior midline. Indications: Cough, asthma, accumulation of phlegm, fullness in the chest and hypochondriac regions, etc. Method: Puncture obliquely or transversely 0. 5-0. 8 cun. Moxibustion is applicable.

御药院 imperial drug institution

掌管帝王和宫廷用药的机构。宋、金、元时期均设此机构。

An imperial organization set up in the Song, Jin and Yuan Dynasties for administrating the use of medicines by emperors and courts.

渊腋 Yuanye (GB22)

经穴名。属足少阳胆经。定位：在侧胸部，当腋中线上，腋下 3 寸，第四肋间隙中。主治：胸满，腋肿，胁痛，上肢痛不可举等。操作：斜刺 0.5～0.8 寸；可灸。

Name of an acupoint. It belongs to the Gallbladder Meridian of Foot-Shaoyang. Location: On the lateral side of the chest, on the midaxillary line when the arm is raised, 3 cun below the axilla, in the 4th intercostal space. Indications: Fullness of the chest, swelling of the axillary region,

pain in the hypochondriac region, pain and motor impairment of the arm, etc. Method: Puncture obliquely 0. 5-0. 8 cun. Moxibustion is applicable.

元儿 Yuaner

膻中穴别名。

The other name of Danzhong (CV17).

元神之府 residence of the original spirit

指脑。人的精神意识、记忆思维、感官机能为元神，皆由脑发生，故称。

It refers to the brain. Consciousness, memory, mental activities and sensory functions are generalized as the original spirit which is controlled by the brain.

元柱 Yuanzhu

攒竹穴别名。

The other name of Cuanzhu (BL2).

原络配穴法 primary-connecting point combination method

配穴法之一。即取病经的原穴为主穴，配以表里经的络穴为辅穴。

One of the point-combining methods, i. e. , the Yuan-Primary point of the corresponding meridians (diseased meridian) are paired with the Luo-Connecting point of the interior-exterior related meridians.

原穴 Yuan-Primary points

特定穴的一种，是脏腑原气经过和留止的部位。十二经脉各有一个原穴。阴经的原穴与五输穴中的输穴相同。原穴主要用于治疗五脏六腑的疾病。

A kind of specific points where the primary qi of zang-organs and fu-organs passes and infuses. There is one Yuan-Primary point in each of the twelve regular meridians. But in the yin meridians the Yuan-Primary point overlaps the Shu-Stream point of the five Shu points. They can be stimulated to treat disease involving zang-fu organs.

圆利针 round-sharp needle

古代九针之一。状如马尾，针尖又圆又尖。多用于治疗痈肿、痹病和某些急性病。

One of the nine needles of the ancient times. Its body is like a ponytail and its tip is sharp and round. It is mainly used for carbuncle and abscess, arthralgia and certain acute conditions.

圆针 round needle

古代九针之一。针体如圆筒状，针尖呈卵圆形。多用于按摩穴位以治疗肌肉疾病。

One of the nine needles of the ancient times. Its body is cylindrical and its tip is oval. It is often used to massage points for muscular diseases.

缘中 Yuanzhong

耳穴名，又称脑点。定位：在对屏尖与轮屏切迹之间。主治：智力低下，遗尿，眩晕，头痛等。

Name of an ear point. Naodian is another name of this point. Location: At the midpoint between antitragic apex and intertragic notch. Indications: Oligophrenia (incomplete development of intelligence), enuresis, vertigo, headache, etc.

远道刺 distant needling

九刺法之一。指身体上部有病时，取下肢部的经穴进行治疗。

One of the nine needling techniques. When a disease occurs in the upper part of the body, it is treated by puncturing the points on the lower limbs.

远近配穴法 distant-adjacent point combination method

即远离和接近病痛部位的穴位配合应用的方法。

A method of combining the points far away form the disease and the ones next to it.

月经病 menopathy

有关月经方面的各种病证，包括月经周期、经量、经色、经质的异常和经期及其前后出现的明显症状。

Menstrual disorders, including the abnormality of its cycle, the amount, colour and characteristics of the menses, as well as the obvious symptoms appearing before, during and after the menstrual cycle.

月经不调 menoxenia

泛指月经周期、经量、经色、经质异常的

各种病症。

A general term for the disorder with abnormality of the amount, colour and characteristics of menses, as well as the irregularity of menstrual cycle.

月经过多 menorrhagia

经期血量过多或行经时间延长超过 7 天以上的病症。多因气虚、血热、劳伤等使冲任不固所致。治宜补气摄血、健脾固冲。取穴:膻中、脾俞、中脘、足三里。

Excessive uterine bleeding occurring at regular intervals of menstruation or the period of flow being longer than usual duration for more than seven days; usually due to debility of Thoroughfare Vessel and Conception Vessel resulting from deficiency of qi, blood-heat, overstrain, etc. Treatment principle: Induce hemostasis by tonifying qi, strengthening the spleen to consolidate the Thoroughfare Vessel. Point selection: Danzhong(CV17), Pishu(BL20), Zhongwan(CV12), Zusanli(ST36).

云门 Yunmen (LU2)

经穴名。属手太阴肺经。定位:在胸前壁的外上方,肩胛骨喙突上方,锁骨下窝凹陷处,距前正中线 6 寸。主治:咳嗽,气喘,胸痛,胸满,肩臂痛等。操作:向外斜刺 0.5~0.8 寸;可灸。

Name of an acupoint. It belongs to the Lung Meridian of Hand-Taiyin. Location: In the superior lateral part of the anterior thoracic wall, superior to the coracoid process of the scapula, in the depression of the infraclavicular fossa, 6 cun la-

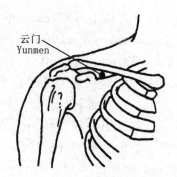

云门
Yunmen

teral to the anterior midline. Indications: Cough, asthma, chest pain, fullness in the chest, shoulder and arm pain, etc. Method: Puncture obliquely 0.5-0.8 cun. Moxibustion is applicable.

云岐子 Yunqizi

金代医学家张壁别号,善针灸,著有《云岐子针法》。

The pen-name of the famous physician Zhang Bi in Jin Dynasty, who was good at acupuncture and moxibustion with the work titled *Yunqizi's Acupuncture Methods*.

运动区 motor zone

以前、后正中线中点后 0.5cm 处为上点,眉枕线和鬓角发际前缘的交点为下点,此两点连线为运动区。其上 1/5 处主治对侧下肢瘫痪,中 2/5 处主治对侧上肢瘫痪,下 2/5 处主治中枢性面瘫、运动性失语、流涎、发音障碍等。

The superior point is located 0.5 cm behind the midpoint of the anterior and posterior midline, while the inferior point is at the intersection of the eyebrow occipital line and the anterior hair line at the temple. The motor zone is the line connecting the two points. Indications:

The upper 1/5 is used for treating paralysis of the lower limb on the opposite side, the mid 2/5, treating paralysis of the upper limb on the opposite side, and lower 2/5, treating central facial paralysis, motor aphasia, salivation, disturbance in phonation.

运用区 praxis zone

从顶部结节至乳突中点，分别引一垂直线及与该线夹角为40°的前后两线，均长约3cm，此三线即为本区。主治精神性失用症。

From the pararietal protuberance to the midpoint of the mastoid draw a line of 3cm long downward, and from the same point draw two oblique lines of 3cm long bilaterally, with an angle of 40° to the first line. It is used for treating mental apraxia.

运针 the manipulation of the needle

指将针刺入人体后施行的各种操作手法。

The variety of techniques of manipulating the inserted needle.

晕灸 fainting during moxibustion

灸治过程中发生的晕厥现象，多因体质虚弱、精神紧张和灸治过度所致。治疗：指压或针刺水沟、素髎、内关、太冲、涌泉。

Fainting or syncope of the patient during moxibustion, mostly due to weakness, nervousness or excessive moxibustion. Treatment principle: Press hard with the finger-nails or puncture Shuigou (GV26), Suliao (GV25), Neiguan (PC6), Taichong (LR3), Yongquan (KI1).

晕针 fainting during acupuncture

针刺异常情况之一。在针刺的过程中，患者突然面色苍白，头晕目眩，心慌气短，出冷汗，胸闷泛恶，脉沉细，严重时可出现四肢厥冷、神志昏迷、二便失禁等。

An abnormal condition during acupuncture. During the acupuncture treatment, the patient is suddenly troubled with pale complexion, dizzness, vertigo, palpitation, shortness of breath, cold sweating, chest stuffiness, nausea, deep and thin pulse, and even cold extremities, loss of consciousness, incontinence of urination and defecation, etc.

熨法 hot medicated compress

把药物粉末或粗粒炒热后，用纱布包裹外敷患部的治疗方法。

An external therapy of applying heated herbal powder or granules wrapped in a cloth to an affected part.

赞刺 repeated shallow needling

十二刺法之一。用于治疗痈肿。刺法是在患处将针直入直出,反复多次地浅刺,使患部出血。

One of the twelve needling techniques for treating carbuncle. It is repeatedly to insert and withdraw the needle vertically and superficially to cause bleeding of the affected part.

脏腑 zang-fu (viscera)

内脏的总称,包括五脏、六腑及奇恒之腑。

The collective name of the internal organs, including the five zang-organs, the six fu-organs and the extraordinary fu-organs.

脏腑辨证 visceral syndrome differentiation

根据脏腑生理、病理特点,对疾病的症状表现进行分析归纳,以判断病变的部位、性质及正邪盛衰状况的一种临床思维方法。它是中医辨证的基本方法之一。

One of the basic methods of differential diagnosis, i. e. , to determine the site and nature of pathological changes and the confliction between the body resistance and the pathogens, based on the analysis and introduction of the clinical manifestations through the observation of the physiological and pathological characeristics of the viscera.

脏腑辨证取穴法 point selection of according to the symptoms of the viscera

通过四诊八纲分辨脏腑、经络之间的联系,选取与疾病有关的穴位进行针灸的一种方法。

To select the points according to the relationship between the viscera and the meridians as determined by means of the four diagnostic methods and the eight principles.

脏会 influential point of zang-organs

即章门穴,为八会穴之一。

It refers to Zhangmen (LR13), one of the eight influential points.

藏俞 zangshu

指五脏各阴经的井、荥、输、经、合各穴,双侧共 50 穴。

The Jing-Well points, Xing-Spring points, Shu-Stream points, Jing-River points and He-Sea points of all the yin meridians of the five zang-organs, fifty points in all on both sides.

藏象学说 visceral manifestation theory

是研究人体脏腑活动规律及其相互关系的学说。它论述脏腑的解剖概念、生理功能和病理现象,对中医诊治疾病有重要的指导意义。

A doctrine on the law of the activities of viscera and their relationships. It not only discuss their anatomical structures, but also on their functional activities and pathological phenomena. It is a guide for the diagnosis and treatment of the diseases in TCM.

早泄 premature ejaculation

性交时排精过早的现象,多由肾虚,相火过旺所致。治宜补益精气、固涩精关。取穴:气海、三阴交、志室、肾俞。

Ejaculation of the semen at the beginning of the sexual act, usually caused by asthenia of the kidney leading to hyperactivity of the minister fire. Treatment principle:Tonify the essential qi so as to control the gate of essence. Point selection:Qihai(CV6), Sanyinjiao(SP6), Zhishi(BL52),Shenshu(BL23).

燥 dryness

①燥邪。六淫之一。其特点是易伤津液,可致目赤,口鼻干燥,干咳,肋痛,便秘等证。②阴津亏损的病症。症见潮热,心烦,唇燥,皮肤干燥,舌干无津。

①Referring to the dryness-evil, one of the six evils, which tends to consume the fluid, and may cause symptoms as conjunctival congestion, dry mouth and nose, non-productive cough, hypochondriac pain, constipation, etc. ②Referring to the dryness syndrome due to consumption of yin-fluid, manifestied as tidal fever, upset, dry lips, skin, and tongue.

躁狂 mania

是神志失常的一种证候。多表现为狂乱不安、手足躁扰等。治宜清肝泻火、清心豁痰。取穴:劳宫、水沟、丰隆、大钟、内庭、行间。

A Syndrome of mental disorder characterized by an expansive emotional state, hyperirritability, increased motor activi-

ty, etc. Treatment principle:Clear the liver-fire,remove heat from the heart and eliminate phlegm for resuscitation. Point selection: Laogong (PC8), Shuigou (GV26), Fenglong(ST40), Dazhong (KI4), Neiting(ST44), Xingjian(LR2).

泽前 Zeqian

经外奇穴名。定位:位于尺泽穴下 1寸。治疗常用直刺或灸治甲状腺肿大,上肢麻痹、痉挛等。

Name of an extra point. Location:1 cun below Chize (LU5). Perpendicular acupuncture or moxibustion is used to cure goiter, upper limb paralysis and cramp.

痄腮 mumps

即流行性腮腺炎。为感受温毒病邪后肠胃积热与肝胆郁火壅遏少阳经脉所致。表现为一侧或两侧腮腺部位肿胀,并有疼痛和压痛。治宜疏风解表、清热解毒。取穴:翳风、颊车、外关、合谷。

Epidemic parotitis caused by the attack of heat-pathogen leading to the accumulation of heat-pathogen in the intestine and stomach and the stagnation of fire pathogen in the liver and gallbladder involving Shaoyang Meridian; marked by swelling of the parotid on one side or on both sides, accompanied with pain and tenderness. Treatment principle:Dispel wind to relieve superficies syndrome and clear heat and toxicity. Point selection:Yifeng (TE17), Jiache(ST6), Waiguan(TE5), Hegu(LI4).

战汗 shiver sweating

即战栗后汗出的症状,是热病过程中正邪相争的表现。如正能胜邪,则疾病随汗而解;如正气不支,则气随汗脱,病趋危重。

A phenomenon indicating the confliction between vital qi and pathogenic evils in the course of a febrile disease. If the vital qi overcomes the evil, the patient recovers after sweating; and if the vital qi cannot overcome the evil, the patient becomes exhausted after sweating.

张从正 Zhang Congzheng

金元四大家之一。因治疗上偏于攻下而被称为攻下派,其学术由麻知己等整理编辑成《儒门事亲》。

One of the four famous physicians in the Jin and Yuan Dynasties, the representative of the school of Purgation or Attack, his learning and experiences were arranged in a book by Ma Zhiji et al, entitled *Confucians' Duties to Their Parents*.

张介宾 Zhang Jiebin

明代医家。编有《类经》《类经图翼》《类经附翼》及《景岳全书》。

A physician of the Ming Dynasty, author of *Classified Canon*, *Illustrated Supplementary to the Classified Canon*, *Subsystematic Classified Canon*, and *Complete Works of Zhang Jingyue*.

章门 Zhangmen (LR13)

经穴名。属足厥阴肝经,脾的募穴,八会穴之一,脏会章门。定位:在侧腹部,当第十一肋游离端的下方。主治:腹胀肠鸣,胁痛,呕吐,泄泻,消化不良等。操作:直刺0.5～1寸;可灸。

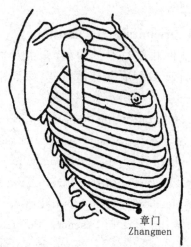

章门
Zhangmen

Name of an acupoint. It belongs to the Liver Meridian of Foot-Jueyin. Front-Mu point of the spleen. Influential point of zang-organs. Location:On the lateral side of the abdomen,below the free end of the 11th rib. Indications:Abdominal distension, borborygmus, pain in the hypochondriac region, vomiting, diarrhea, indigestion, etc. Method:Puncture perpendicularly 0.5-1 cun. Moxibustion is applicable.

掌 palm

手指与手腕之间之内侧面。心包经与心经过掌中。掌心是劳宫穴。

Inner part of the hand between the wrist and fingers through which the Heart and Pericardium meridians pass. The point Laogong (PC8) is located at the center of the palm.

爪切进针法 nail pressure insertion method

进针法之一。其法:两手配合,用左手拇指或示指的指甲切住穴位,右手持针沿着指甲旁迅速刺入。

One of the insertion techniques which consists in cooperative manipulation of the two hands during the insertion, i. e., the thumb nail or index nail of the left hand is used to press incisively on the point while the right hand holding the needle inserts swiftly into the point closely to the pressing nail.

赵学敏 Zhao Xuemin

清代医药学家。著有《本草纲目拾遗》。他搜集和整理民间医生经验,编成《串雅内篇》和《串雅外篇》。

A physician and pharmacist of the Qing Dynasty, author of *A Supplement to the Compendium of Materia Medica*. He summed up the folk healers and experience and systematized it in his works *Internal treatise on Folk Medicine* and *External Treatise on Folk Medicine*.

照海 Zhaohai (KI6)

经穴名。属足少阴肾经,八脉交会穴之一,通于阴跷脉。定位:在足内侧,内踝尖下方凹陷处。主治:月经不调,带下,阴挺,阴痒,尿频,癃闭,便秘,癫痫,失眠,咽喉肿痛,气喘等。操作:直刺 0.5～1 寸;可灸。

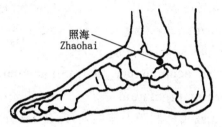

照海
Zhaohai

Name of an acupoint. It belongs to the Kidney Meridian of Foot-Shaoyin. One of the eight confluence points, communicates with Yin Heel Meridian. Location: On the medial side of the foot, in the depression below the tip of the medial malleolus. Indications: Irregular menstruation, leukorrhea, prolapse of uterus, pruritus of vulvae, frequency of micturition, retention of urine, constipation, epilepsy, insomnia, sore throat, asthma, etc. Method: Puncture perpendicularly 0.5-1 cun. Moxibustion is applicable.

折针 breaking of inserted needle

指针法操作时,刺入体内的针突然被折断的异常情况。

An abnormal condition that the needle inserted into the body may accidently be broken during acupuncture treatment.

辄筋 Zhejin (GB23)

经穴名。属足少阳胆经。定位:在侧胸部,渊腋前 1 寸,平乳头,第四肋间隙中。主治:胸满,胁痛,气喘等。操作:斜刺 0.5～0.8 寸;可灸。

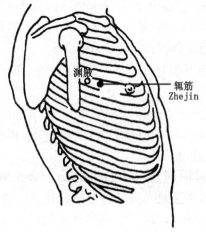

渊腋

辄筋
Zhejin

Name of an acupoint. It belongs to the

Gallbladder Meridian of Foot-Shaoyang. Location:On the lateral side of the chest, 1 cun anterior to Yuanye(GB22), level with the nipple,and in the 4th intercostal space. Indications:Fullness of the chest, pain in the hypochondriac region, asthma etc. Method:Puncture obliquely 0. 5-0. 8 cun. Moxibustion is applicable.

针柄灸 warm needling

即温针灸。

It refers to the warm acupuncture.

针刺补泻 reinforcing and reducing manipulations of acupuncture therapy

指应用不同手法,产生不同刺激强度与特点的针刺方法。如"开阖补泻""迎随补泻""呼吸补泻""疾徐补泻""提插补泻""捻转补泻"等。

Different manipulations of acupuncture generate different intensities and characteristics of stimulation, e. g. "open-closed reinforcing-reducing""directional reinforcing-reducing""respiratory reinforcing-reducing""quick-slow reinforcing-reducing" " lifting-thrusting reinforcing-reducing " "twirling reinforcing-reducing", etc.

针刺感应 needle sensation

患者接受针刺时局部出现的酸、胀、重、麻的感觉。

Patient's local sensation of soreness, distension, pressure or numbness during needling.

针刺后遗感 post-needling sensation

针刺后局部或针刺肢体有酸、麻、胀、重等感觉,一般在出针后数小时自行消失。

Lingering sensation of either soreness, numbness, distension, or pressure felt by the patient following removal of the needle, which usually disappears within se-veral hours.

针刺角度 angle of needle insertion

指针刺时针体与穴位皮面所呈的夹角,一般采用直刺(90°)、斜刺(30°～60°)或平刺(10°～20°)。采用何种角度取决于穴位的解剖特点和刺法的要求。

The angles formed between the needle and the body surface of the point. Perpendicular (90°), oblique(30°-60°)or horizontal(10°-20°)acupunctures are usually adopted according to the anatomical features of the point and to the requirements of the acupuncture.

针刺麻醉 acupuncture anaesthesia

即用针刺进行麻醉的方法。用毫针刺入选定穴位后,通过手法操作(或用电流)进行诱导,使手术区域处于一定的麻醉状态,使患者在神志清醒状态下能够接受各种手术治疗。

The method to induce analgesia by acupuncture. After filiform needles are inserted into the selected points, analgesia of the operative area is induced by manipulating the needles or by applying electric current to the needles. The patient remains fully conscious and can undergo various surgical procedures.

针法 acupuncture therapy; acupuncture mainpulation

①指用针刺激人体经穴(穴位)或敏感点(阿是穴),通过经络的调整作用,达到治疗目的的方法。②各种针具针刺操作

方法的总称。

①To stimulate a certain acupoint or a trigger point (Ashi point) by a needle so as to treat diseases through the regulating action of meridians and collaterals. ②A general term of all kinds of acupuncture manipulations with all kinds of needles.

针感 needle sensation

又称针刺感应。指患者对针刺所产生的酸、胀、重、麻等感觉,以及医生手指所感到的针下沉紧的反应。

Also known as acupuncture reactions, i. e. , the sensations of soreness, distention, pressure, numbness, etc. of the patient during acupuncture as well as the adsorbing reaction of the needle felt by the doctor's fingers.

针灸 acupuncture and moxibustion

针刺法和艾灸法的合称。

A collective term for acupuncture therapy and moxibustion therapy with Chinese mugwort.

针灸大成 Compendium of Acupuncture and Moxibustion

书名。明代杨继洲撰。该书全面总结了明代以前的针灸学术成就。

A comprehensive summing-up of experiences and achievements in acupuncture and moxibustion up to then, collected by Yang Jizhou in the Ming Dynasty.

针灸大全 Complete Guinness of Acupuncture and Moxibustion

书名。明代徐凤撰,是一部综合性的针灸著作。

The complete work on acupuncture and moxibustion compiled by Xu Feng in the Ming Dynasty.

针灸逢源 Feng Yuan of Acupuncture and Moxibustion

书名。清代李学川撰。

The work on acupuncture and moxibustion compiled by Li Xuechuan in the Qing Dynasty.

针灸甲乙经 A-B Classic of Acupuncture and Moxibustion

晋代皇甫谧撰,是中国现存最早、内容较完整的针灸专著。

The earliest more complete work on acupuncture and moxibustion extant in China, compiled by Huangfu Mi in the Jin Dynasty.

针灸聚英 Collection of Gems in Acupuncture and Moxibustion

又名《针灸聚英发挥》。明代高武撰。

Also known as An Elucidation of the Collection of Gems in Acupuncture and Moxibustion, written by Gao Wu in the Ming Dynasty.

针灸铜人 bronze acupuncture figure

我国宋代著名医官司王惟一设计,并用铜铸造的刻有标准经络腧穴的人体模型,常用作教学和医生考试的教具。铜人外涂黄蜡,内盛清水,如果针法准确,刺中穴位,水即从孔中流出。

Bronze human model designed by Wang Weiyi, which was engraved with the standardized meridian and collateral and acupuncture points, as the teaching model for teaching and examination of practitioner. The figure was coated with a layer of wax and filled with water. If the point was punctured accurately, the water would flow out from the point immediately, if not, the water could not flow out.

针灸资生经 *Classic of Nourishing Life with Acupuncture and Moxibustion*

宋代王执中撰。该书包括人体各部腧穴及作者的临床心得,并附图46幅。

A systematic presentation of acupuncture and moxibustion, including the location of points of various parts of the body, the author's experiences of clinical practice and 46 illustrations, written by Wang Zhizhong in the Song Dynasty.

针挑疗法 needle-pricking method

针刺疗法之一,选一定的腧穴或某些体表部位出现的异点,用粗针挑刺出血或使渗出少量液体,或挑出少量白色纤维样物。

A form of needling therapy, using large-gauge needle to prick the skin at selected point or the affected part until blood or tissue fluid appears, or until whitish fiber-like substance are picked up.

针尾 needle end

针柄末端。

Upper end of the needle handle.

针向补泻 directional reinforcing-reducing

指以针芒顺逆分补泻,即迎随补泻。

Method of reinforcing-reducing by the directions of the needle point along or against the channel moving directions, as is the same as the method of meeting and following reinforcing-reducing.

诊法 diagnostic methods

诊断疾病的方法。一般是指四诊。

The methods used for diagnosing disease, generally referring to the four diagnostic methods.

枕 Zhen

耳穴名。在对耳屏外侧面后上方。主治:头晕,头痛,失眠,神经衰弱,哮喘,癫痫。

Name of an ear point. It is at the posterior superior corner of the lateral aspect of antitragus. Indications: Dizziness, headache, insomnia, neurasthenia, asthma, epilepsy, etc.

枕骨 Zhengu

头窍阴穴别名。

The other name of Touqiaoyin (ST8).

震颤法 trembling technique

针刺手法名。捏持针柄做上下震颤的动作,以加强针感。

Name of the acupuncture technique, i. e. , holding the needle handle and vibrating the needle upward and downward at a high frequency and small amplitude to promote the needling sensations.

怔忡 severe palpitation

自觉心跳剧烈的证候。多由阴血亏损,心失所养;或心阳不足,水饮上逆;或突受惊恐所致。以虚证为多。治宜益心安神、养血定惊。取穴:心俞、巨阙、间使、神门、膈俞、通里。

A symptom due to heart disorder resulting from consumption of yin-blood, or insufficiency of heart-yang with fluid retention, or sudden frightening; mostly seen in deficiency syndrome. Treatment principle: Supplement qi and tranquilize mind, enrich blood and arrest convulsion. Point selection: Xinshu (BL15), Juque (CV14), Jianshi (PC5), Shenmen (HT7), Geshu(BL17), Tongli(HT5).

蒸脐治病法 medicinal partition moxibustion on the navel

间隔灸法之一。以多种中药配合成膏状,涂于脐内,上施以随年壮。

One kind of the partition moxibustion with traditional Chinese drugs paste put into the navel and with the number of the moxa cones on the navel in accordance with the patient's age.

正经 regular meridians

指十二条直接与内脏相联络的主要经脉。包括手太阴肺经、手阳明大肠经、足阳明胃经、足太阴脾经、手少阴心经、手太阳小肠经、足太阳膀胱经、足少阴肾经、手厥阴心包经、手少阳三焦经、足少阳胆经、足厥阴肝经。

They are the twelve meridians connecting directly with the viscera, including the Lung Meridian of Hand-Taiyin, the Large Intestine Meridian of Hand-Yangming, the Stomach Meridian of Foot-Yangming, the Spleen Meridian of Foot-Taiyin, the Heart Meridian of Hand-Shaoyin, the Small Intestine Meridian of Hand-Taiyang, the Urinary Bladder Meridian of Foot-Taiyang, the Kidney Meridian of Foot-Shaoyin, the Pericardium Meridian of Hand-Jueyin, the Sanjiao Meridian of Hand-Shaoyang, the Gall-bladder Meridian of Foot-Shaoyang, and the Liver Meridian of Foot-Jueyin.

正气 vital qi; normal climate

①又称真气。指机体生命功能和抗病能力。②指四季正常气候。即春温、夏热、秋凉、冬寒。

①The vital function of the body and the body resistance against diseases; also termed genuine qi. ②The proper climate matched with the four seasons, i. e., warm in spring, hot in summer, cool in autumn and cold in winter.

正邪相争 counteraction between vital qi and pathogens

即致病因素侵入人体后与机体抗病功能的互相作用。一般地说,一切疾病都是这种作用的反映,拿个别症状来说,如恶寒发热,就是正邪斗争的反映。

A condition of the invaded pathogenic agents and the body resistance acting against each other, generally representing the process of all diseases, as an individual symptom, for example, chilliness and fever signify this counteraction.

正虚邪实 deficiency of vital qi and excessive of evil

指正气不足或邪气过盛的病理现象,通常以正虚为本、邪实为标。

A morbid condition of low body resistance and hyperactivity of the pathogenic factor, in which the deficiency of vital qi is primary or causative, while the sthenia of evil is secondary or resultant.

正穴 regular acupoints

指十四经腧穴,与经外奇穴相对而言。

The acupoints of the fourteen meridians as contrasted with the extra points.

正营 Zhengying (GB17)

经穴名。属足少阳胆经。定位：在头部，当前发际上 2.5 寸，头正中线旁开 2.25 寸。主治：偏头痛，眩晕等。操作：平刺 0.5～0.8 寸；可灸。

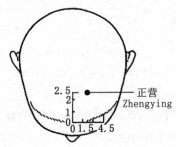

Name of an acupoint. It belongs to the Gallbladder Meridian of Foot-Shaoyang. Location：On the head, 2.5 cun above the anterior hairline and 2.25 cun lateral to the midline of the head. Indications：Migraine, vertigo, etc. Method：Puncture horizontally 0.5-0.8 cun. Moxibustion is applicable.

证候 symptoms and signs

根据临床表现，对疾病发展过程中的某一阶段的病因、病位、病性、邪正盛衰等所做的病理概括。

A pathological synthesis of cause, location, nature of disease at certain stage in the course of development together with waxing-waning of pathogenic factor and vital qi according to clinical manipulations.

支沟 Zhigou (TE6)

经穴名。属手少阳三焦经，本经经穴。定位：在臂背侧，当阳池与肘尖的连线上，腕背横纹上 3 寸，尺骨与桡骨之间。主治：耳鸣，耳聋，胁痛，呕吐，便秘，热病，瘰疬，暴喑。操作：直刺 0.5～1 寸；可灸。

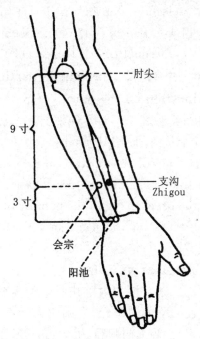

The acupoint, Jing-River point, belongs to the Sanjiao Meridian of Hand-Shaoyang. Location：On the dorsal side of the forearm and on the line connecting Yangchi(TE4) and the tip of the olecranon, 3 cun proximal to the dorsal crease of the wrist, between the radius and ulnar. Indications：Tinnitus, deafness, pain in hypochondriac, vomiting, constipation, febrile diseases, scrofula, sudden hoarseness of voice, etc. Method：Puncture perpendicularly 0.5-1 cun. Moxibustion is applicable.

支节 zhijie

支，指四肢；节，指骨节。支节又泛指穴位。

Zhi means four extremities; jie means joints. In the extensive meaning they also refer to the acupoints when used together.

支正 Zhizheng (SI7)

经穴名。属手太阳小肠经，本经络穴。定位：在前臂背面尺侧，当阳谷与小海的连线上，腕背横纹上 5 寸。主治：项强，头痛，头晕，癫痫，热病，肘臂酸痛。操作：直刺或斜刺 0.5～0.8 寸；可灸。

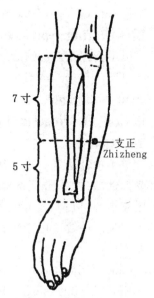

7寸

5寸

支正
Zhizheng

The acupoint, Luo-Connecting point, belongs to the Small Intestine Meridian of Hand-Taiyang. Location: On the ulnar side of the posterior side of the forearm and on the line connecting Yanggu(SI5) and Xiaohai(SI8), 5 cun proximal to the dorsal crease of the wrist. Indications: Neck rigidity, headache, dizziness, mania, febrile diseases, pain in the elbow and arm, etc. Method: Puncture perpendicularly or obliquely 0.5-0.8 cun. Moxibustion is applicable.

肢节痛 arthralgia of extremities

指肢体关节疼痛不适的症状。多因风湿、寒湿、痰饮、瘀血留滞经络或因血虚不能养筋所致。治宜通经活络。取穴：肩髃、曲池、合谷、阳溪、髀关、梁丘、足三里、解溪。

A disorder mostly due to the retention of wind-damp, cold-damp, phlegm or blood stasis in the meridians, or due to blood deficiency failing to nourish the tendon. Treatment principle: Clear and activate the meridians and collaterals. Point selection: Jianyu (LI15), Quchi(LI11), Hegu(LI4), Yangxi (LI5), Biguan(ST31), Liangqiu(ST34), Zusanli(ST36), Jiexi(ST41).

直肠 Zhichang

耳穴名。又称直肠下段。在耳屏上切迹的耳轮处。主治：便秘，脱肛，痔疮等。

Name of an ear point, also named Zhichangxiaduan. It is on the end of the helix approximate to superior tragic notch. Indications: Constipation, anus prolapse, hemorrhoids, etc.

直刺 perpendicular acupuncture

指针体与穴位皮肤面呈 90°角左右的刺法。适用于肌肉丰厚部及四肢部。

Acupuncture with an angle of 90° between the needle and the point skin surface, suitable for the fleshy parts and the extremities.

直接灸 direct moxibustion

指将艾炷直接放在体表穴位的皮肤上进行灸治的方法。

To administer moxibustion with a burning moxa cone directly on the skin of the point.

直针刺 perpendicular needling

十二刺法之一。用于治疗病位较浅的寒痹。刺法是提起皮肤，刺入皮下，不需深刺。

One of the twelve needling techniques for treating cold bi in a relatively shallow area. It is to lift the skin and puncture subcutaneously but not deeply.

指 Zhi

耳穴名。在耳舟的上端。主治手指麻木疼痛。

Name of an ear point. It is at the top of scapha. It is used for treating numbness and pain of fingers.

指拨法 plucking technique with a finger

针刺手法名。进针后,拇、示指捏持针柄,以中指轻轻拨动针体,以增强针感。

Name of the manipulating technique, i. e. , after insertion, the thumb and the index finger firmly hold the needly handle while the middle finger pluck the needle to increase the sensations.

指寸 finger cun

以患者的手指作为取穴的比例寸。包括中指寸、拇指寸和横指寸。

Using the patient's fingers as the proportional measurement units for locating acupoints, including the middle finger cun, the thumb cun and the transverse finger cun.

指根 Zhigen

经外奇穴名。定位:位于第二、三、四、五指指掌横纹之中点,左右共计 8 穴。三棱针点刺出血,主治手部疔疮、指痛、腹痛、呕吐,并可解热。此穴又称四横纹、下四缝。

Name of extra points. Location:At the midpoints of the four palm phalangeal creases except the thumb crease,8 points in all. Letting out blood with a three-edged needle can cure hand sores, finger pain, abdominal pain, vomiting and to relieve fever. The point is also known as "Sihengwen" and "Xiasifeng".

指压法 finger-press method

以手指按压穴位的治疗方法。

Therapeutic method of pressing the point with finger.

指压进针 fingernail-pressing needle insertion

单手进针法之一。一般是右手拇、示指紧捏针柄,中指或无名指直抵穴位,针身紧靠指旁,以拇、示指的压力将针迅速刺入穴位。一般适用于短针进针,不需左手按压。

One of the needle inserting techniques with only one single hand, i. e. , the thumb and the index finger firmly grip the needle handle and the middle or ring finger directly presses on the point, closely against the middle or ring finger, the needle will be swiftly inserted into the point by the thrusting force of the gripping fingers. The technique is usually adopted for short needle insertion without the help of the left hand.

指针 finger acupuncture

指用手指按压、揉摩体表的穴位以代替针刺的治疗方法。

Using the finger to press and knead the points on the body surface instead of using needles.

趾 Zhi

耳穴名。定位:在对耳轮上脚的外上角。主治肢体相应部位的疼痛及功能障碍。

Name of an ear point. Location:At the superior and lateral corner of the superior antihelix crus. It is used for treating pain and dysfunction of corresponding area of the body.

至阳 Zhiyang (GV9)

经穴名。属督脉。定位:在背部,当后正中线上,第七胸椎棘突下凹陷中。主治:黄疸,咳嗽,气喘,脊强,胸背痛等。操作:向上斜刺 0.5~1 寸;可灸。

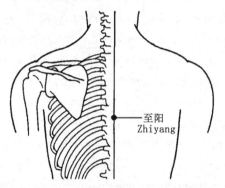

至阳
Zhiyang

Name of an acupoint. It belongs to the Governor Vessel. Location:On the back and on the posterior midline, in the depression below the spinous process of the 7th thoracic vertebra. Indications:Jaundice, asthma, cough, stiffness of the back, pain in the chest and back, etc. Method:Puncture obliquely upward 0.5-1 cun. Moxibustion is applicable.

至阴 Zhiyin (BL67)

经穴名。属足太阳膀胱经,本经井穴。定位:在足小趾末节外侧,距趾甲角 0.1 寸。主治:头痛,鼻塞,鼻衄,目痛,胎位不正,难产,胞衣不下等。操作:浅刺 0.1 寸;可灸。

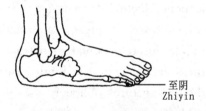

至阴
Zhiyin

The acupoint, Jing-Well point, belongs to the Bladder Meridian of Foot-Taiyang. Location:On the lateral side of the distal segment of the little toe, 0.1 cun from the corner of the toenail. Indications:Headache, nasal obstruction, epistaxis, eye pain, malposition of fetus, difficult labour, retention of placenta, etc. Method:Puncture shallowly 0.1 cun. Moxibustion is applicable.

志室 Zhishi (BL52)

经穴名。属足太阳膀胱经。定位:在腰部,当第二腰椎棘突下,旁开 3 寸。主治:遗精,阳痿,遗尿,尿频,水肿,小便不利,月经不调,腰脊强痛等。操作:斜刺 0.5~0.8 寸;可灸。

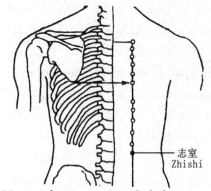

志室
Zhishi

Name of an acupoint. It belongs to the Bladder Meridian of Foot-Taiyang. Location:On the lower back, below the spinous process of the 2nd lumbar vertebra,

3 cun lateral to the posterior midline. Indications:Nocturnal emission, impotence, enuresis, frequency of urination, edema, dysuria, irregular menstruation, stiffness and pain of the lumbar spine. Method:Puncture obliquely 0.5-0. 8 cun. Moxibustion is applicable.

治腑者取其合 treat the fu-organs diseases with the He-Sea points

取穴法则之一。即治疗六腑病要取位在足三阳经上的六腑合穴。

One of the point-selecting principles, i. e. , in order to cure the diseases of the six fu-organs, the He-Sea points of the three Foot-Yang Meridians should be selected.

治痿独取阳明 treat the atrophy specifically with Yangming Meridian

取穴法则之一。即治痿证应专取阳明经的穴位,兼取受病之经的穴位。

One of the point-selecting principles, i. e. , to treat atrophic diseases, the points of Yangming Meridians should be adopted with the points of the diseased meridians as adjuvant.

治脏者取其输 treat the visceral diseases with the Shu-Stream points

取穴法则之一。即治疗五脏的病症要取相应经脉的输穴。

One of the point-selecting principles, i. e. , in order to cure the diseases of the five viscera, the Shu-Stream points of the corresponding meridians should be adopted.

秩边 Zhibian (BL54)

经穴名。属足太阳膀胱经。定位:在臀部,平第四骶后孔,骶正中嵴旁开 3 寸。主治:腰骶痛,下肢痿痹,小便不利,阴肿,痔疾,便秘等。操作:直刺 1.5～2 寸;可灸。

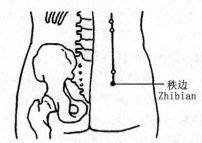

Name of an acupoint. It belongs to the Bladder Meridian of Foot-Taiyang. Location:On the buttock,level with the 4th posterior sacral foramen, 3 cun lateral to the median sacral crest. Indications:Pain in lumbosacral region, muscular atrophy, motor impairment of the lower extremities, dysuria, swelling around external genitalia, hemorrhoids, constipation, etc. Method: Puncture perpendicularly 1. 5-2 cun. Moxibustion is applicable.

痔核点 Zhihedian

耳穴名。定位:在与对耳轮上脚前缘相对的耳轮处。主治痔疮。

Name of an ear point. Location:On the helix, on the anterior border of superior antihelix crus. It is used for treating hemorrhoid.

滞针 stuck needle

针刺治疗时,刺入人体内的针出现的不能捻转、提插或手法操作困难等现象。多因患者精神紧张,肌肉痉挛;或捻转幅度过大,肌纤维缠绕针尖所致。一般在滞针部位周围轻度按摩,并将针轻轻提出;或在附近再刺一针,使肌肉松弛后,再将针拔出。

An abnormal condition occurring in the acupuncture therapy due to emotional stress and muscular spasm of the patient or fixation of the needle by fibrous tissues resulting from over-rotating. The needle can be withdrawn by gentle massage or giving another puncture nearby to relieve the muscular spasm.

中病傍取 central diseases treated with the peripheral points

《内经》取穴法之一。指中部的病症取用其周围穴。

One of the point-selecting principles in *Huangdi's Canon of Medicine*, i. e., the central diseases can be cured with peripheral points.

中冲 Zhongchong (PC9)

经穴名。属手厥阴心包经,本经井穴。定位:在手中指尖端的中央。主治:心痛,心悸,昏迷,舌强肿痛失语,热病,小儿惊风,掌中热等。操作:浅刺0.1寸,或点刺出血;可灸。

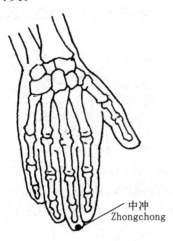

中冲
Zhongchong

The acupoint, Jing-Well point, belongs to the Pericardium Meridian of Hand-Jueyin. Location: At the center of the tip of the middle finger. Indications: Cardialgia, palpitation, loss of consciousness, aphasia with stiffness and swelling of the tongue, febrile diseases, infantile convulsion, feverish sensation in the palm, etc. Method: Puncture shallowly 0.1 cun or prick with a three-edged needle to cause bleeding. Moxibustion is applicable.

中都 Zhongdu (LR6)

经穴名。属足厥阴肝经,本经郄穴。定位:在小腿内侧,当足内踝尖上7寸,胫骨内侧面的中央。主治:腹痛,胁痛,泄泻,疝气,崩漏,恶露不尽等。操作:平刺0.5～0.8寸;可灸。

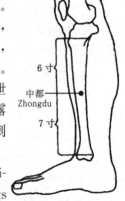

6寸

中都
Zhongdu

7寸

The acupoint, Xi-Cleft point, belongs to the Liver Meridian of Foot-Jueyin. Location: On the medial side of the leg, 7 cun above the tip of the medial malleolus, in the middle of the medial aspect of the tibia. Indications: Abdominal pain, hypochondriac pain, diarrhea, hernia, metrorrhagia and metrostaxis, prolonged lochia, etc. Method: Puncture horizontally 0.5-0.8 cun. Moxibustion is applicable.

中渎 Zhongdu (GB32)

经穴名。属足少阳胆经。定位:在大腿

外侧,当风市下 2 寸,或在腘横纹上 5 寸,股外侧肌与股二头肌之间。主治:膝腿酸痛,痿弱,半身不遂等。操作:直刺 1～2 寸;可灸。

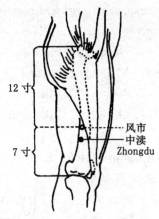

12 寸

7 寸

风市
中渎
Zhongdu

Name of an acupoint. It belongs to the Gallbladder Meridian of Foot-Shaoyang. Location:On the lateral side of the thigh, 2 cun below Fengshi(GB31)or 5 cun above the poplifeal crease,between the vastus lateralis and biceps femoris. Indications:Pain and soreness of the thigh and knee, numbness and weakness of the lower limbs, hemiplegia. Method:Puncture perpendicularly 1-2 cun. Moxibustion is applicable.

中耳背 Zhongerbei

耳穴名。主治:皮肤病,坐骨神经痛,背痛等。

Name of an ear point. Indications:Dermatosis, sciatica, back pain, etc.

中封 Zhongfeng (LR4)

经穴名。属足厥阴肝经,本经经穴。定位:在足背侧,当内踝前,商丘与解溪连线上,胫骨前肌肌腱的内侧凹陷处。主治:疝气,外阴痛,遗精,小便不利,胁胀痛等。

操作:直刺 0.5～1 寸;可灸。

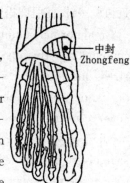

中封
Zhongfeng

The acupoint, Jing-River point, belongs to the Liver Meridian of Foot-Jueyin. Location:On the instep of the foot, anterior to the medial malleolus, on the line connecting Shangqiu(SP5) and Jiexi(ST41), in the depression medial to the tendon of the anterior tibia muscle. Indications:Hernia, pain in the external genitalia, nocturnal emission, retention of urine, distending pain in the hypochondrium, etc. Method:Puncture perpendicularly 0.5-1 cun. Moxibustion is applicable.

中府 Zhongfu (LU1)

经穴名。手太阴肺经募穴。定位:在胸前壁的外上方,云门下 1 寸,平第一肋间隙,前正中线旁开 6 寸。主治:咳嗽,气喘,胸痛,肩背痛,胸胁胀满等。操作:可向外斜刺0.5～0.8 寸,不宜过深,以免伤及肺脏。

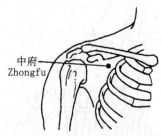

中府
Zhongfu

The acupoint, Front-Mu point, belongs to the Lung Meridian of Hand-Taiyin. Location:In the superior lateral part of the anterior thoracic wall, 1 cun below Yunmen(LU2), level with the 1st intercostal space, 6 cun lateral to the anterior midline. Indications: Cough, asthma, pain in the chest, shoulder and back, fullness of the chest, etc. Method: Puncture obliquely 0. 5-0. 8 cun towards the lateral aspect of the chest. To avoid injuring the lung, never puncture deeply towards the medial aspect.

中国针灸学概要 *An Outline of Chinese Acupuncture and Moxibustion*

北京中医学院、南京中医学院、上海中医学院、中医研究院针灸研究所合编,1964 年成书。分上、中、下三篇:上篇讲中医基础理论,中篇介绍经络及腧穴,下篇介绍针灸治疗 52 种常见病的方法。

A book dealing with the basic theory of traditional Chinese medicine, meridians, collaterals, and acupoints, the methods of acutherapy in 52 common diseases, compiled by Beijing, Nanjing and Shanghai Colleges of Traditional Chinese Medicine, Institute of Acupuncture and Moxibustion of the Academy of Traditional Chinese Medicine in 1964.

中极 Zhongji (CV3)

经穴名。属任脉,膀胱的募穴。定位:在下腹部,前正中线上,当脐中下 4 寸。主治:遗精,遗尿,阳痿,疝气,崩漏,月经不调,痛经,白带,尿频,小便不利,少腹痛,阴挺,阴道炎等。操作:直刺 0. 5～1 寸;可灸。

Name of an acupoint. It belongs to the Conception Vessel. Front-Mu point of the bladder. Location: On the lower abdomen and on the anterior midline, 4 cun below the

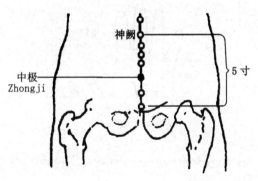

centre of the umbilicus. Indications: Nocturnal emission, enuresis, impotence, hernia, metrorrhagia and metrostaxis, irregular menstruation, dysmenorrhea, leukorrhea disease, frequency of urination, dysuria, lower abdomen pain, uterine prolapse, vaginitis, etc. Method: Puncture perpendicularly 0. 5-1 cun. Moxibustion is applicable.

中焦 middle jiao

三焦的中部,膈以下、脐以上的部位,脾胃位于其中。主要功能是消化、吸收、传输营养物质。

The middle part of sanjiao, corresponding to the body cavity below the diaphragm and above the level of the umbilicus, where the stomach and spleen are located. Its main function is to digest the food, to absorb and transport the nutrients.

中魁 Zhongkui (EX-UE4)

经外奇穴名。定位:在手背中指近端指间关节的中点。主治:恶心,呕吐,呃逆等。

Name of an extra point. Location: On the midpoint of the proximal interphalangeal joint of the middle finger at dorsum

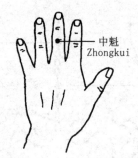

中魁
Zhongkui

aspect. Indications：Nausea， vomiting， hiccup, etc.

中髎 Zhongliao（BL33）

经穴名。属足太阳膀胱经。定位：在骶部，当次髎下内方，适对第三骶后孔处。主治：腰痛，便秘，泄泻，小便不利，月经不调等。操作：直刺 1～1.5 寸；可灸。

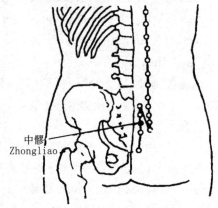

中髎
Zhongliao

Name of an acupoint. It belongs to the Bladder Meridian of Foot-Taiyang. Location：On the sacrum, medial and inferior to Ciliao(BL32), just at the 3rd posterior sacral foramen. Indications：Lower back pain, constipation, diarrhea, dysuria, irregular menstruation, etc. Method：Puncture perpendicularly 1-1.5 cun. Moxibustion is applicable.

中膂俞 Zhonglüshu（BL29）

经穴名。属足太阳膀胱经。定位：在骶部，当骶正中嵴旁 1.5 寸，第三骶后孔。主治：泄泻，疝气，腰脊强痛等。操作：直刺 1～1.5 寸；可灸。

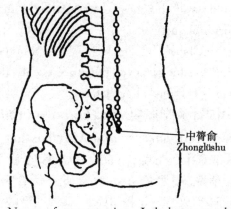

中膂俞
Zhonglüshu

Name of an acupoint. It belongs to the Bladder Meridian of Foot-Taiyang. Location：On the sacrum, level with the 3rd posterior sacral foramen, 1.5 cun lateral to the median sacral crest. Indications：Diarrhea, hernia, stiffness and pain of the lower back, etc. Method：Puncture perpendicularly 1-1.5 cun. Moxibustion is applicable.

中平 Zhongping

经外奇穴名。定位：位于中指指掌横纹之中央。主治口腔炎。直刺或灸治。

Name of an extra point. Location：At the center of the crease between the middle finger and the palm. Main indication is stomatitis using perpendicular acupuncture or moxibustion.

中气不足 deficiency of middle qi

脾胃之气虚弱，引起消化吸收功能减退的病理。症见食欲不振、面色淡白、眩晕、怠倦乏力、大便稀烂、声低、气短、脉虚等。治宜补气养血。取穴：脾俞、胃俞、足三里、三阴交、关元、气海。

A morbid condition caused by the debility of the spleen-qi and stomach-qi leading to the disturbance of digestive function; manifested as poor appetite, pallor, dizziness, fatigue, discharge of loose stools, low voice, shortness of breath, feeble pulse, etc. Treatment principle: Tonify qi and nourish blood. Point selection: Pishu (BL20), Weishu (BL21), Zusanli (SP36), Sanyinjiao (SP6), Guanyuan(CV4), Qihai(CV6).

中泉 Zhongquan(EX-UE3)

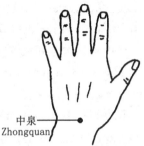

经外奇穴名。定位：在腕背横纹中，当指总伸肌腱桡侧凹陷处。主治：胸满，胃痛，吐血等。

Name of an extra point. Location: On the dorsal transverse crease of the wrist, in the depression on the radial side of the tendon of the common extensor muscle of the fingers. Indications: Stuffiness of chest, gastric pain, spitting of blood, etc.

中守 Zhongshou

水分穴别名。

The other name of Shuifen (CV9).

中枢 Zhongshu (GV7)

经穴名。属督脉。定位：在背部，当后正中线上，第十胸椎棘突下凹陷中。主治：腰脊强痛，上腹痛等。操作：向上斜刺0.5～1寸；可灸。

Name of an acupoint. It belongs to the

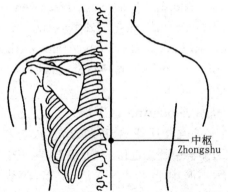

Governor Vessel. Location: On the back and on the posterior midline, in the depression below the spinous process of the 10th thoracic vertebra. Indications: Stiffness and pain of the lower back, pain in the epigastric region, etc. Method: Puncture obliquely upward 0.5-1 cun. Moxibustion is applicable.

中庭 Zhongting (CV16)

经穴名。属任脉。定位：在胸部，当前正中线上，平第五肋间，即胸剑联合部。主治：胸胁胀满，恶心，呃逆等。操作：平刺0.3～0.5寸；可灸。

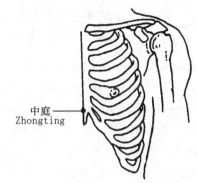

Name of an acupoint. It belongs to the Conception Vessel. Location: On the chest and on the anterior midline, level with the 5th intercostal space, i. e., the xiphisternal synchondrosis. Indications: Distension and fullness in the chest and hypochondrium, nausea, hiccup, etc. Method: Puncture horizontally 0. 3-0. 5 cun. Moxibustion is applicable.

中脘 Zhongwan (CV12)

经穴名。属任脉,胃的募穴,八会穴之一,腑会中脘。定位:在上腹部,前正中线上,当脐中上 4 寸。主治:胃痛,腹胀肠鸣,恶心呕吐,吞酸,泄泻,痢疾,黄疸,消化不良,失眠等。操作:直刺 0. 5～1 寸;可灸。

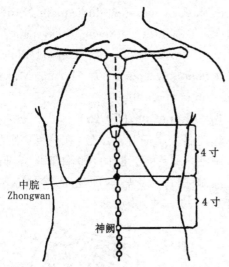

中脘
Zhongwan

4寸

4寸

神阙

Name of an acupoint. It belongs to the Conception Vessel. Front-Mu point of the stomach. Influential point of the fu-organs. Location: On the upper abdomen and on the anterior midline, 4 cun above the center of the umbilicus. Indications: Stomach pain, abdominal distension, borborygmus, nausea, vomiting, acid regurgitation, diarrhea, dysentery, jaundice, indigestion, insomnia. Method: Puncture perpendicularly 0. 5-1 cun. Moxibustion is applicable.

中郄 Zhongxi

①中都穴别名。②委中穴别名。

①The other name of Zhongdu (LR6). ②The other name of Weizhong (BL40).

中指节 Zhongzhijie

经外奇穴名。位于手中指背侧,远端指节横纹中点稍前之凹陷中。灸治牙痛有奇效。

Name of an extra point. Located at the depression slightly before the midpoint of the distal interphalangeal joint crease on the back of the middle finger. Moxibustion is effective in treating toothache.

中指内间 inner web of the middle toe

足中趾与次趾间之缝隙。

The web region between the middle and the second toes.

中指同身寸法 oneself middle finger measurement、中指寸 middle finger cun

针刺取穴法之一。以患者中指中节桡侧两端纹头间距离为 1 寸(拇、中指屈曲成环形),常用于四肢和背部的取穴。

One of the method of locating acupoints. 1 cun is equivalent to the distance between the two radial end of the transverse creases of the interphalangeal joints of the patient's middle finger when it is fixed. It is usually used in locating points on the back and limbs.

中指外间 outer web of the middle toe

足中趾与第四趾之间的缝隙。

The web region between the middle and the fouth toe.

中渚 Zhongzhu (TE3)

经穴名。属手少阳三焦经,本经输穴。定位:在手背部,当环指本节的后方,第四、五掌骨间凹陷处。主治:

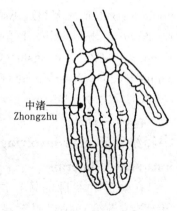

头痛,目赤,耳聋耳鸣,咽喉肿痛,热病,臂肘痛,手指不能屈伸等。操作:直刺0.3~0.5寸;可灸。

The acupoint, Shu-Stream point, belongs to the Sanjiao Meridian of Hand-Shaoyang. Location: On the dorsum of the hand, posterior to the 4th metacarpophalangeal joint, in the depression between the 4th and the 5th metacarpal bones. Indications: Headache, red eyes, deafness, sore throat, febrile diseases, pain in the elbow and arm, motor impairment of finger, etc. Method: Puncture perpendicularly 0. 3-0. 5 cun. Moxibustion is applicable.

中注 Zhongzhu (KI15)

经穴名。属足少阴肾经。定位:在中腹部,当脐中下1寸,前正中线旁开0.5寸。主治:月经不调,腹痛,便秘等。操作:直刺1~1.5寸;可灸。

Name of an acupoint. It belongs to the Kidney Meridian of Foot-Shaoyin. Location: On the medial abdomen, 1 cun below the center of the umbilicus and 0. 5 cun lateral to the anterior midline. Indica-

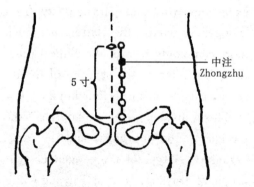

tions: Irregular menstruation, abdominal pain, constipation, etc. Method: Puncture perpendicularly 1-1. 5 cun. Moxibustion is applicable.

中柱 Zhongzhu

中枢穴别名。

The other name of Zhongshu (GV7).

踵 zhong

部位名。指足跟部。

Name of a body part, i. e. , the heel.

中风 apoplexy; wind-stroke

①猝然昏倒,伴口眼歪斜、言语不利、半身不遂的病证。古代医家将其分为真中风与类中风两大类,临床所见多为类中风。按其病情轻重又分为中络、中经、中腑、中脏。常见于脑血管意外。②外感风邪的病证。是太阳表证的一个类型,见于太阳中风(外感风寒病邪侵袭太阳经的病证)。症见头项强痛,发热,恶风,自汗,脉浮缓等。治宜醒脑开窍、通经活络。取穴:内关、水沟、极泉、委中、太冲、十二井。

① Sudden syncope accompanied with deviation of mouth and eyes, dysphasia and hemiplegia, usually seen in cerbrovascular accidents. There are two kinds of apoplexy, i. e. , true apoplexy from exogenous wind and paraapoplexy from endogenous wind, the latter is much more commonly seen in the clinical practice. According to the severity of the disease, it is divided into four kinds, i. e., apoplexy involving the collaterals, the meridians, the fu-organs, and the zang-organs. ②A type of the exogenous-syndrome of Taiyang; seen in Taiyang wind-stroke syndrome (a disease caused by the attack of wind-cold pathogens to the Taiyang Meridian); manifested as stiffness and pain of the neck, headache, fever, aversion to wind, spontaneous sweating, floating and slow pulse, etc. Treatment principle: Activate the brain and regain consciousness, clear and activate the meridians and collaterals. Point selection: Neiguan (PC6), Shuigou (CV26), Jiquan (HT1), Weizhong (BL40), Taichong (LR3), the twelve Jing-Well points.

中风不语 Zhongfengbuyu

经外奇穴名。定位：位于第二、五胸椎棘突上。主治中风不语。灸治。

Name of an extra points. Location: Above the 2nd and the 5th spinous processes of thoracic vertebra. Main indication is aphasia from apoplexy by using moxibustion.

中风七穴 seven points for apoplexy

指治疗中风的七个经验穴：百会，耳前发际，肩井，风市，足三里，悬钟，曲池。对侧灸治。

Seven empirical effective points for a-poplexy: Baihui (GV20), Erqianfaji (extra point at the hairline before the ear), Jianjing (GB21), Fengshi (GB31), Zusanli (ST36), Xuanzhong (GB39), Quchi (LI11). Moxibustion is applicable on the opposite side.

中经络 apoplexy involving the meridians and collaterals

病在经脉和络脉的较轻型的中风证。以无神志改变而见口眼歪斜、半身不遂、言语不利为特征。治宜醒脑开窍、通经活络。取穴：内关、水沟、极泉、委中、太冲、十二井。

A milder type of apoplexy involving the meridians and collaterals, marked by deviation of mouth and eyes, hemiplegia and dysphasia, but no impairment of consciousness. Treatment principle: Activate the brain and regain consciousness, clear and activate the meridians and collaterals. Point selection: Neiguan (PC6), Shuigou (CV26), Jiquan (HT1), Weizhong (BL40), Taichong (LR3), the twelve Jing-Well points.

中暑 sunstroke

炎热高温环境中感受暑邪而突然昏厥的病证。多伴见身热烦躁、气喘、大汗或无汗、牙关紧闭、四肢抽搐等。治宜清泄暑热、醒神。取穴：水沟、十宣、曲泽、委中、曲池。

A condition of sudden syncope caused by the attack of summer-heat pathogen under an environment with high temperature, usually accompanied with fever, restlessness, dyspnea, profuse perspiration or lack of perspiration, trismus, spasm of the extremities, etc. Treatment principle: Clear summer-heat and regain consciousness. Point selection: Shuigou (CV26), Shixuan (EX-UE11), Quze (PC3), Weizhong(BL40), Quchi(LI11).

周荣 Zhourong (SP20)

经穴名。属足太阴脾经。定位:在胸外侧部,当第二肋间隙,距前正中线 6 寸。主治:胸胁胀痛,咳嗽,呃逆等。操作:斜刺或向外平刺 0.5～0.8 寸;可灸。

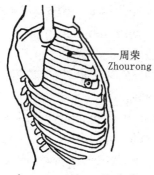

周荣
Zhourong

Name of an acupoint. It belongs to the Spleen Meridian of Foot-Taiyin. Location: On the lateral side of the chest and in the 2nd intercostal space, 6 cun lateral to the anterior midline. Indications: Pain and fullness in the chest and hypochondriac, cough, hiccup, etc. Method: Puncture obliquely or horizontally outward 0.5-0.8 cun. Moxibustion is applicable.

肘 Zhou

耳穴名。在腕穴与肩穴之间。主治肢体相应部位的疼痛及功能障碍。

Name of an ear point. Located between Wan and Jian. It is used for treating pain and dysfunction of the corresponding area of the limbs.

肘尖 Zhoujian (EX-UE1)

经外奇穴名。定位:屈肘,在尺骨鹰嘴的尖端。主治:瘰疬。

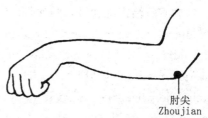

肘尖
Zhoujian

Name of an extra point. Location: On the tip of the ulnar olecranon when the elbow is flexed. Indication: Scrofula.

肘髎 Zhouliao (LI12)

经穴名。属手阳明大肠经。定位:在臂外侧,屈肘,曲池上方 1 寸,当肱骨边缘处。主治:肘臂疼痛、麻木、拘挛等。操作:直刺 0.5～1 寸;可灸。

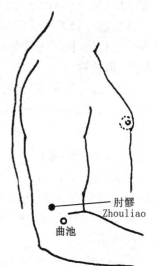

肘髎
Zhouliao

曲池

Name of an acupoint. It belongs to Large Intestine Meridian of Hand-Yangming. Location: On the lateral side of the upper arm, 1 cun above Quchi(LI11) and on the border of the humerus with the elbow flexed. Indications: Elbow and arm diseases, such as pain, numbness, and contracture, etc. Method: Puncture perpendicularly 0.5-1 cun. Moxibustion is applicable.

肘椎 Zhouzhui

经外奇穴名。定位：患者俯卧，伸臂贴身，两肘尖连线与脊中线交点旁开 1 寸为穴。斜刺或灸治霍乱、吐泻、腹痛等。

Name of an extra point. Location: 1 cun lateral to the crossing point of the posterior midline and the two elbow tips joining line when the patient lies in prone position and puts the two arms closely to the body. Oblique acupuncture or moxibustion is used to cure cholera, vomiting, diarrhea, abdominal pain, etc.

诸阳之会 convergence of all yang-qi

指头部。因人体清阳之气皆上注于头；而十二经脉中手三阳经和足三阳经也均经头部，故称。

The head. It is so called because the body yang-qi converges into the head, and all yang meridians pass through the head.

竹杖 Zhuzhang

经外奇穴名。定位：位于后正中线，与脐相对之脊骨上是穴。灸治腰痛、便血、吐血、衄血、痔疮、脱肛、阴挺、慢性肠炎及脊髓疾患等。

Name of an extra point. Location: On the posterior midline, at the vertebra just opposite to the navel. Moxibustion is used to cure lumbago, hemafecia, hematemesis, epistaxis, hemorrhoids, rectal and uterine prolapse, chronic enteritis, and spinal cord diseases.

主配 main and matching

配穴用语。针灸选穴，以远离病痛部穴为主，邻近病痛部穴为配。

A term of combining points in acupuncture and moxibustion, i. e., selecting the points distal from the diseases as the main points and the points proximal to the diseases as matching points.

主客 host and guests

配穴用语。针灸配穴中称主要穴为"主"，相配伍穴为"客"。

A term used in combining points. During acupuncture and moxibustion, the principal points are called "host" while the associate points are called "guest".

主客原络配穴法 host-guest combination of Yuan and Luo points

配穴法之一。即根据各经所属病症，取其本经的原穴为主，配用与其相表里经脉的络穴为客。

Method of combining points according to principle Yuan-Primary points methods, namely, selecting the Yuan-Primary points of the meridian affected by the disease as the principle points and the Luo-Connecting points of the meridian correlated interiorly or exteriorly with the affected meridian as associate points.

主穴 main points

指针刺配方中起主要治疗作用的穴位。

The points play a major role in prescription of acupuncture.

煮针法 needle-boiling technique

古代为解铁毒及增强疗效，用中药煮针一日而后用之。

In ancient China, the needles were boiled with the traditional Chinese drugs for one day to eliminate the iron toxicity and increase the effect.

注射进针 injecting insertion

进针法之一。又称快插进针法。以拇指、示指夹住针下段，稍露出针尖，对准穴位，快速插入。

One of the insertion techniques, also called fast insertion, i. e. , gripping firmly the lower part of the needle with the thumb and index finger to show the needle point slightly and then aiming at the acupoint to insert quickly.

注市 Zhushi

经外奇穴名。定位：腋窝下方。第七、八肋间处。主治痜夏、胸胁痛、腹痛等。治疗常用斜刺或灸。

Name of an extra point. Location：At the 7th and 8th intercostal spaces below the axillary fossa. Oblique acupuncture or moxibustion is used to cure summer non-acclimation, thoracic and hypochondric pain, abdominal pain, etc.

柱骨 zhugu

①指锁骨。②指颈椎。

① The clavicle. ② The cervical vertebrae.

痜夏 Zhuxia

经外奇穴名。定位：在掌侧与合谷穴相对处。直刺或灸治夏令食欲不振、消化不良、呕吐、腹泻等。

Name of an extra point. Location：At the palm just opposite Hegu (LI4). Perpendicular acupuncture or moxibustion is used to cure loss of appetite in summer, indigestion, vomiting, diarrhea, etc.

筑宾 Zhubin (KI9)

经穴名。属足少阴肾经，阴维脉郄穴。

定位：在小腿内侧，当太溪与阴谷的连线上，太溪上 5 寸，腓肠肌肌腹内下方。主治：神志失常，足跟痛，疝气等。操作：直刺 1～1.5 寸；可灸。

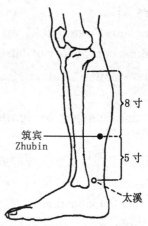

Name of an acupoint. It belongs to the Kidney Meridian of Foot-Shaoyin, Xi-Cleft point of Yin Link Vessel. Location：On the medial side of the leg, on the line connecting Taixi(KI3) and Yingu(KI10), 5 cun above Taixi(KI3), medial and inferior to the gastrocnemius muscle belly. Indications：Mental disorders, heel pain, hernia, etc. Method：Puncture perpendicularly 1-1. 5 cun. Moxibustion is applicable.

转谷 Zhuangu

经外奇穴名。定位：位于腋前皱襞直下，当第三肋间隙处。主治胸胁支满、食欲不振、呕吐、肋间神经痛等。治疗常用斜刺或灸治。

Name of an extra point. Location：At the 3rd intercostal space directly below the anterior axillary fold. Oblique puncture or moxibustion is adopted to cure thoracic and hypochondrial fullness, poor appetite, vomiting, intercostal neuralgia, etc.

壮 zhuang

①指艾炷。②艾炷灸的计量单位,每灸1艾炷称1壮。

①The moxa cone. ②A unit measurement of moxa cone in moxibustion. Each moxa cone burned out is counted as 1 zhuang.

壮数 the number of ignited moxa cones

指每次施灸时所点燃艾炷的数目。

The number of the moxa cones ignited during each moxibustion.

浊浴 Zhuoyu

经外奇穴名。定位:位于中枢穴旁各2.5寸处。治疗常用斜刺灸治胆病惊恐、胸满无力、口苦无味、食欲不振、癔病等。

Name of an extra point. Location:2.5 cun lateral to Zhongshu (GV7). Oblique puncture or moxibustion is used to cure panic and fear due to gallbladder diseases, thoracic fullness and weakness, bitterness and tastelessness in the mouth, loss of appetite, hysteria, etc.

子盗母气 illness of a child-organ may involve its mother-organ

用五行(相生的)母子关系说明五脏病变的相互影响。具有(相生的)母子关系的两个脏,当子(脏)发生病变时,常可以累及母(脏)。如肺气虚弱,可导致脾脏虚弱。

The pathological changes in one organ may involve another because of their connection. According to the five-phase theory, the two organs bear a generative re-

lationship, the one which is considered as son-organ may involve the mother-organ, e. g., insufficiency of lung-qi may cause asthenia of the spleen.

子宫 Zigong (EX-CA1)

经外奇穴名。定位:在脐下4寸,前正中线旁开3寸处。主治:阴挺,月经不调等。

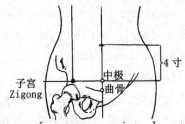

Name of an extra point. Location:4 cun below the umbilicus,3 cun lateral to the anterior midline. Indications:Uterine prolapse, irregular menstruation, etc.

子宫脱出 uterine prolapse

又称子宫脱垂。子宫从正常位置沿阴道下降到坐骨棘水平以下,甚至脱出阴道外口。多由劳倦、多产损伤脾肾,致中气下陷,肾气亏损,带脉失去约束,冲任不固引起。治宜益气升阳、固摄胞宫。取穴:百会、气海、维道、足三里、三阴交。

Uterine prolapse occurs when the uterus sags or slips from its normal position and into vagina, or protrudes out of the vagina; caused by overstrain and multiparous, which damage the spleen and kidney, leads to the collapse of middle qi, deficiency of kidney-qi, dysfunction of the Belt Vessel, and insecurity of the Thoroughfare Vessel and the Conception Vessel. Treatment principle:Supplement qi, elevate yang and consolidate the uterus. Point selection:Baihui (GV20), Qihai

（GV6）， Weidao （GB28）， Zusanli
(ST36)，Sanyinjiao(SP6).

子母补泻 reinforcing and reducing with mother acupoints and son acupoints

针刺补泻法之一。补法选用五输穴中的母穴,泻法选用其子穴。

One of the acupuncture methods for reinforcing or reducing. The mother acupoints of the five Shu points are selected to reinforce while the corresponding son acupoints are selected to reduce.

子午八法 eight midnight-midday methods

子午流注针法和灵龟八法的合称。

The collective name of the midnight-midday ebb flow acupuncture method and the eight methods of the intelligent turtle.

子午补泻 ziwu reinforcing and reducing

即左右捻转补泻法。据时间、性别、病情等的不同,补泻也是相对性的。

One of the reinforcing and reducing methods by twisting the needle leftward or rightward. Reinforcing or reducing in the method are relative to the time, sex, state of illness, etc.

子午捣臼 ziwudaojiu

针刺手法名。子午指左右捻转,捣臼指反复上下提插。这是一种捻转与提插相结合的针刺手法。

Name of a needle-manipulating method. Ziwu means twisting the needle leftward and rightward; daojiu means lifting and thrusting the needle repeatedly. This is an acupuncture method combining the twisting and lifting-thrusting manipulations.

子午流注针法 midnight-midday ebb flow acupuncture method

按时配穴法的一种。是以日、时、干支推算人体气血流注盛衰的时间,据此进行配穴和针刺治疗。子午表示昼夜的时间变化,流注表示气血的运行。

One of the point-combinating methods according to time. The point combination and acupuncture are based on the time when qi and blood flow increasingly or decreasingly through different parts of the human body and this time is calculated according to the date, the hour, the heavenly stem and the earthly branch. Ziwu means the passing time in the day and night while liuzhu means the movement of qi and blood in the human body.

子肿 pregnancy swelling

怀孕后期全身水肿的病证。因孕妇平素脾肾阳虚,胎儿日渐长大后,母体的运化输布功能失调,以致水湿泛滥所致。治宜健脾益肾、调气行水。取穴:脾俞、肾俞、水分、复溜、公孙。

A disorder occurring in the pregnant women with deficiency of spleen-yang and kidney-yang, caused by the retention of fluid resulting further functional disorder. Treatment principle: Strengthen the spleen and tonify the kidney, promote qi and fluid circulation. Point selection: Pishu(BL20), Shenshu(BL23), Shuifen

(CV9), Fuliu(KI7), Gongsun(SP4).

紫宫 Zigong (CV19)

经穴名。属任脉。定位：在胸部，当前正中线上，平第二肋间隙。主治：胸痛，气喘，咳嗽等。操作：平刺 0.3～0.5 寸；可灸。

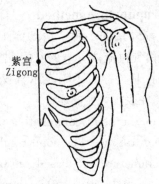

紫宫
Zigong

Name of an acupoint. It belongs to the Conception Vessel. Location: On the chest, on the anterior midline, level with the 2nd intercostal space. Indications: Pain in the chest, asthma, cough, etc. Method: Puncture horizontally 0.3-0.5 cun. Moxibustion is applicable.

紫外线穴位照射法 ultraviolet irradiation of the acupoints

用紫外线照射穴位，周围可进行适当防护。主治慢性支气管炎、哮喘、流感、丹毒等。

Irradiate the points with ultraviolet rays with the surrounding skin protected to cure chronic bronchitis, asthma, influenza, erysipelas, etc.

自汗 spontaneous sweating

在清醒状态下，不因劳动、厚衣或发热而汗自出的一种症状。多因气虚、阳虚所致，痰阻或伤湿也可引起。

Excessive sweating in a conscious state, which is not induced by physiological factor, such as labour, over clothing, heating, etc.; mostly caused by qi deficiency and yang deficiency, and also by the retention of phlegm and dampness.

宗筋 zongjin

①指前阴部。②指阴茎。

① The external genitals. ② Referring to the penis.

宗经 major meridian

数条经脉汇集处形成的主脉或大脉。

A major or large meridian formed by convergence of several meridians.

宗脉 converging meridian

由许多经脉汇聚而成的主脉或大脉，通常分布于眼、耳等重要器官上。

The major meridian or large meridian formed by the convergence of small meridians, which usually distributes over the vital organs, such as eyes, ears, etc.

宗气 pectoral qi

由水谷精微化生的营卫之气与吸入之清气相结合而成，积于胸中，出咽喉，贯心脉，蓄于丹田，经气街注于足阳明经。能助呼吸、行气血。

It is made of nutrient qi and defensive qi generated from nutritive essense as well as inhaled fresh air, which accumulates in the chest, then goes through throat and Heart Meridians, stores in Dantian and pours into the Stomach Meridian of Foot-Yangming. It can promote respiration and activate qi and blood flowing.

走罐法 movable cupping

拔罐法的一种。先在皮肤上涂润滑油，

拔上罐以后,向邻近部位移动。

A cupping method performed by moving the cup to the adjacent area with application of lubricant oil on the skin prior to the cupping.

足跗 dorsum of foot

即脚背部。

The dorsal side of the foot.

足跟痛 heel pain

即脚跟痛。多由肾亏,精血不足所致。症见足跟一侧或两侧疼痛,不红不肿,行走不便。治宜通经活络。取穴:合谷、足三里、解溪、水泉。

A symptom due to kidney deficiency and insufficiency of essence and blood; manifested as pain in one or two sides of the heel and difficulty in walking, but neither local redness nor swelling. Treatment principle: Clear and activate the meridians and collaterals. Point selection: Hegu (LI4), Zusanli (ST36), Jiexi (ST41), Shuiquan(KI5).

足厥阴肝经 the Liver Meridian of Foot-Jueyin

十二正经之一。它的循行路线是:在体内,属肝,络胆,并与生殖器、胃、横膈膜、咽喉、眼球相连;在体表,由足大趾经下肢内侧(由前部转向中部)、外阴部、腹部,止于侧胸部。本经患病时,主要表现为胸满、呕逆、腰痛、下利、疝气、遗尿、小便不通、月经不调、子宫出血、口咽干燥、面色晦暗等症状,以及本经循行部位的局部症状。

One of the twelve regular meridians. Its circulating path is as follows: Inside

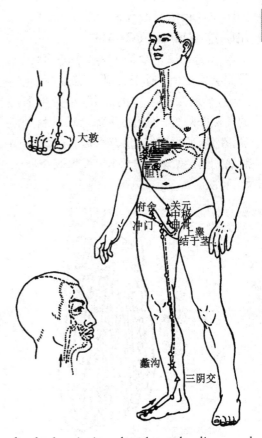

the body, it is related to the liver and connected with the gallbladder, genital organs, stomach, diaphragm, throat, and eyeballs; on the body surface, it runs from the big toe, along the medial side of the lower limbs(from the anterior to the medial), external genitalia and abdomen, ends at the lateral aspect of the chest. When this meridian is diseased, the main symptoms are fullness in the chest, hiccup, lumbago, diarrhea, hernia, enuresis, retention of urine, abnormal menstruation, metrorrhagia, dryness of the mouth and throat, dusky complexion, etc. , as well as the local symptoms of the parts along its pathway.

足临泣 Zulinqi (GB41)

经穴名。属足少阳胆经,本经输穴,八脉交会穴之一,通于带脉。定位:在足背外侧,当足四趾本节的后方,小趾伸肌腱的外侧凹陷处。主治:头痛,眩晕,目外眦痛,瘰疬,胁肋痛,乳胀痛,月经不调,足背肿痛,足趾痹痛等。操作:直刺 0.3～0.5寸;可灸。

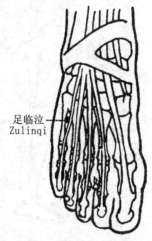

足临泣
Zulinqi

The acupoint, Shu-Stream point, belongs to the Gallbladder Meridian of Foot-Shaoyang. One of the eight confluential point, communicate with the Belt Vessel. Location: On the lateral side of the instep of the foot, posterior to the 4th metatarsophalangeal joint, in the depression lateral to the tendon of the extensor muscle of the little toe. Indications: Headache, vertigo, pain in the outer canthus, scrofula, pain in the hypochondriac region, distending pain of the breast, irregular menstruation, pain and swelling of the dorsum of foot, spastic pain of the toes, etc. Method: Puncture perpendicularly 0.3-0.5 cun. Moxibustion is applicable.

足窍阴 Zuqiaoyin (GB44)

经穴名。属足少阳胆经,本经井穴。定位:在足第四趾末节外侧,距趾甲角 0.1寸。主治:偏头痛,耳聋,耳鸣,失眠,热病,目痛等。操作:直刺 0.1～0.2 寸;可灸。

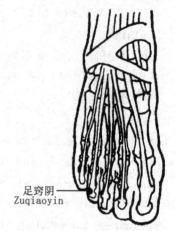

足窍阴
Zuqiaoyin

The acupoint, Jing-Well point of the Gallbladder Meridian of Foot-Shaoyang. Location: On the lateral side of the 4th toe, 0.1 cun from the corner of the toenail. Indications: Migraine, deafness, tinnitus, insomnia, febrile disease, eye pain. Method: Puncture perpendicularly 0.1-0.2 cun. Moxibustion is applicable.

足三里 Zusanli (ST36)

经穴名。属足阳明胃经,本经合穴。定位:在小腿前外侧,当犊鼻下 3 寸,距胫骨前缘一横指。主治:胃痛,呕吐,呃逆,腹胀,肠鸣,泄泻,痢疾,便秘,乳痈,膝腿痛,脚气,水肿,咳嗽,气喘,头晕,消化不良,癫狂等。操作:直刺 1～1.5 寸;可灸。

The acupoint, He-Sea point, belongs to Stomach Meridian of Foot-Yangming.

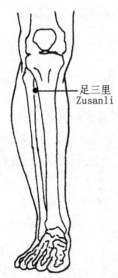

Location: On the anterior lateral side of the leg, 3 cun below Dubi(ST35), one finger breadth from the anterior crest of the tibia. Indications: Gastric pain, vomiting, hiccup, abdominal distension, borborygmus, diarrhea, dysentery, constipation, acute mastitis, aching of the knee joint and leg, beriberi, edema, cough, asthma, dizziness, indigestion, mania, etc. Method: Puncture perpendicularly 1-1.5 cun. Moxibustion is applicable.

足三阳经 the three yang meridians of the foot

指足部的三条阳经。即足阳明胃经、足太阳膀胱经、足少阳胆经。

The Stomach Meridian of Foot-Yangming, the Bladder Meridian of Foot-Taiyang, and the Gallbladder Meridian of Foot-Shaoyang.

足三阴经 the three yin meridians of the foot

指足部的三条阴经。即足太阴脾经、足少阴肾经、足厥阴肝经。

The Spleen Meridian of Foot-Taiyin, the Kidney Meridian of Foot-Shaoyin, and the Liver Meridian of Foot-Jueyin.

足少阳胆经 the Gallbladder Meridian of Foot-Shaoyang

十二正经之一。它的循行路线是：在体内，属胆，络肝；在体表，由眼部经侧头部、耳、面颊、后颈部、肩、胸外侧、腹部、下肢外侧，止于第四趾端。本经患病时，主要表现为疟疾、恶寒、汗出、头痛、颔痛、目痛、口苦、锁骨部及腋窝部肿痛、胸及侧胸部痛使身体转侧困难、甲状腺肿大、淋巴结结核等症状，以及本经循行部位症状。

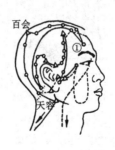
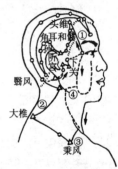

One of the twelve regular meridians. Its circulating path is as follows: Inside the body, it is related to the gallbladder and connected with the liver; on the body surface, it runs from the eyes, along the lateral aspect of the head, ear, cheek, posterior aspect of the neck, shoulder, lateral aspects of the chest, the abdomen, and the lateral side of the lower limb, and terminates at the tip of the 4th toe. When this meridian is diseased, the main symptoms are malaria, aversion to cold, sweating, headache, pain of the

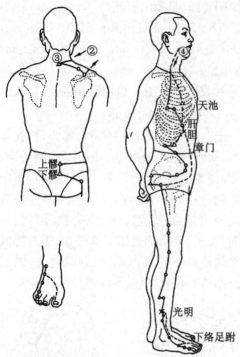

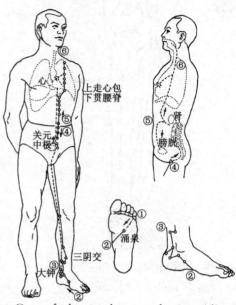

chin, pain of the eyes, bitterness in the mouth, swelling and pain in the clavicular and axillary region, difficulty to turn the body around due to pain of the chest and the lateral side of the chest, enlargement of the thyroid, lympy node tuberculosis, etc., as well as the local symptoms of the parts along its pathway.

足少阴肾经 the Kidney Meridian of Foot-Shaoyin

十二正经之一。它的循行路线是:在体内,属肾,络膀胱,并与脊髓、肝、膈膜、喉部、舌根、肺、心、胸腔等相连;在体表,由足小趾,经足心、内踝、下肢内侧后面、腹部,止于胸部。本经患病时,主要表现为口中热、舌干、咽喉痛、饥饿而不欲食、羸瘦、咯血、哮喘、心悸、胸痛、烦躁、黄疸、腹泻、面色暗黑、视物不清、精神萎靡、嗜睡、痿厥等症状,以

One of the twelve regular meridians. Its circulating path is as follows: Inside the body, it is related to the kidney and connected with the urinary bladder, spinal cord, liver, diaphragm, throat, the root of the tongue, lung, heart, chest, etc.; on the body surface, it runs from the little toe along the sole of the foot, medial malleolus, postero-medial aspect of the lower limb, the abdomen, and terminates at the chest. When this meridian is diseased, the main symptoms are warmth of the mouth, dryness of the tongue, sore throat, hunger with poor appetite, emaciation, hemoptysis, asthma, palpitation, chest pain, restlessness, jaundice, diarrhea, dusky complexion, blurred vision, listlessness, somnolence, atrophy and coldness of the hands and feet, etc., as well as the local symptoms of the parts along its pathway.

足太阳膀胱经 the Bladder Meridian of Foot-Taiyang

十二正经之一。它的循行路线是：在体内，属膀胱，络肾，并与脑相连。在体表，由眼部向上越过头顶，向后向下，经过颈部、背部一侧、臀部、下肢后面，止于小趾端。本经患病时，主要表现为疟疾、癫狂、目黄、流泪、鼻衄、头项强痛、腰背痛、痔疮、尿频、排尿疼痛、小便不利等症状，以及在本经循行部位的局部症状。

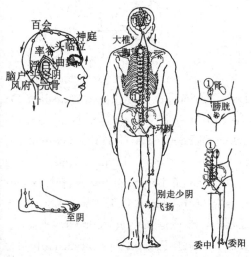

One of the twelve regular meridians. Its circulating path is as follows: Inside the body, it is related to the urinary bladder and connected with the kidney and brain; on the body surface it runs from the eyes upwards, over the vertex of the head, then backwards down, along the nape and back, lateral side of the spinal column, the buttock, the posterior aspect of the lower limb and terminates at the tip of the small toes. When this meridian is diseased, it will cause malaria, mania, yellowish sclera, epiphoria, epistaxis, stiffness and pain of the neck and head, pain of the lower back, hemorrhoids, frequent urination, painful micturition, dysuria, etc. , as well as the local symptoms of the parts along its pathway.

足太阴脾经 the Spleen Meridian of Foot-Taiyin

十二正经之一。它的循行路线是：在体内，属脾，络胃，并与心及舌根相连；在体表，由足大趾沿下肢内侧（由中部转向前部）、腹部、胸部，止于侧胸部。本经患病时，主要表现为胃痛、呕吐、肠炎、腹胀、噫气、黄疸、水肿、自觉身体沉重、行动困难、不能平卧、舌痛、舌根强直、小便不通等症状，以及本经循行部位的局部症状。

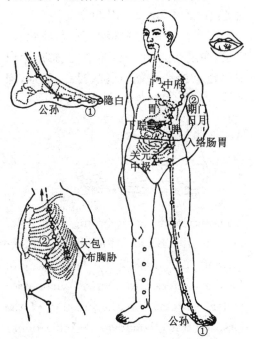

One of the twelve regular meridians. Its circulating path is as follows: Inside the body, it is related to the spleen and connected with the stomach, heart, and the root of the tongue; on the body surface, it runs from the big toe along the medial aspect of the lower limb(from the medial to the anterior), abdomen, and chest, and terminates in the lateral aspect of the chest. When this meridian is diseased, it will cause gastralgia, vomiting, enteritis, abdominal distension, belching, jaundice, edema, feeling of bodily heaviness, difficulty in walking, being unable to lie flat, pain of the tongue, stiffness of the root of the tongue, retention of urine, etc., as well as the local symptoms of the parts along its pathway.

足通谷 Zutonggu (BL66)

经穴名。属足太阳膀胱经,本经荥穴。定位:在足外侧,足小趾本节的前方,赤白肉际处。主治:头痛,项强,目眩,鼻衄,癫狂等。直刺 0.3～0.5 寸;可灸。

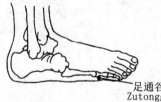

足通谷
Zutonggu

The acupoint, Xing-Spring point, belongs to the Bladder Meridian of Foot-Taiyang. Location: On the lateral side of the foot, anterior to the 5th metatarso-phalangeal joint, on the junction of the dorso-ventral boundary. Indications: Headache, neck rigidity, dizziness, epistaxis, mania, etc. Method: Puncture per-

pendicularly 0.3-0.5 cun. Moxibustion is applicable.

足五里 Zuwuli (LR10)

经穴名。属足厥阴肝经。定位:在大腿内侧,当气冲直下 3 寸,大腿根部,耻骨结节的下方,长收肌的外缘。主治:小腹胀满,小便不利等。操作:直刺 1～2 寸;可灸。

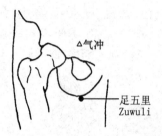

△气冲

足五里
Zuwuli

Name of an acupoint. It belongs to the Liver Meridian of Foot-Jueyin. Location: On the medial side of the thigh, 3 cun directly below Qichong(ST30), at the proximal end of the thigh, below the pubic tubercle and on the lateral border of the long abductor muscle of the thigh. Indications: Lower abdominal distension and fullness, dysuria, etc. Method: Puncture perpendicularly 1-2 cun. Moxibustion is applicable.

足心 Zuxin

经外奇穴名。定位:位于足底第二趾尖端至足跟后缘连线之中点。主治崩漏、头痛、眩晕、癫痫、足底痛、休克等。治疗常用直刺或温灸。

Name of an extra point. Location: At the midpoint of the line between the 2nd toe tip and the posterior heel margin. Perpendicular acupuncture or warm moxibustion is used to cure metrorrhagia and metrostaxis, headache, vertigo, epilepsy, sole pain, shock, etc.

足阳明胃经 the Stomach Meridian of Foot-Yangming

十二正经之一。它的循行路线是:在体内,属胃,络脾;在体表,由鼻部经过侧头部、面部、颈部、胸腹部、下肢外侧的前面,止于第二趾端。本经患病时,主要表现为胃肠炎、胃痛、腹胀、肠鸣、腹水、咽喉炎、鼻衄、口眼歪斜、唇生疱疹、颈部肿大、恶寒战栗、呻吟不舒、面色微黑、精神失常、热病发狂等病症,以及本经循行部位的局部症状。

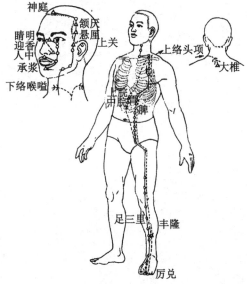

One of the twelve regular meridians. Its circulating path is as follows: Inside the body, it is related to the stomach and connected with the spleen; on the body surface, it runs from the nose, along the lateral aspect of the head, face, neck, chest, abdomen, anterolateral aspect of the lower limb, terminates at the tip of the 2nd toe. When this meridian is diseased, it will cause gastroenteritis, gastralgia, abdominal distension, borborygmus, ascites, sore throat, epistaxis, deviation of mouth and eyes, herpetic and pustular lesions on the lips, swelling of the neck, chills and shivering, groaning due to discomfort, dusky complexion, delirium, acute pyrexial mania, as well as the local symptoms of the parts along its pathway.

足针 foot-acupuncture

将足底部划分为一定的区域进行针刺以治疗疾病的方法。

To divide the sole of the foot into zones and puncture a certain zone to treat a related disease.

足之三阳头外足 the three yang meridians of the foot from head to foot

指足之三阳经的体表循行路线均是从头部沿躯干外侧、腿外侧到足部。

The circulating routes of the three yang meridians of the foot are from the hand along the lateral aspects of the trunk and the lower limb to the foot.

足之三阴足内腹 the three yin meridians of the foot from foot to abdomen

指足之三阴经的体表循行路线均是从足部沿腿内侧到腹部。

The circulating routes of the three yin meridians of the foot are from the foot along the medial aspects of the foot and the lower limb to the abdomen.

左右配穴法 left-right point combination

配穴法之一,指左右两侧相对穴位的配合应用。十二经脉的穴位左右对称,两侧同源。临床上对内脏疾病,一般左右两侧同取,以增强治疗作用。

One of the point-combining methods, i. e. , the combination of the bilateral corresponding points. The points of the twelve meridians are symmetrical and of the same source both on the left and on the right, so while treating the diseases in the viscera, the bilateral points are usually taken at the same time to enhance the effect.

坐骨神经　Zuogushenjing

耳穴名。定位:在对耳轮下脚前 2/3 处。主治坐骨神经痛。

Name of an ear point. Location:At anterior 2/3 of the inferior antihelix crus. It is used for treating sciatica.